Healing Logics

Culture and Medicine

in

Modern Health Belief Systems

Healing Logics

Culture and Medicine

in

Modern Health Belief Systems

Edited by
Erika Brady

UTAH STATE UNIVERSITY PRESS
Logan, Utah

Utah State University Press
Logan Utah 84322-7800

Cover design by Barbara Yale-Read
Cover illustration: Santería shrine for saints/spirits. Courtesy of Patrick A. Polk and the
Folklore and Mythology Archives, University of California, Los Angeles

Manufactured in the United States of America
Printed on acid-free paper

10 9 8 7 6 5 4 3 2 1   01 02 03 04 05 06 07 08 09 10

Library of Congress Cataloging-in-Publication Data

Healing logics : culture and medicine in modern health belief systems /
edited by Erika Brady.
    p. cm.
Includes bibliographical references and index.
    ISBN 0-87421-411-4 (hard : alk. paper) — ISBN 0-87421-410-6 (pbk. :
alk. paper)
    1. Traditional medicine. 2. Healing. 3. Medical anthropology. I.
Brady, Erika, 1952– II. Title.
    GR880 .H43 2001
    398'.353—dc21
                            00-013261

Contents

Acknowledgments   VII

prologue

1   Introduction   3
    Erika Brady

2   Understanding Folk Medicine   13
    Bonnie B. O'Connor and David J. Hufford

places and practitioners

3   Invisible Hospitals: Botánicas in Ethnic
    Health Care   39
    *Michael Owen Jones and Patrick A. Polk, with
    Ysamur Flores-Peña and Roberta J. Evanchuk*

4   *The Poor Man's Medicine Bag:* The Empirical
    Folk Remedies of Tillman Waggoner   88
    *Richard Blaustein, Anthony Cavender, and Jackie
    Sluder, with comments by Tillman Waggoner*

communication and the interplay of systems

5   Integrating Personal Health Belief Systems:
    Patient-Practitioner Communication   115
    Shelley R. Adler

6   Competing Logics and the Construction of Risk   129
    Diane E. Goldstein

the new age dilemma

7   The New Age Sweat Lodge   143
    William M. Clements

8   Evergreen: The Enduring Voice of a
    Nine-Hundred-Year-Old Healer   163
    Frances M. Malpezzi

taking it in: the observer healed

9   Reflections on the Experience of Healing:
    Whose Logic? Whose Experience?   183
    Bonnie Glass-Coffin

10 The Hózhó Factor: The Logic of Navajo Healing   197
    Barre Toelken

further investigation

Bibliography of Folklore and Medicine   211
    *Michael Owen Jones and Erika Brady, with Jacob
    Owen and Cara Hoglund*

Contributors   278

Index   284

Acknowledgments

This collection grew out of Utah State University's 1996 Fife Conference on folk medicine, in which contributors Bonnie B. O'Connor, David Hufford, Bonnie Glass-Coffin, Barre Toelken, and I participated as faculty. During an intense week of conferences and informal discussion, we realized that the direct involvement of humanities scholars in various aspects of institutional biomedicine—such as medical education, clinical pastoral care, and negotiation of transcultural issues—now informs work in folklore and medicine as never before. Old models of investigation that artificially isolate "folk medicine," "complementary and alternative medicine," and "biomedicine" as mutually exclusive conduits of information were proving too limited in our exploration of the real-life complexities of health belief systems as they observably exist and are applied by contemporary Americans. Our own work as well as recent research in medical publications strongly suggests that individuals construct their health belief systems from diverse sources of authority, including community and ethnic tradition, education, spiritual beliefs, personal experience, influence of popular media, and perception of the goals and means of formal medicine. What is less evident is *how* these health belief systems of authority interact—sometimes competing, sometimes conflicting, sometimes remarkably congruent. We agreed that it was time for a publication exploring this new integrative (dare I say "holistic"?) dimension in our observation and research.

It was evident from the beginning that to do justice to the current scholarship we would need to include many more scholars than those who had been present at the conference; there are yet other scholars not represented here whose work is adding important insights to our understanding of the cultures of medicine, vernacular and otherwise. Two important "shadow contributors" to this publication are Margaret Brady of the University of Utah and Patrick Mullen of Ohio State University, our fellow participants in the

1996 conference, whose comments and support then and since have been invaluable to the project.

The staff at Utah State make participation in the Fife Conference a memorable event in any folklorist's career. Special thanks go to Barbara Walker, Randy Williams, and their helpers for transforming us into family for our week in Logan. Barre Toelken's engagement in this project has been pervasive, from his organization of Fife 1996 to his fine contribution to this volume. It was a casual conversation with him at a subsequent meeting of the American Folklore Society that suggested to me the title for this work.

It is my personal pleasure as editor to thank my colleagues, students, and friends at Western Kentucky University. Release time and a sabbatical leave made my work on the project possible, thanks to the generosity of Dean David D. Lee, former and current department heads Thomas Baldwin and Linda Pickle, and former folk studies program director Michael Ann Williams. My graduate assistants Cara Hoglund and Jacob Owen were indomitable comrades, offering excellent organizational ideas as well as basic editorial "grunt work." Work-study students Scott Sisco and Jennifer Englert were prompt, accurate, and unfailingly cheerful.

Finally, warm thanks to John Alley of Utah State University Press, who combines two rare and wonderful qualities in an editor: patience and optimism.

for Nolan

A friend is the medicine of life.
—Aelred of Rielvaux

prologue

1

INTRODUCTION

ERIKA BRADY

Sometimes the attraction of a field of study emerges naturally and predictably within the ivied structure of an academic setting; sometimes it ambushes you from an unanticipated stronghold. In the course of many years of academic training in folklore, I never regarded medical folklore as a specialty. Although my office as a graduate student at UCLA adjoined that of Wayland Hand, the distinguished American taxonomist of medical folklore, his room-length boxes of file cards and the boundless store of arcane tidbits painstakingly organized struck me at the time as more exotic than relevant to contemporary ethnography. It was not until the early 1980s, when I unexpectedly assumed the duties of a part-time chaplain associate at a midsize hospital in southeast Missouri that I began to see the implications of my training for work in a hospital setting, and grasped the emerging significance of efforts by folklorists and anthropologists in other medical institutions nationwide.

Cape Girardeau, Missouri, is located on the Mississippi River, at the intersection of several cultural regions marked by distinctive vernacular health systems: to the west, the richly diverse biome of the Ozark Plateau has produced a notable heritage of herbal treatment; to the south, the Missouri Bootheel is an economic and social extension of the Mississippi Delta, with flourishing practice of rootwork derived from West African patterns. Most consistent of all, so deeply taken for granted that it escapes notice as a traditional health belief system, is the profound, almost universal assumption that soul and body are linked in some larger pattern of meaning that should be acknowledged, and can even be altered, by prayer. As a chaplain specializing in oncology, I learned to recognize the verbal rhythms that preceded ecstatic trance in Pentecostal patients. I lit candles for Catholics, and obtained permission for holy medals to accompany them into surgery. From patients of all social backgrounds I heard the many supernatural and natural, folk and "new age" remedies that had been tried and discarded before so-called "primary" care had been sought, and learned also of these nonconventional practices being surreptitiously or openly continued concurrent with official biomedical care—some of which knowledge posed delicate ethical issues for me as mediator between patient, family, and hospital. I came to realize the cures so aggressively and ingeniously sought, and the palliation of acute pain when a cure was past hope, were not necessarily goals most highly valued by patients and families. In corridors and waiting rooms following a death, many times the agonized question posed to me was not "Did he suffer?" but rather, "Was he saved?"

There was nothing out of the ordinary about these experiences in themselves—they could be replicated in various forms in any hospital at any time. Few people, medical professionals included, self-treat illness exclusively within strict biomedical protocols. Just as social practices deriving from folk custom rather than scientific method govern many aspects of hospital behavior (Hufford 1989; Stein 1980; George and Dundes 1978), nonconventional models for healing and wellness quietly and stubbornly coexist with the official allopathic approach, even in a hospital setting. What was unusual and new in my experience was the responsiveness of the staff to the possibilities of an ethnographic approach to patient and family issues my training offered, and their interest in learning more about making sense of the practices and beliefs they observed—not necessarily to suppress them, but, like folklorists and anthropologists, to understand them well enough from the patient's standpoint to grasp their persuasive power. Their interest reflected a much larger trend in contemporary medicine: the incomplete but growing recognition that the four-hundred-year-old enterprise to institutionalize medicine and place health care on a fully secular, professional, and scientific footing can never—and perhaps should never—entirely succeed.

The dominant theme in the social history of U.S. medicine in the twentieth century has been the emergence of allopathic treatment—the lineal descendent of nineteenth-century "heroic" medicine—as preeminent, virtually excluding all competing modalities from participation in official status. Allopathic medicine enjoys all the privileges of what social scientists label "formal" or "elite" institutions. It is administered by a limited number of carefully credentialed specialists, change in practice is elaborately controlled, and the whole is supported by complex interrelationships with similarly "formal" institutions such as the legal, medical, and economic systems in this country. As is often the case with well-established formal institutions, the predominance of allopathic medicine has been so pronounced as to suggest an almost Olympian extracultural inevitability: it has achieved a superorganic mystique, as though it exists outside the social, cultural, and historic contingencies that shape other aspects of custom and practice—a kind of secular religion. This process has been fueled by the dramatic advances of biomedicine, especially in treatment of physical trauma; bacterial, fungal, and parasitic infections; and hormonal deficiencies.

This privileged role, and the infallible status accorded formal medicine, can lead to a kind of biomedical absolutism which has been labeled "medico-centrism" (O'Connor 1995, 4), which finds expression in ways that overreach even the immense credibility accorded the practice. The official guide to alternative medical practices published by the American Medical Association defines "quackery" as the promotion of a scientifically unproven practice or remedy, regardless of intent (Zwicky 1993, 5). This definition would make a "quack" of a mother administering any nonscientific home remedy, no matter how amply supported by generations of informal empirical observation, not to mention any hospital chaplain who "promotes" the healing benefits of prayer.

Despite its aura of timeless mastery, the predominance of allopathic medicine in this country is relatively recent. The publication of Abraham Flexner's famous report in 1910 on the state of medical education in the U.S. provides a convenient terminus a quo from which to date its ascendance. Using German universities and the European-influenced curriculum then current at Johns Hopkins as models, he outlined a system in which training of physicians would take place within relatively few research-centered institutions emphasizing scientific method first and foremost, with clinical skills developed later and somewhat secondarily. The consequence is now a comprehensive and lengthy process which in practice now involves nothing less than a full transformation of a would-be doctor's way of knowing—as total an acculturative conversion experience as Roman Catholic seminary or military boot camp.

The Flexner report struck a responsive chord because his recommendations were both timely in terms of emergent economic and social forces of the period, and consistent with long-standing cultural values, practices, and preferences deriving historically from a much larger frame of reference than medicine alone. From the time of the ancient Greeks and the subsequent influence of Islamic thought, the Western European intellectual tradition has generally favored inductive, empirical processes of inquiry over deductive and metaphysical models. Regarding two essential methods of investigation and treatment in Western medicine, dissection and surgery, this attraction to inductive, empirical process was assisted (or at least relatively unimpeded) by the Christian theological division of soul from organism, permitting procedures which in other cultures would have violated a sacred unity of the being. In the application of these observations to therapeutic problem solving, the Western fascination with cause and effect and its accompanying spirit of invention have driven investigators to devise ingenious pharmaceutical and mechanical innovations in treatment—techniques specific enough in intended action to be effectively tested in a controlled setting. Finally, these techniques of treatment have proven well suited for dissemination by means of yet another feature of Western culture shaping its formal medicine: the talent for constructing elaborate bureaucratic organizations, which now research, test, regulate, and administer the therapeutic product. The organizational commodification of healing in the West is one of its most striking characteristics: it is no linguistic accident that the term "medicine" describes both the broad field of endeavor, and its product.

These observations concerning Western official medicine as a social construct are by no means news to social scientists (Glaser 1968, 94–95). But their expression in recent *medical* literature is something new. The characterization of contemporary biomedicine as "a highly refined form of folk medicine . . . [which is] the traditional practice in industrialized Western nations" (Harrison 1992, 2594) would not be astonishing in a social sciences text, but it *is* striking to encounter it in the most recent edition of *The Merck Manual of Diagnosis and Therapy*, a standard desk reference published for physicians. This open recognition of formal medicine by its practitioners as a culturally contingent institution not only suggests a reevaluation of many of the assumptions underlying its teaching methods and practice, but also a reevaluation of attitudes toward nonconventional health belief systems with which it coexists and sometimes competes.

To some degree, pragmatic concerns motivate this self-critique on the part of the medical establishment. In 1993, the prestigious *New England Journal of Medicine* published an eye-opening article titled "Unconventional Medicine in the United States: Prevalence, Costs, and Patterns of Use," in which the authors reported the results of a national survey conducted in 1990. One in three respondents had in the previous year made use of at least one of sixteen biomedically unproven modalities such as acupuncture, relaxation techniques, spiritual healing, et cetera. The estimated number of visits to providers of nonconventional therapy exceeded visits to primary care physicians by almost 10 percent, and the out-of-pocket expenditures for these visits was $10.3 billion—an amount comparable to out-of-pocket expenditures for all hospitalizations in the United States during the same period. What is more, the individuals seeking nonconventional treatment during the period in question were generally those who were more affluent and better educated. This study represented a significant heads-up to anyone assuming that the institutional authority of biomedicine is currently unchallenged.

But perhaps more importantly, acknowledgment of the de facto inter-play between diverse healing systems in the U.S. has been seen as a call for a more introspective self-critique, especially among practitioners of primary care. In a thoughtful essay now required reading in some family practice residencies, physician G. Gayle Stephens observes:

> From where I sit, the philosophical beliefs and attitudes of medical educators, the problems of clinical practice, and the organization and structures of medical care have common root defects that were contained in Flexner's famous report. They are the preoccupation with the human body as the only proper object of medical knowledge and the faith in experimental biology as the solution to all problems of health and illness. Until we take the whole human person in his or her social and cultural dimensions as the proper object of knowledge, until we expand our notions of science to include forms of rationality other than the logical, we will continue to depersonalize and fragment medical care, increase its costs beyond all calculation, and fail to make its benefits equally available to the whole population. (1988, 187)

Clearly both medical consumers and medical providers are asking for a careful evaluation of the relational as well as institutional patterns of medicine and healing—an evaluation in which specialists in medical folklore are playing an increasing role.

Intrinsic to the practice of "Flexnerian" medicine is the importance of institutional authority: from a patient's standpoint, the credibility and accountability of a practitioner of official medicine depend to a significant degree on the validity of credentials that guarantee that he or she is a participant in good standing in the formal medical community. But there are other forms of authority to which a patient may turn when in need of medical assistance. Experiential authority—personal recall and application of what has worked in the past—is persuasive but limited. Far more extensive is the realm of relational authority: the credibility of those individuals and resources whose accountability lies not with a remote institutional affiliation, but exists within the community. The healing practices and customs supported by relational authority represent just a portion of the affective linkages that bind a community through many shared forms of expression, including linguistic patterns, foodways, music, and other cultural manifestations. These expressive forms derive strength not only from the ways in which they fulfill the immediate needs of community members, but also from the ways in which they embody larger patterns of shared beliefs and values. Relational authority may extend horizontally to influence health-related practices of a group at a given time—"everyone does it"—or it may extend vertically to invoke generations of past practice—"we have always done it."

The concepts of institutional and relational authority are not absolute or mutually exclusive when applied to contemporary conventional and non-conventional medicine. No physician, however impressively credentialed, would care to suggest that his or her accountability lies only toward the state licensure bureau, and many nonconventional areas of practice such as chiropractic and acupuncture have official or quasi-official levels of institutional education and control. The very complexity of medicine and culture in this society invites analysis in relational and institutional terms. Observe, for example, how commercial medicine depends on one model or the other in its advertising to the general public, depending on the nature and effect of the product: television viewers are either lectured by actors in white coats gravely citing research results, or are entertained by commercial minidramas in which Dr. Mom is rewarded for her recommendation of an over-the-counter medication for yeast infection by her daughter's fervent "Gee, Mom, you're swell."

Riddling through the complex interplay of health belief systems in the U.S. is a task well suited to the skills of medical ethnography. Most of the contributors to this collection are medical folklorists, or medical anthropologists with close ties to the related field of medical folklore. For nonspecialist readers who are curious about the distinctions between the fields of medical folklore, anthropology, and sociology, it may be helpful to observe that folklore as an academic discipline has tended to address cultural aspects of behavior which, though informal and not protected from change, have nonetheless demonstrated a certain consistency of form over time and which are particular to a specific community or group within a larger society. Central is the concept of "traditional" forms of expressive behavior, both stable and dynamic, which satisfy basic human needs at the immediate levels of subsistence (food, shelter, healing), and which also reflect and maintain deeper beliefs and values within a social group. The method of inquiry into these patterns of behavior has always been qualitative, setting the discipline apart from sociology, and has tended to concentrate investigation in communities and cultures existing within the society of the investigator, rather than pursuing research in more exotic faraway locals, as has often been the practice historically in the field of anthropology.

The tendency of folklorists to examine discrete expressive forms—in the case of medical folklore, specific remedies—has been both a liability and an asset to the discipline. At its best, the study of folklore incorporates what is most valuable in both the social sciences and the humanities, interpreting traditional practices as texts as dense in meaning as poetry. Early folk-medical scholarship was decidedly "item-centered," resulting in ambitious cross-cultural comparative bibliographies such as the magisterial work produced from those long file boxes by Wayland Hand, in which practices common to many different communities and cultures could be examined and commonalities adduced. But the item-centered approach—not unlike the extreme forms of allopathic practice—removes the object of their study from the rich matrix of social context, leaving behind much of what may be relevant to an understanding of the whole picture. In this volume, Bonnie B. O'Connor and David J. Hufford, both pioneers in the area of medical folklore, offer a comprehensive introduction to a contemporary approach to medical folklore centered on an understanding of folk belief systems, examining the ways in which these systems draw on bodies of knowledge and belief, support specific means of knowledge production, provide explanatory models for causation and treatment, and supply evaluative strategies to determine efficacy.

If effectively pursued, the methods necessary for the quantitative interviews customary among folklorists tend to undermine a purely item-centered approach. So-called "participant observation" has been at the methodological core of anthropology and folklore for decades, a process in which the investigator acquires an experiential understanding of social process by actually engaging in the activities of a community while simultaneously observing them with an eye to making sense of them in disciplinary terms. The consequences of this process of engagement have been pervasive. Readers whose background is medical may be surprised at the extent to which contributions to this collection are presented in the first person, unabashedly presenting "consciousness of self" as an integral part or the presentation of research. What may appear to be a radical (and unnerving) subjectivity reflects a current tendency in the ethnographic disciplines toward a radical empiricism—an experience-centered approach which not only attempts to take into account the full complexity of experience of individuals in the community being studied, but also the full complexity of the subjective and objective experience being reported by the investigator. Thus readers of the article concerning Los Angeles *botánicas* by Michael Owen Jones and his colleagues can expect not only an analysis of the meaning of these "invisible hospitals" in the communities they serve, but also an impressionistic evocation of their sights and smells.

When a field worker sets about studying a traditional healer, for example, he or she becomes a student, figuratively and sometimes literally an apprentice to that individual. The native preceptor may in fact become an active collaborator in the publication of the research, and, not surprisingly, an increasing number of researchers in the ethnographic disciplines are or become participants in the cultures which they study. A collaborative model for research is becoming increasingly common in folklore and anthropology. The articles "Invisible Hospitals: Spiritual Herbal Centers in Ethnic Communities" and

"*The Poor Man's Medicine Bag:* Empirical Folk Remedies of Tillman Waggoner of Knoxville, Tennessee" both represent such a cooperative model; in the latter the informality of the relationship between authors and practitioner is suggested by their references to the subject of the article by his first name, "Tim." Addressing the communicative conduits, both personal and commercial, in which folk medicine may be shared in a community, the authors raise old questions concerning the role of the practitioner as both healer and entrepreneur in impoverished, underserved, or "biomedically resistant" communities. These are issues which go back at least to the herbal publications of Nicholas Culpeper in the seventeenth century.

A common stereotype of folklore culture views it as existing in isolation from both academic, elite culture and from profit-driven and media-promulgated influences. "Folk" communities in which traditional ways predominate are scarce today, both in the U.S., and to an increasing extent, worldwide. A more useful model suggests that each individual within complex contemporary cultures appropriates systematic elements of health belief from a number of sources: communal and traditional, journalistic, commercial, and institutional. In "Competing Logics and the Construction of Risk," Diane Goldstein examines the subtle cultural contextualization of even "objective" information conduits concerning risk factors in AIDS, raising powerful questions concerning the consequences of policy based on such data. Shelley Adler examines the bases on which breast cancer patients evaluate conventional and nonconventional treatment choices, and the implied consequences for biomedical practitioners in addressing these patient choices. Both essays remind us that any approach to communication in health care is shaped at least in part by culture-based terms and parameters.

The so-called "new age" movement in health and spirituality has been something of a headache for folklorists and physicians alike. It is a loose term referring to a quickening of interest dating from the late 1960s in religious and health belief systems characterized by a perceived integration of body, mind, and spirit and attunement of cosmic or natural forces; an eclectic appropriation of American Indian, Eastern, and self-constructed systems of healing and spirituality; and an appreciation of the therapeutic spiritual effects of altered states of consciousness (Levin and Coreil 1986). Physicians are frustrated by the critique of institutional medicine both implied and directly expressed by many devotees of "new age" modalities. Accustomed to identifying and interpreting community-based traditional behavior, folklorists are annoyed by the cavalier popular appropriation of traditional practices in a manner that can be insensitive and even potentially exploitative, and are frustrated as well by the challenge to the traditional tools of investigation of cultural behavior, especially when the "community" of practice is a virtual one often linked only by electronic means. William Clements and Frances Malpezzi discuss the dynamics supporting two areas of new age interest: the borrowing of practices relating to the American Indian sweat lodge rituals, and the attribution of authority to the medical recommendations of the German medieval mystic Hildegard of Bingen.

The final two articles in this collection raise powerful questions for both ethnographers and practitioners of formal medicine, both at the phenomenological and the epistemological levels. "Participant observation" as a methodological technique is relatively straightforward for the field worker when "participation" involves practices that do not challenge basic assumptions, values, and beliefs. Mastering the steps of a social dance or learning to pat a tortilla into shape may provide valuable experiential insights that have implications for much higher levels of meaning. But for investigators who accidentally or intentionally place themselves in the way of experiences that are uninterpretable within their native frameworks of understanding, the consequences of participant observation can demand not just an empathic grasp of the beliefs of others, but a radical transformation of one's own beliefs and understandings and a concomitant distance placed between the researcher and his or her constituency of colleagues and students, not to mention friends and family. When it is the body as well as the mind that has undergone an experience uninterpretable save through "other" ways of knowing—when the investigator of healing practice is unexpectedly healed—the issues go to the core of what it means to know and to observe. Bonnie Glass-Coffin's discussion of the questions crystallized by the challenge she faces in teaching ethnographic courses based both on the Western critical tools of inquiry and on her own experience of shamanistic practice and healing provocatively frames many of the tensions faced by medical ethnographers, whether or not they have the courage to address the tensions as directly and publicly as she does here. Pursuing related themes, Barre Toelken explores the meaning of a personal experience in which, in Navajo terms, his survival required of his adopted family a series of immediate personal sacrifices followed by tragic consequences extending to the present—a price with which he is only beginning to come to grips professionally and personally decades later.

Most of the contributors to this volume have worked directly with formal medical institutions, applying their ethnographic expertise to contemporary problems in medical education and practice—a relatively new area of "applied folklore" which has special relevance to those who look forward to an era in which a "post-Flexnerian" approach to primary care is an honorable and honored companion to purely scientific medicine. At the close of the above-quoted essay in *The Task of Medicine*, Gayle Stephens recalls Abraham

Flexner's likening of the role of the physician to that of an engineer who makes life and death decisions. Stephens suggests that "a physician also needs the creativity and intuitiveness of the novelist," the same qualities of observation that also make for good interpretive ethnography. The contributors to this volume look forward to updating colleagues on the status of research in this rapidly developing area of our discipline. We also hope that the results of our research will have a larger consequence, perhaps "ambushing" a few readers who as yet fail, as I too once failed, to see the dynamic, emergent nature of nonconventional health belief systems, and the importance of understanding, and when appropriate, honoring the diversity of healing logics.

REFERENCES

Flexner, Abraham. [1910] 1973. *Medical education in the United States and Canada: A report to the Carnegie Foundation for the Advancement of Teaching.* Reprint, Buffalo, New York: Heritage Press.

George, Victoria, and Alan Dundes. 1978. The Gomer: A figure of hospital folk speech. *Journal of American Folklore* 91: 224–81.

Glaser, William A. 1968. Ethnomedicine: Social aspects. In *International encyclopedia of the social sciences.* Vol. 10, 87–95. New York: Macmillan.

Harrison, William R. 1992. Cross-cultural issues in medicine. In *The Merck manual of diagnosis and therapy.* 16th ed. Rahway, New Jersey: Merck Research Laboratories.

Hufford, David. 1989. Customary observances in medicine. *Western Folklore* 48: 129–43.

Levin, Jeffrey S., and Jeannine Coreil. 1986. "New age" healing in the U.S. *Social Science and Medicine* 23: 889–97.

O'Connor, Bonnie Blair. 1995. *Healing traditions: Alternative medicine and the health professions.* Philadelphia: University of Pennsylvania Press.

Stein, Leonard I. 1980. Male and female: The doctor-nurse game. In *Conformity and conflict: Readings in cultural anthropology,* ed. James P. Spradley and David W. McCurdy. Boston: Little, Brown.

Stephens, G. Gayle, M.D. 1988. Reflections of a post-Flexnerian physician. In *The task of medicine: Dialogue at Wickenburg,* ed. L. Kerr White, 172–89. Menlo Park, California: Henry J. Kaiser Family.

Zwicky, John F. 1993. *Reader's guide to alternative health methods.* Chicago: American Medical Association.

2

Understanding Folk Medicine

Bonnie B. O'Connor and David J. Hufford

Introduction

Both the term "folk medicine" and the conceptual category to which it refers are academic constructs that identify a particular subset of healing and health care practice. The most common interpretation of folk medicine in both popular and professional thought is that it represents a body of belief and practice isolated in various ways from the social and cultural "mainstream" and intriguingly unaffected by "modern" knowledge, with which it is frequently compared on the apparent presumption that "folk" and "modern" are mutually exclusive classifications. Folk medicine thus tends to be conceptualized within a hierarchical model of knowledge and sophistication of thought, in which it is typically located in a sort of lower midsection between official, scientific medicine at the hierarchical pinnacle and "primitive" medicine on the bottom stratum.

In part this schema is a product of the widely influential nineteenth-century Anglo-European theory of cultural evolution. From this perspective, medicine, like the rest of culture, was presumed to have developed "upward" in a largely linear and unidirectional progression from its crudest, most primitive form into its modern, Western, highly sophisticated state. All that was most effective, according to this theory, was retained and improved upon during this ascent, while discarded and obsolete ideas and practices drifted "downward" and were preserved in the "lower layers" of culture (somewhat tautologically identified by their difference from or incongruence with the social class and cultural heritage membership of those who articulated the theory). This model remains very influential in current popular and professional thought, despite the fact that the evolutionary view of culture on which it was based has been largely dismissed by most modern scholars of culture.

The simple evolutionary model leads almost inevitably to the erroneous conclusion that folk medical resources are by definition outdated and uninformed, and to the equally erroneous presumption that they are likely to be replaced by conventional biomedicine through improved access, together with the processes of education and acculturation. (Until quite recently this was the typical medical and academic perception of all the health care resources now gaining increasing popularity and legitimacy, under the general heading of complementary and alternative medicine, and it remains most persistent with respect to those nonbiomedical systems and modalities classified as "folk.") On the other hand, there are also those who romanticize folk medicine, inverting the value structure to portray it as an important repository of once-universal human knowledge and talents abandoned or forgotten in the push for progress and increasingly complex technological development (Fulder 1982; Grossinger 1982). The romantic view leads to misattributions to, and misinterpretations of, folk medical traditions. Neither of these models is an accurate or sufficient depiction of the nature of folk medicine, of its robust persistence in modern times, or of the complexity of the interactions between folk medicine and other health and healing resources— both through history and in the present day.

DEFINING FOLK MEDICINE

What makes some medicine "folk" is not the particular content of the system of knowledge and practice, but the mode of transmission together with the status of the system by comparison with whatever other medical system is recognized as "official" in the local context (Yoder 1972; Press 1978). Folklorists generally consider a heavy reliance on oral transmission to be a definitive feature of all aspects of folk culture. By this standard, folk medical systems are those learned and maintained primarily through oral channels. Because in the United States there is at present practically no cultural or identity group that is entirely independent of print and other technological media, the criterion of oral transmission is relative; that is, folk healing traditions have greater reliance on orality by comparison with other healing systems that rely primarily on (usually fairly standardized) printed information sources. Unofficial status, with respect to "official" dominant cultural forms, is another defining feature of folk knowledge and practice. These two characteristics—unofficial status and strong reliance on oral transmission—therefore interact in defining folk medicine.

Oral traditions involve relatively direct communication among individuals who share enough values and meanings for the communication to be accurately and easily interpreted, and for responses to have a direct and immediate impact. Thus folk medical traditions tend to show regional variation and to accommodate specific local conditions, as well as to be closely tied to groups or populations who share important identity-defining features such as a particular ethnicity (for example, the Pennsylvania German *Bräuche* or powwow tradition), a broadly shared cultural heritage (like the recognition by many distinct Latino populations of a hot/cold classificatory index for foods, medicines, and bodily states), or common regional influences (for instance, both blacks and whites in the Appalachian South share many aspects of regional folk herbalism and its related worldview and theories of disease causation).

Particularly in the present day, oral traditions often supplement direct, face-to-face speech with additional communicative media. In the United States these occasionally include use of telephones and circulation of audio- and videotapes to disseminate and maintain the vigor of traditional knowledge and practice and to accomplish or facilitate diagnostic and therapeutic ends, as well as exchanges of self-care information and recommendations by phone, fax, and internet. In addition, most do include some written source materials. For example, many refer closely to various religious scriptural sources and several include handwritten or printed books of recipes, formulae, verbal charms and prayers, and interpretive dicta.

PRAGMATIC AND SYSTEMATIC NATURE OF FOLK MEDICINE

Several significant oversights have characterized the study of folk medicine until quite recently. For example, although folk medicine, like all medicine, carries both benefits and risks, the effectiveness of folk medical practices has seldom been studied (with the exception of some ethnobotanical studies of medicinal plants), tending rather to be dismissed a priori as improbable. (One consequence of this persistent academic blind spot is that we have no independently verifiable record of the benefits or detriments of the majority of folk medical practices, or of their effects on health outcomes.) The precepts and practices of folk medicine have usually been presumed to be erroneous, and therefore thought to survive mainly through unexamined habitual usage or cultural custom. However, it is precisely the health promoting capacities of any system or therapeutic modality that are of greatest importance to its proponents and users. People dealing with health problems are typically quite pragmatic in approaching and evaluating any form of treatment or remedy: if it seems not to work, or produces effects that are too unpleasant, it tends to be rejected; if it seems to work, it tends to be supported and retained in the repertoire of healing resources likely to be tried again (and recommended to others). This pragmatism operates at both individual and collective levels. Folk healing traditions' reputations for efficacy, based on aggregate observation and experience, are central to their persistence and continued vitality.

Folk medicine has historically been viewed as a rather random aggregation of disparate ideas and practices. The presumed randomness and fragmentation, however, are attributions based largely on insufficient depth of study and unexamined assumptions. In fact, folk medical beliefs and practices are typically organized into complex and coherent systems of thought, action, and content (Hufford 1988a, 1992, 1994). Folk medical systems encompass, for example, complex bodies of knowledge and belief, specific modes of knowledge production (intuition, introspection, experimentation), evaluative processes applied in assessing the effectiveness of interventions and the qualifications of practitioners, definitions and categories of health and illness, explanatory models (Kleinman 1975, 1984) of disease etiology and human function, theories relating cause and nature of illness to preventive and therapeutic choices, specific repertoires of diagnostic and therapeutic actions and materia medica, generalist and specialist practitioners and the means to their training and legitimation within the system (apprenticeship, cross-gender training, supernatural selection), self-care modalities, and generative principles for formulating system-consistent responses to new input arising from confronting novel situations (O'Connor 1995a) and from interactions with other systems, including biomedicine.

One significant reason that the systematic organization of folk medicine has been overlooked for so long is the fact that in modern Western society systematization is a characteristic explicitly associated with official status. In conventional biomedicine, for example, the use of textbooks and specified curricula; the development of professional societies, standardized practice guidelines, licensure requirements, and regulatory legislation; the establishment of third-party payor systems following minutely articulated reimbursement criteria; and a host of other features of official culture foster the development and articulation of explicit systematization. In addition, these interconnecting features cause the systematization to be socially visible and prominently displayed in institutional forms—clearly enough, in fact, that ordinary people commonly refer to the entire aggregate as "the [health care] System."

Folk medicine, by contrast, generally relies more heavily on oral than printed transmission; is passed on more by observation and apprenticeship than by collective instruction in institutional settings; does not follow specific curricular formulations; does not seek or generate formal licensure or legal sanctions; does not give rise to professional publications or practitioner associations, or establish ties with external payors; and functions without internal or external requirements of standardization. These characteristics do not generate the explicit display of a systematic framework of organization. However, the lack of such visible expression is not an indication that no systematization exists. Within any folk healing tradition, the ways in which practitioners are selected, trained, and recognized as legitimate and qualified are interconnected, and are articulated with such other aspects of the system as help-seeking patterns (from self-care to seeking the services of a practitioner), understandings of illness causation, modes of recompense for services, and so forth.

For example, in spiritist healing traditions, practitioners are often identified initially through some form of supernatural indication or selection, and acquire their specialized knowledge through a combination of apprenticeship with recognized healers and mystically or intuitively acquired knowledge. Their "credentials," consisting of their communities' collective evaluations of them, derive in part from the reputations of those with whom they have trained, and in part from their cumulative personal reputations for proper and successful practice. Clients dealing with health problems are aware of a range of possible causes of illness, from environmental factors to spiritual or supernatural ones. The client or patient who believes an illness to be mild, or to have only material causes, typically begins with self-treatment through widely familiar home remedies, may move to consultation with an herbalist who has more specialized knowledge if results are not satisfactory, and upon suspecting that the illness has a spiritual cause, then may seek the services of the spiritist healer. The healer, having acquired his or her abilities as supernatural or divine gifts, may refuse to charge for services rendered, though the patient or a close relative may nevertheless leave an offering of goods or money in exchange or in gratitude. All of these features are systematically linked through shared bodies of knowledge and principles of action that form a coherent and integrated whole. Members of the system may nevertheless be unable to describe it in much detail, to identify its many components, or to articulate the principles by which these features are interconnected: they can *do* it, even if they cannot *say* precisely how and why.

The most useful explanatory analogy is language. Official ("correct") English has a rigorous and highly complex systematic structure that is codified in books. There are official English speakers and teachers who can recite the rules and correct inaccurate usages. Practically all American children are exposed to much of this official system, and some even learn it, though most do not achieve proficiency in articulating its structural elements and principles. Folk language (for instance local dialects and vernaculars, or slang) does not have such a prominent codified system, but linguists have amply demonstrated that a complex system is nonetheless present and is consistently acted upon. Speakers speak their particular linguistic forms correctly (with varying degrees of individual competence) and recognize errors, but they generally find it difficult to state the rules behind the distinctions. A linguist can infer the rules, however, through observation, analysis, and the questioning of speakers, and can construct an accurate descriptive grammar on the basis of these inferences.

Systems of folk medical belief and practice operate in the same fashion. Believers vary both in the scope of their traditional knowledge and in their competence to act within the system. Some, for example, folk healers, may be able to state the theoretical basis or directly describe substantial portions of the system, but the entire system is rarely available for direct inspection. The natural form for the expression of folk medical knowledge is in actions and in narratives about events. The theories and complex content of the systems must therefore at least in part be inferred from observing and listening to those who act within them. Then, like linguistic inferences, they can be checked with "insiders" for validity and situational applicability.

Core Concepts and Characteristics

Folk medicine in the United States comprises a very large and diverse array of health practices and beliefs. Because of the ethnic and cultural heterogeneity of the U.S. population, American folk medicine bears the influences of healing traditions and practices from all over the world. Although the range of distinct folk medical systems and modalities in the United States is enormous, many of these systems do share a number of fundamental concepts that can be broadly identified—so long as one bears in mind that the fine points of specific interpretations and the precise combinations in which they are found vary from system to system.

Characteristics of folk medical systems

- Transmission primarily through oral means, coupled with unofficial status
- Health as harmony or balance
- Interrelation of body, mind, spirit
- Vitalism
- Magical or supernatural elements
- Thoughts and emotions as etiologic factors
- Concern with underlying causes
- Positive/negative energies; transference of energies
- Moral tone; meaning of illness

Health as harmony or balance.   Most folk medical systems define health in terms of some form of harmony or balance. This balance can be among bodily humors or regulatory substances; innate properties such as heat and cold or yin and yang; forces such as upward and downward or inward and outward motion; states of the blood or other vehicles of internal bodily nourishment and cleansing; or periods of activity and rest. The spectrum of health practices is informed by this concept of balance. Many Latino, Caribbean, Asian, and Southeast Asian folk traditions, for example, incorporate a balance between hot and cold properties of foods, medicaments, and symptoms or bodily states. Cold conditions are offset with hot foods and medicines; hot conditions with cool ones. The goal of preventive and therapeutic actions is to maintain or restore health by moving toward a neutral center, usually with a preference for remaining slightly on the warm side (Harwood 1971, 1981; Schreiber and Homiak 1981; Duong 1987; LaGuerre 1987; Assanand et al. 1990; Gleave and Manes 1990).

In addition to internal states of equilibrium, harmony between the individual and external factors such as social, environmental, spiritual, and cosmological elements may affect health. For example, times of seasonal change are typically regarded as times of particular vulnerability to illness, and may require special protective steps such as seasonal "tonics," specific foods to be taken or avoided, and attention to health-promoting dress. Protection from exposure to cold, particularly in the form of cold air, drafts, and wind is a common preventive measure against ill health (indeed, it is difficult to find a person of *any* background or persuasion who did not grow up with some form of routine familial advice concerning protection from cold for reasons of health maintenance and disease prevention). This concern accompanies a pervasive conviction that cold can enter the body and accumulate, causing or contributing to a large variety of illnesses both immediately and in the (even quite distant) future (Snow 1974; Helman 1978; Ragucci 1981; Duong 1987). Cosmological factors such as lunar and astrological cycles may also be identified as affecting health or vitality in a variety of ways. These may call for behavioral adjustments to maintain a healthful balance or reduce health risk, and may be factored into the planting, harvesting, and preparation of medicinal plants and other substances (Snow 1977; Crellin and Philpott 1990).

Interrelation of body, mind, and spirit.   Most folk healing systems assume a complex interconnectedness of body, mind, and spirit (Harwood 1977; Trotter and Chavira 1981; Reimensnyder 1982; Hufford 1985, 1993; Duong 1987; LaGuerre 1987; Hufford and Chilton 1996). The balance and harmony that define health incorporate all of these aspects of persons, and disturbances in any of the aspects can produce sickness and symptoms in any of the others. Physical injury or sickness may bring about mental, emotional, or spiritual unwellness; emotional disturbance and mental unrest or worry may cause or exacerbate physical illness and disease. Spiritual well-being and harmony may be crucial aspects of health, and are variously defined in terms of an individual's inner state as well as in terms of relationships between human individuals and spiritual entities understood to interact with the material world and to influence personal health and more general well-being (success, prosperity, happiness, social relations) in a variety of ways.

Vital force or essence.   The human body is understood in most folk medical systems to be animated and sustained by a special type of force, energy, or essence whose presence and proper activity are essential to life and health. The nature, source, behavior, and manipulability of this life-sustaining force are variously defined across systems. There is a wide range of spiritual and metaphysical interpretations of this vital force, including, in some systems, connection of each individual's vital force with universal or cosmological fonts or reservoirs (Davis 1988). Damage to or disturbance, obstruction, or capture of the vital force leads to illness; restoration of its proper embodiment, freedom, and function promotes healing.

Magical and supernatural elements.   A significant number of folk medical systems recognize magical and supernatural elements in disease etiology. These may include, for example, sin as a direct cause of illness and disharmony; interventions by deities or spirit entities causing illness as retribution or reminder; undesirable states of spirit possession or intrusion (Duong 1987); spiritual causes such as soul loss or capture (Harwood 1981; Trotter and Chavira 1981; Rubel et al. 1984; Davis 1988; Dinh et al. 1990; Stephenson 1995); and malign human agency such as cursing, hexing witchcraft, and sorcery (Harwood 1977, 1981; Ragucci 1981; Reimensnyder 1982; LaGuerre 1987; Davis 1988; Brainard and Zaharlick 1989).

In some systems there are illness types that are specific to supernatural or magical causation. In addition, many systems recognize the possibility of variable causation, including supernatural elements, for *any* type of disease or illness (mental illnesses, infectious diseases, cancers, et cetera). Particular developments or details of an illness episode may suggest that supernatural causal factors are involved. In Haitian and Haitian-American folk healing tradition, for example, a magical or supernatural origin for disease may be suggested by sudden and severe onset, or by an unusually protracted course (LaGuerre 1987); in many Latino cultures, by either lengthy duration or failure to respond to standard (folk or conventional) treatment (Harwood 1977, 1981; Schreiber and Homiak 1981; Trotter and Chavira 1981); in African-American folk healing, by inability of a medical doctor to arrive at a diagnosis or identify a cause for troubling symptoms, or by a continual worsening of symptoms in spite of medical treatment (Snow 1974).

Treatment of illnesses that have supernatural or magical causal factors may involve simultaneous use of conventional biomedicine and one or more folk healing systems. Herbal remedies or conventional medicine may be the system used for symptom relief or to handle illnesses that seem serious. Whenever magical or supernatural causes are determined to be involved, however, these must also be properly addressed in the healing effort or else illness can be expected to recur, even if symptoms abate for the near term. Some of these types of healing measures can be carried out on one's own or in the context of the family, for example, through prayer, offerings, ritual baths and cleansings, use of specific medicaments and other protective and therapeutic substances, and so forth. Others require the interventions of a specialist practitioner, such as a *curandera*, shaman, rootworker, powwow, religious authority, or spiritual healer.

Thoughts and emotions as etiologic factors.   Obsessive, fearful, or negative thoughts, mental unrest and worry, and extremes of emotion (especially strong and negative emotions, such as anger or envy) are regarded as direct etiologic factors for illness in a number of systems. These factors too may be considered contributory in any type of disease or illness process (not just in mental and emotional illness), and again require that appropriate therapeutic action be taken to address them in order for healing to be complete or lasting.

One example common to many systems is envy as a possible etiologic factor in illness, both for the envious person and for those who are objects of the envy. Symptoms (for either person) may include headache, sleep disturbance, nightmares, fatigue or lassitude, loss of appetite, and gastric distress, among others. Envy as a direct cause of illness in others may be mediated through the envious or covetous gaze or the evil eye, which may be cast both intentionally and unintentionally (Foulks et al. 1977; Dundes 1981; Harwood 1981; Ragucci 1981; Assanand et al. 1990). Evil eye beliefs form a part of many American folk medical systems. Babies and children may be considered especially susceptible, and protective charms and amulets are commonly worn by children and adults alike as a preventive measure.

Concern with underlying causes.   Most folk medical systems seek to identify and treat underlying as well as immediate causes of disease. Underlying causes help to establish the conditions under which illness may develop or disease take hold, and may represent some type of fundamental imbalance or disharmony. This view generally accommodates conventional medical views quite readily, for example, accepting medical etiologies as identifying certain immediate causes. Thus, a germ may be accepted as the immediate cause of a disease, but it is understood to have caused it in a particular person at a particular time because of, for example, internal disequilibrium (hot/cold, or yin/yang), a buildup of toxins in the body, individual sinfulness, violation of dietary requirements (which in some instances may itself be a sin), diminished vital energy, and so forth (Hufford 1993; O'Connor 1995a). From the perspective of the folk medical system, diseases, and the body's susceptibility to their pathological agents, are often considered to be symptoms of underlying imbalances that require redress. This attention to underlying causes commonly leads proponents to feel that folk medicine treats the *causes* of ill health, while conventional medicine addresses itself primarily or exclusively to the *symptoms*. This view furnishes a conceptual framework in which the two kinds of healing systems can readily be integrated together in treating disease and promoting health.

Energies and transference.　　An emphasis on various kinds of "energy" is almost universal in folk medical systems, beginning, as previously noted, with the recognition of an animating energy or vital force. Folk medicine often involves several kinds of positive energies in promoting healing, and these are frequently contrasted with negative, life-destroying energies. Disease may result from imbalances in or the loss or theft of vital energy, but it may also be caused by the presence or intrusion of negative energies. These energies may be implicated in both natural and supernatural concepts of disease etiology. For example, improper preparation or cooking of foods may destroy their energetic vitality (natural), or witchcraft may steal it (supernatural), resulting in food that appears good but cannot nourish. Either circumstance can lead to illness.

　　A transference of positive energy from healer to patient is a characteristic of those systems in which a practitioner's hands are used therapeutically on or near the patient's body. In secular interpretations, this healing energy may be understood to come from within the healer's own vital energy stores or to pass through the healer from a cosmic source. In religious or spiritual interpretations, the healing energy is usually considered to be of divine origin; healers stress that it is God (or another powerful spiritual figure, depending on the system) who does the actual healing, while the practitioner is but an intermediary.

　　Many of the folk beliefs interpreted by scholars as based on the principle of "magical contagion" imply the exchange of such energies. Material objects may be endowed with negative energies and placed in the victim's environment; or the residue of a victim's unique life force in hair, nail parings, or an object long worn on his or her body may serve to focus the transmission of negative force, as in malign magical assault using figurines or magical packets. (These techniques are found, for example, in rootwork, a part of African-American folk tradition, and in some forms of Pennsylvania-German hexing.) In some traditions of prayer healing and psychic healing, conversely, personal objects still resonant with the sick person's life force serve to focus "distant healing." Disease, as a negative energy, may be transferred out of a person and into another living organism (such as a tree or an animal), or onto another object—as a wart is transferred onto a potato or a silver coin in some folk wart cures, later to wither away as the potato decays, or to be transferred to a new host along with the coin (Hand 1980). Conversely, positive energies and innate qualities (serenity, courage, vigor) may be imbibed with specific therapeutic substances and contribute in this nonpharmacologic way to the restoration or maintenance of health.

Moral tone. Folk healing systems generally incorporate a strong moral element such as a presumption of the inherent goodness of Nature, or a sense of personal responsibility for right behavior and health-protecting actions. Together with the high value placed on harmony and balance, these moral elements underscore the interconnectedness of personal health with the community, the physical environment, and the cosmos, and integrate the experience of sickness and health within a comprehensive and meaningful view of the world. This accounts for the characteristic way in which folk medical systems address the meaning of disease and suffering alongside attention to causation and cure, helping to furnish explanations for the always urgent questions that seriously sick people have of why (in the moral or metaphysical sense) they are sick, why in this way, and why now.

DISEASE AND ILLNESS CLASSIFICATIONS

Folk medical systems include illness taxonomies which tend, on the whole, to classify illnesses according to causation. In systems that incorporate a hot/cold index, one way of classifying diseases (or specific symptoms) is by their hot or cold type. Folk medical systems of Southeast-Asian historical origin may classify diseases and syndromes as caused primarily by "wind," "fire," or other elements in the body. Across a number of systems, two broad categories indicate natural or supernatural causation. In several systems, as mentioned, any disease or illness may entail natural and/or supernatural causality, and features of the particular illness episode and its progression will help to determine which factors are implicated and in which ways.

In African-American folk tradition, sickness can be broadly classified as natural or unnatural. Natural illnesses occur in accordance with the proper workings of Nature (or, in a religious interpretation, in accordance with God's laws); unnatural ones are brought on by means that in some way violate God's will (in religious terms) or the natural order (in secular terms), such as sickness caused by sorcery or by excessive worry or mental unrest (Snow 1974, 1977). Both natural and unnatural sicknesses may have material causes (such as germs), or may have divine causal elements such as punishment for sin, or illness sent as a test or reminder of faith and religious duty.

Across folk medical systems, some types of illness may be specific to one category while for others a variable type of causation is possible, and etiology may differ in specific instances of the same disease. Causality may also be mixed, or one type may establish the imbalance or disharmony (underlying cause) that makes a person vulnerable to another form of (immediate) causal agent or circumstance. Treatment is in accordance with the nature and causes of the disease. As new information is gained in the course of the illness, or as prior treatment strategies are deemed ineffective or inappropriate, substitutions or additions will be made in the treatment strategy—both within the folk medical system and by incorporation of other treatment forms such as elements from other systems, including conventional medicine.

Folk Illnesses

Folk healing systems generally include recognition of some types of illness that are not recognized as disease categories in the biomedical diagnostic canon. These illnesses are referred to by scholars and health professionals as "folk illnesses," sometimes also called "culture-bound syndromes" (Simons and Hughes 1985; Hufford 1988b; Pang 1990; American Psychiatric Association 1994). The concept of "folk illness" is an academic construct which takes the diagnostic and etiological categories of biomedicine as its reference point. The implication of the label is that an illness so referenced is not "real," or at least is not "really" what people who accept it as real believe it to be. This is an etic viewpoint that is of course not shared by members of and believers in the folk medical systems in which these illness categories are found. Cultural insiders likewise do not use the term "folk illness," referring instead to each such illness by its own culturally supplied name (Snow 1977; Harwood 1981; Schreiber and Homiak 1981; Trotter and Chavira 1981; Hufford 1982; Rubel et al. 1984; Duong 1987).

Folk illnesses, like other illnesses, have recognized etiologies, particular constellations of symptoms, diagnostic criteria, identified sequelae, and specified preventive and therapeutic measures. Some folk illnesses appear to represent local names or varied symptom patterns of currently recognized medical disorders (Rubel et al. 1984; Hufford 1992), while others do not seem to have medical correlates (although they are frequently—and often erroneously—reinterpreted in psychiatric terms by health professionals and researchers). In either case, some aspects of the explanatory model of folk illnesses will depart from the conventional medical model, and treatment will follow the system-congruent reasoning: cooling excess heat, restoring proper motion of vital force, dispelling cold or toxins accumulated in the body, extirpating evil influences, and so on. Folk medical causality and therapeutics are not confined solely to folk illnesses, however, but are also applied to medically recognized diseases. This is another element that helps to account for the fact that folk healing traditions are frequently combined as therapeutic options both with biomedicine and with other unofficial systems or modalities with which particular individuals may be familiar.

Some folk illnesses are closely tied to specific populations or healing traditions, while others are widely recognized across cultures and systems. Of these, perhaps the most ubiquitous is soul loss, called by a variety of system-specific names, and sometimes academically referred to as "magical fright" or "fright illness" (Simons and Hughes 1985). The fundamental pathogenic factor in soul loss is inappropriate, undesirable, or unintentional separation of a living person's soul from the body. Soul loss (perhaps most familiar to academics and researchers by its Spanish name, *susto* [Rubel et al. 1984]) is recognized across a number of systems as most commonly being caused by severe fright, trauma, or emotional shock. This may be precipitated by experiencing (or even witnessing) a frightening accident or incident of violence or brutality, receiving sudden bad news for which one is unprepared, experiencing extended extreme hardship, or being caught up in terrifying natural events such as earthquakes and other natural disasters. Some systems also recognize the possibility of soul loss through capture by human sorcerers (Davis 1988) or malicious spirits (Geddes 1976).

Like many medically recognized conditions, soul loss is considered both a sickness in itself, and a contributing factor in other illnesses. Soul loss is always serious, and if not properly treated can lead to death. Indications are that treatment outcomes for at least some folk illnesses, including susto, are best when the appropriate traditional remedies are used or the indicated folk healers provide the treatment (Rubel et al. 1984). It is important that health professionals not dismiss or trivialize folk illnesses since, for at least some of them, there is also evidence that their sufferers are at increased risk for general morbidity and mortality (Rubel et al. 1984), and in some cases traditional treatments may also have important clinical consequences, both positive and negative (Trotter 1981a, 1981b, 1985; Lazar and O'Connor 1997).

FOLK PRACTITIONERS

Self-care or family care and home-based first aid account for a great proportion of health behavior in both folk tradition and "mainstream" practice. Household staples such as eggs, lemons, garlic, chicken soup, rice, and other foodstuffs are used preventively and therapeutically across populations and traditions, together with common medicinal plants and herbs; and their proper preparation and applications tend to be matters of general knowledge. Many households maintain a small herb or medicine garden, or keep a few of the "standards" potted indoors. Dietary and behavioral patterns may or may not explicitly be considered parts of "health care," yet still may constitute important health behaviors within the system and follow system-consistent organizing principles.

Generalist and specialist practitioners are also found in most folk medical systems. Across several traditions these include midwives, massagers, bonesetters, blood stoppers, wart curers, thrush or "thrash" doctors (for infants and children), healers of burns and other skin conditions, religious, magical, and spiritual specialists of various kinds, and herbalists. Selection as a practitioner occurs in a number of ways. Common among these are birth order or other birth circumstances; conferring of divine or other supernaturally bestowed gifts and callings; special life circumstances; transformative personal experiences, including experiences of serious illness and healing; familial inheritance; and of course self-selection for reasons of personal desire or interest (Hand 1980).

Seventh children—especially seventh sons—are widely believed to be born with special powers and abilities, and among these may be the gift of healing. (Variations on this theme include the seventh same-sex child with no intervening opposite sex births, or the seventh son of a seventh son.) The gift does not usually become active until near adulthood, though there are instances of child healers in many folk systems. Twins may have innate healing abilities, and if one twin dies the "left twin" (the one left behind) is especially likely subsequently to be able to heal. Posthumous children (those born after the death of their mothers—usually a death in childbirth, but also deaths from other circumstances such as illness or accident, following which the child is taken alive from the womb) are often considered born healers, either with general healing abilities, or with a particular capacity to heal thrush and other diseases of infancy and childhood (Hand 1980). Children born with a veil or caul (a portion of the amniotic membrane covering the face or eyes) may be believed destined to be healers, and sometimes also to have "second sight" or clairvoyant abilities, which may also be used in their healing vocations.

Ordinary individuals may be singled out to become healers by receipt of a divine or other supernatural gift or calling. The indication of this calling can come in a number of ways, including mystical experience, notification in dreams or visions, direct cognitive awareness, human messenger (often another person with special abilities), or a series of subtle signs whose cumulative import gradually becomes clear. It is common in a number of traditions for individuals singled out in this way to find the gift or calling burdensome, and to try to ignore or reject it—especially as acting on it may require substantial changes in behavior and lifestyle. Typically the attempt to refuse such a calling results in an escalating series of illnesses and other misfortunes that befall the designee, until he or she reaches the point of determining that the gift or calling is truly an imperative and must be accepted. Acceptance and the accompanying change in life direction resolve the preceding state of disruption of the healer's life.

Special life circumstances such as widowhood or childlessness may confer healing ability or simply make a (potential) healer readily identifiable (Hand 1980). Transformative life experiences, including mystical and visionary experiences, religious conversion, and instances of sudden and extreme good or bad fortune may prompt a person to become a healer, or provide a sign of a calling. Serious illness which subsequently resolves or is healed by specific means (including biomedical ones), together with accidents that leave the victim permanently changed in some way, also figure prominently among these transformative experiences. In some cases this may be simply because harsh personal experience yields insight and empathy and a desire to help others; in others, the illness experience includes receipt of special information or mystical insight. Shamanic healers may in the course of their illness enter the spirit world and there be instructed, tested, assaulted, or even spiritually killed and resurrected, and return to consciousness and the material world redirected to become healers (Eliade 1964). Supernatural selection may be implied in the occurrence of any transformative experience, including illness. The likelihood of such selection may or may not run in families. Selection or calling to become a healer may itself bestow healing abilities directly upon the designee, or these may have to be acquired through a period of apprenticeship—sometimes quite long and arduous—with an established healer.

COMMON THERAPEUTIC PRACTICES

The enormous diversity of American folk medicine makes it impossible to enumerate every therapeutic practice found in every system. There are, however, broad common categories of preventive and therapeutic modalities in use across systems, including physically applied therapies, medicinal herbs and other naturally derived substances, sacramental objects, and prayers and other religious and spiritual actions. It is important to note that these are not mutually exclusive categories. Indeed, it is most common to find considerable overlap among them, for example, medicinal herbs used in a mash physically applied to the body, with accompanying prayer, for the purpose of bringing about spiritual purification as a step in the healing process.

Of course, particular theories of the modes of action of these therapies, and of the relationship between a particular therapy and the specific health condition or individual illness episode for which it is applied, vary across healing traditions in keeping with system-specific explanatory models of health and illness and care. Because standardization is not a feature of folk medicine, it is also quite common to find significant variation from region to region, or from healer to healer, in the interpretation and applications of even those practices most fundamental to a given system.

Religious, spiritual, and magical actions and sacramental objects.   Spiritual and magicoreligious actions commonly used to promote health and healing include prayer; reading or recitation of sacred texts; pious ejaculations (for example "Ave María" among Spanish-speaking Catholics, or "Good Saint Anne, protect us!"); recitation of verbal charms and brief formulaic utterances (such as "knock wood" or "*kain ein horeh*") to ward off misfortune or evil influences; protective gestures such as making the sign of the cross, or spitting between the first two fingers or extending the index and little fingers to ward off the evil eye; meditation and spiritual contemplation of a variety of types; laying on of hands or use of the hands near the body to remove illness and negative influences or energies; petitions and offerings to or bargaining with spiritual entities; visits to holy sites and healing shrines; temporary internment in places of worship or spiritual contemplation; burning of incense and of "spirit money" or joss paper; spiritual cleansings of a variety of types (including herbal baths, and "sweepings" with plant and animal substances); soul callings and restorations; preparation of figurines and magical packets; and use of amulets and other protective items, among innumerable other possibilities. Prescription or administration of botanical and other natural medicaments, as mentioned, may occur in a religious healing setting, with spiritual instruction or guidance, or with spiritual or metaphysical health outcomes in mind.

Natural substances.   Ethnic and regional cultures almost without exception have developed a materia medica of locally available natural substances—botanical, animal, and mineral. Therapeutic goals and modes of use of these natural medicines are determined by the tenets of a wide variety of theoretical models, and pharmacological and biochemical models do not necessarily apply (O'Connor 1986). Herbs and other natural medicinals are used for their physical actions and effects, but also (among other purposes) for metaphysical properties such as hot and cold or yin and yang qualities and effects; for spiritual qualities with which they are associated, such as purity, patience, inner strength, or calm; for effects they will have on the quality and function of the body's vital energy; or for their capacity to absorb and carry away negative influences.

Natural medicants are taken orally as teas or soups and are cooked into foods, both primarily as medicines, and as culinary herbs intended to provide both gustatory and salutary benefits. They are used as inhalants and as ingredients in baths, sweats, and steamings; in ointments, linaments, and salves, ear and eye drops, douches and enemas, poultices, wet or dry packs, massage compounds; and in moxibustion (the burning on or very near the skin surface of tiny amounts of dried compressed plant material). Specific substances may be used to "sweep" the body in ritual cleansings, drawing out disease-causing malignancies. Eggs or small live animals are also used for this purpose in many settings, because their life force may successfully substitute for the vital essence of the patient as a target for malign forces, possessing spirits, and other agents of ill health which may be transferrable out of the patient.

Any natural substances, in any of their multitudinous modes of use, may be used to achieve physical, mental, emotional, or spiritual healing objectives. An herb taken internally is as likely to be intended to bring about changes in the state or motion of vital energy, to imbue a quality of character or state of mind, or to enhance or restrain specific bodily functions, for example, as it is to alleviate a physical symptom. An herbal rubdown or sweeping may be used to draw out a fever or put an end to respiratory distress as well as to deal with spiritual or metaphysical aspects of illness.

Physical therapies.   Various forms of massage, stroking, and rubbing are physical therapies found in numerous folk medical traditions. As with herbs and other natural medicinals, the therapeutic goals are varied. For example, abdominal massage is used in Mexican-American folk healing to achieve specific physical ends: alleviation of intestinal gas or of muscle pain and cramping, or release of "stuck" digestive products that are thought to adhere to the stomach lining, causing the folk illness *empacho* (Schreiber and Homiak 1981; Trotter 1981a, 1985). Pinching and lifting of the skin may serve a similar purpose, while other forms of massage and physical manipulation are intended to ameliorate the flow and functional status of vital energy, or to promote states of physical relaxation or mental or emotional calm or clarity. In some Southeast-Asian traditions, dermabrasive techniques such as rubbing the skin with a lubricated metal utensil or coin (hence the English name, "coining") have as their goal the release of "wind" (Yeatman and Dang 1980; Duong 1987), an etiologic factor in a variety of illness states. Cupping is used in folk medical traditions of a wide range of ethnic and cultural origins. This entails placing on the skin (most commonly on the back and upper shoulders) small cups or jars which adhere by means of a vacuum created when they are first heated. Depending on the tradition within which this treatment is undertaken, it is intended to draw impurities, excess humors, "bad blood," or "wind" out of the body; if blood is specifically to be released, small cuts may be made in the skin before placement of the cups.

A number of folk medical traditions also include physical actions which are intended to achieve their therapeutic ends through essentially magical or metaphysical means. These include such practices as "measuring" (sometimes using a specific type or color of ribbon or string), and "passing through," a practice in which the sick person (most often a child) is passed through a fork or other opening in a tree, during which process it is intended that the sickness or other negative energy or undesirable influence will be drawn out (Hand 1980).

Interactions with Other Systems

Most people—even those for whom a single health care system is dominant—use a wide variety of home treatment and prevention strategies far more often than they seek the services of any kind of practitioner (Levin et al. 1976; Dean 1981). If they do consult a doctor or other healer, these self-care practices often continue in some way to be used together with newly prescribed regimens. The herb teas taken to promote relaxation or sleep during an episode of disabling back pain, for example, are not necessarily replaced by the treatments of a chiropractor, the prescriptions of a physician, or the ministrations of a religious healer, but used concurrently with the practitioner's services. Indeed, *all* of these resources may be used simultaneously without causing any sense of dissonance or conflict for the patient: each may be seen to address a specific aspect of the problem, or all may be felt to complement and support each other in a well-rounded therapeutic plan (Hufford 1992; O'Connor 1995a, 1995b).

Self-care efforts are typically informed by a mixture of folk and "official" belief, gleaned during an individual's life through a variety of exposures and experiences. These are incorporated together into a coherent, if sometimes quite eclectic, personal system (Hufford 1988a), and involve beliefs that shape the manner in which any practitioner's advice is interpreted and pursued. For example, for adherents of a folk healing system incorporating a hot-cold theory, use of a medical doctor or other healer is common. If an herbal or pharmaceutical medication classified according to the folk taxonomy as "hot" is prescribed for a disease or symptom classified as "cold," it is likely to be accepted readily because its use is consonant with the patient's model of healthful balance. If "hot" symptoms or side effects then develop, however, it is likely that the dosage will be reduced or the medication discontinued: the hot medicine may be thought to be creating too much internal heat in the body (Harwood 1971), or the hot symptoms may be an indication that the body's balance has shifted and it is time to stop the treatment. If other types of treatments provided by a folk or "alternative" practitioner produce symptoms or reactions indicating disturbance of hot/cold balance, these too are likely to be suspended or amended to become congruent with the individual's dominant model.

For different patients the number of resources and the order in which they are brought to bear will vary depending on the availability of each option and other features of the sickness context, including the advice and opinions of trusted others and the nature and severity of the illness. The same person is likely to activate different health resources, or to come to them in a different order, for each particular health problem. Many people will try a folk remedy or have a folk healer treat them for warts much more readily than they will seek out a physician for the same purpose. The same individual may see a chiropractor for neck pain or chronic headaches but never for severe gastrointestinal symptoms, which are instead presented to a medical doctor. The services of the folk healer may be (re-)added if other treatments seem not to be working. If a diagnosis or prognosis is sufficiently alarming, it may move the patient to use modalities or practitioners which have been a part of his or her broader cultural repertoire, but of which he/she was previously fearful or skeptical. Entirely new and previously unfamiliar options may be sought out if new information has recently been acquired through the media, or through the patient's social network—a source of abundant health-related information and advice at almost any time, but especially so when one is known to have a health problem.

The precise patterns of folk medical use are highly individualized and case-specific. Folk medical systems have constant interactions with conventional medicine, though often without the knowledge of the medical profession. Many folk healers freely refer clients to medical doctors, even insist that they go, and they sometimes come into hospitals to continue to provide treatments for their patients (Hufford 1988a). The conventional medical model can be incorporated rather easily along with folk models of illness, and in some instances may even serve to reinforce them (Helman 1978).

Predictions that folk medicine would (even "should") die out in the face of scientific medical advances have been made in the United States for well over a century. They clearly have not been borne out to date, and there is no reason to suppose that they will be realized in the future. These healing systems are dynamic and flexible, readily incorporating new content and adapting to changing conditions while preserving many traditional elements, including some ideas and practices considered outmoded in parallel healing traditions. Folk medicine remains vigorously active in the United States, continually attracting new proponents who find the systems effective, broadly accessible, and often comfortably consonant with their general worldviews. It is fair to say that folk medicine is an important part of the total pool of health care resources upon which people draw for both therapeutic and preventive purposes. From herbalism to food customs to the use of prayer in preserving and restoring health, folk medicine is in fact the most basic and persistent dimension of the pluralistic health culture of the United States.

REFERENCES

American Psychiatric Association. 1994. *Diagnostic and statistical manual of mental disorders (DSM-IV).* Washington, D.C.: American Psychiatric Association.

Assanand, S., M. Dias, E. Richardson, and N. Waxler-Morrison. 1990. The south Asians. In *Cross-cultural caring: A handbook for health professionals in western Canada,* ed. N. Waxler-Morrison, J. M. Anderson, and E. Richardson, 141–80. Vancouver: University of British Columbia Press.

Brainard. J., and A. Zaharlick. 1989. Changing health beliefs and behaviors of resettled Laotian refugees: Ethnic variation in adaptation. *Social Science and Medicine* 29: 845–52.

Crellin, J. K., and J. Philpott. 1990. *Herbal medicine past and present.* Vol. 1, *Trying to give ease.* Durham, North Carolina: Duke University Press.

Davis, E. W. 1988. *Passage of darkness: The ethnobiology of the Haitian zombie.* Chapel Hill: University of North Carolina Press.

Dean, K. 1981. Self-care responses to illness: A selected review. *Social Science and Medicine* 15A: 673–87.

Dinh, D.-K., S. Ganesan, and N. Waxler-Morrison. 1990. The Vietnamese. In *Cross-cultural Caring: A handbook for health professionals in western Canada*, ed. N. Waxler-Morrison, J. M. Anderson, and E. Richardson, 181–213. Vancouver: University of British Columbia Press.

Dundes, A., ed. 1981. *The evil eye: A folklore casebook*. New York: Garland Publishing.

Duong, V. H. 1987. The Indochinese patient. In *Urban family medicine*, ed. R. B. Birrer, 238–42. New York: Springer-Verlag.

Eliade, M. 1964. *Shamanism: Archaic techniques of ecstasy*. Princeton, New Jersey: Princeton University Press.

Foulks, E., D. Freeman, F. Kaslow, and L. Madow. 1977. The Italian evil eye: *Mal occhio. Journal of Operational Psychiatry* 8 (2): 28–34.

Fulder, S. 1982. *The tao of medicine: Ginseng, Oriental remedies, and the pharmacology of harmony*. New York: Destiny Books.

Geddes, W. R. 1976. *Migrants of the mountains: The cultural ecology of the Blue Miao (Hmong Njua) of Thailand*. Oxford: Clarendon Press and Oxford University Press.

Gleave, D., and A. S. Manes. 1990. The Central Americans. In *Cross-cultural caring: A handbook for health professionals in western Canada*, ed. N. Waxler-Morrison, J. M. Anderson, and E. Richardson, 36–67. Vancouver: University of British Columbia Press.

Grossinger, R. 1982. *Planet medicine: From Stone Age shamanism to post-Industrial healing*. Revised edition. Boston: Shambhala Publications.

Hand, Wayland D. 1980. *Magical medicine: The folkloric component of medicine in the folk belief, custom, and ritual of the peoples of Europe and America. Selected essays of Wayland D. Hand*. Berkeley and Los Angeles: University of California Press.

Harwood, A. 1971. The hot/cold theory of disease: Implications for the treatment of Puerto Rican patients. *Journal of the American Medical Association* 216: 1153–58.

———. 1977. *Rx: Spiritist as needed: A study of a Puerto Rican community mental health resource*. Ithaca: Cornell University Press.

———. 1981. Mainland Puerto Ricans. In *Ethnicity and medical care*, ed. A. Harwood, 397–481. Cambridge, Massachusetts: Harvard University Press.

Helman, C. G. 1978. "Feed a cold, starve a fever": Folk models of infection in an English suburban community, and their relationship to medical treatment. *Culture, Medicine, and Psychiatry* 2: 107–37.

Hufford, David J. 1982. *The terror that comes in the night: An experience-centered study of supernatural assault traditions*. Philadelphia: University of Pennsylvania Press.

———. 1985. Sainte Anne de Beaupré: Roman Catholic pilgrimage and healing. *Western Folklore* 44: 194–207.

———. 1988a. Contemporary folk medicine. In *Other healers: Unorthodox medicine in America*, ed. N. Gevitz, 228–64. Baltimore: Johns Hopkins University Press.

———. 1988b. Inclusionism vs. reductionism in the study of the culture bound syndromes. *Culture, Medicine, and Psychiatry* 12: 503.

———. 1992. Folk medicine in contemporary America. In *Herbal and magical medicine: Traditional healing today*, ed. James Kirkland, Holly F. Mathews, C. W. Sullivan III, and Karen Baldwin, 14–31. Durham, North Carolina: Duke University Press.

———. 1993. Epistemologies of religious healing. *Journal of Medicine and Philosophy* 18: 175–94.

———. 1994. Folklore and medicine. In *Putting folklore to use: From health to human welfare*, ed. Michael Owen Jones, 117–35. Lexington: University Press of Kentucky.

Hufford, David J., and M. Chilton. 1996. Politics, spirituality, and environmental healing. In *The ecology of health: Issues and alternatives*, ed. J. Chesworth, 59–71. Thousand Oaks, California: Sage.

Kleinman, A. 1975. Explanatory models in health care relationships. In *Health of the family*, 159–72. Washington, D.C.: National Council for International Health.

———. 1984. Indigenous systems of healing: Questions for professional, popular, and folk care. In *Alternative medicines: Popular and policy perspectives*, ed. J. W. Salmon, 251–58. New York: Tavistock.

LaGuerre, M. S. 1987. *Afro-Caribbean folk medicine*. South Hadley, Massachusetts: Bergin and Garvey Publishers.

Lazar, J. S., and Bonnie Blair O'Connor. 1997. Talking with patients about their use of alternative therapies. *Primary Care: Clinics in Office Practice* 24 (4): 699–714.

Levin, L. S., A. H. Katz, and E. Holst. 1976. *Self-care: Lay initiatives in health*. New York: Prodist.

O'Connor, Bonnie Blair. 1986. Material and immaterial essences in herbal healing. Unpublished paper, delivered at the American Folklore Society annual meeting, Baltimore, Maryland.

———. 1995a. *Healing traditions: Alternative medicine and the health professions*. Philadelphia: University of Pennsylvania Press.

———. 1995b. Vernacular health care responses to HIV and AIDS. *Alternative Therapies in Health and Medicine* 1 (5): 35–52.

———. 1998. Healing practices. In *Handbook of immigrant health*, ed. S. Loue. New York: Plenum Press.

Pang, K. Y. C. 1990. *Hwabyung*: The construction of a Korean popular illness among Korean elderly immigrant women in the United States. *Culture, Medicine, and Psychiatry* 14: 495–512.

Press, I. 1978. Urban folk medicine: A functional overview. *American Anthropologist* 80: 71–84.

Ragucci, A. J. 1981. Italian Americans. In *Ethnicity and medical care*, ed. A. Harwood, 211–63. Cambridge, Massachusetts: Harvard University Press.

Reimensnyder, B. 1982. Powwowing in Union County. Ph.D. diss. Philadelphia: University of Pennsylvania.

Rubel, A. J., C. O'Nell, and R. Collado-Ardon. 1984. *Susto: A folk illness.* Berkeley: University of California Press.

Schreiber, J. M., and J. P. Homiak. 1981. Mexican Americans. In *Ethnicity and medical care*, ed. A. Harwood, 264–336. Cambridge, Massachusetts: Harvard University Press.

Simons, R. C., and C. C. Hughes. 1985. *The culture-bound syndromes: Folk illnesses of psychiatric and anthropological interest.* Dordrecht: D. Reidel Publishing Company.

Snow, L. 1974. Folk medical beliefs and their implications for care of patients: A review based on studies among black Americans. *Annals of Internal Medicine* 81: 82–96.

———. 1977. Popular medicine in a black neighborhood. In *Ethnic medicine in the Southwest*, ed. E. Spicer, 19–98. Tucson: University of Arizona Press.

Stephenson, P. H. 1995. Vietnamese refugees in Victoria, B.C.: An overview of immigrant and refugee health care in a medium-sized Canadian urban centre. *Social Science and Medicine* 40 (12): 1631–42.

Trotter, R. T., III. 1981a. Folk remedies as indicators of common illnesses: Examples from the United States-Mexican border. *Journal of Ethnopharmacology* 4: 207–21.

———. 1981b. *Remedios caseros:* Mexican American home remedies and community health problems. *Social Science and Medicine* 15B: 107–14.

———. 1985. Folk medicine in the Southwest: Myths and medical facts. *Postgraduate Medicine* 78 (8): 167–79.

Trotter, R. T., III, and J. A. Chavira. 1981. *Curanderismo: Mexican American folk healing.* Athens: University of Georgia Press.

Yeatman, G. W., and V. V. Dang. 1980. *Cao gio* (coin rubbing): Vietnamese attitudes towards health care. *Journal of the American Medical Association* 244: 2748–49.

Yoder, D. 1972. Folk medicine. In *Folklore and folklife: An introduction*, ed. Richard M. Dorson, 191–215. Chicago: University of Chicago Press.

places and practitioners

3

Invisible Hospitals: Botánicas in Ethnic Health Care

Michael Owen Jones and Patrick A. Polk, with Ysamur Flores-Peña and Roberta J. Evanchuk

The extent to which folk medicine is practiced today by Hispanics is not clearly established. Probably its popularity varies in different regions of the country. . . . But the one thing that is definite is that faith healers are a part of the Hispanic culture and that some Hispanics do utilize their services. This alone should be reason enough to look to faith healers as a potential reserve when considering the most effective ways for providing help to Hispanics. (LeVine and Padilla 1980, 150, 186)

Their existence scarcely noted by medical and cultural researchers, *botánicas* have burgeoned in recent years not only in Los Angeles but throughout the country (principal works on the subject include Borrello and Mathias 1977; Fisch 1968; George 1980; Murphy 1988; and Suro 1991). For many Latinos and African Americans in Los Angeles, they are a point of entry into the community, the source of familiar sacramental items, a mainstay of spiritual, family, and personal counseling, and the provider of crucial herbal preparations for various illnesses. Associated with such ethnomedical and spiritual systems as Santería, folk Catholicism, Curanderismo, Espiritismo, and Hoodoo (also called "conjure" or "rootwork"), botánicas sell herbal products, ritual implements, and sacramental goods as well as provide medical and spiritual consultations. As such, they are an urban, community-based resource serving a variety of immigrant and migrant groups. Botánicas also attract those from the general populace dissatisfied with conventional medicine, in search of holistic healing, or seeking alternative therapies.

Botánicas as an alternative health care provider are important because of several facts about the population of southern California. First, the families of nearly half of Los Angeles County's 8.8 million residents came from Latin America, the Caribbean, and the American South. According to the 1990 census, some cities consist almost entirely of Latinos, African Americans, or both. The first account for three-fourths of El Monte's population of 106,209. Huntington Park's 56,065 residents include 51,496 Mexicans, Cubans, Salvadorans, Guatemalans, Nicaraguans, and Puerto Ricans. A quarter of a century ago Compton was 5 percent Hispanic and 93 percent black; among the 90,454 individuals now dwelling there, 39,510 are Latinos and 49,598 are African Americans, about one-third of whom migrated from southern states. Many African American businesses in Compton have yielded to Latino storefront churches as a result of these changing demographics (Weightman 1993, 8). More than one-fourth of California's population is foreign born, most of whom are from Mexico and Asia. The Legislative Analyst's Office estimates that between 1990 and 2010, California's Hispanic population will double and the state's Asian population will grow by two-thirds (www.lao.ca.gov).

Another reason botánicas need to be studied is that according to public health surveys 6.6 million Californians lack health insurance, 1.8 million of whom are children. Those without insurance include 38 percent of the state's nonelderly Latino residents and 22 percent of African Americans. Los Angeles County has the largest portion of uninsured residents, most of whom work in menial jobs with no fringe benefits or at a wage too low to afford premiums when available. Without insurance, they have limited access to preventive medicine and often must delay professional treatment (Edelman, Lazarus, and Salisbury 1998; Maugh 1998; Pyle 1999; also see www.ph.ucla.edu).

Given these two sets of conditions, it is crucial to consider the services that botánicas provide to the many people who rely on them in the absence of other health care resources. How, exactly, do botánicas and healers associated with them address the medical, spiritual, and social needs of clients? The purpose of this chapter is to explore ways that many immigrant as well as some mainstream populations in southern California utilize spiritual and herbal healing centers for a wide variety of problems. Knowledge of traditional precepts and practices can help health care professionals better understand the orientation of many of their clients with a view toward enhancing the care extended to them. Information about alternative ethnomedical and spiritual approaches also has ramifications for public health programming, including the utilization of community-based, traditional practitioners as important resources and helpful intermediaries.

RESEARCH ON ETHNIC HEALTH

The medical literature on Latinos and African Americans in Los Angeles ranges widely. Some of the 250 or so articles, based largely on quantitative and clinical research, indicate the need for more intensive, qualitative research on ethnic health status and community-based healing traditions. For example, a number of epidemiological works that point to ethnic differences and ethnic-specific patterns of behavior associated with morbidity urge further exploration of linkages (see Newell and Mills 1986 on cancer; Norris et al. 1993 on heart disease; Zambrana and Scrimshaw 1997 on substance use during pregnancy; and Brekke and Barrio 1997, Shrout et al. 1992, and Vega et al. 1998 on mental illness). Some studies present statistics on differential rates in the use of screening, diagnosis, and treatment apparently related to ethnicity; they often report underutilization by Latino and African American populations for reasons not yet determined, for example, mammography (Carlisle, Leake, and Shapiro 1995; Bastani et al. 1995), psychiatric diagnosis (Flaskerud and Hu 1992; Sue et al. 1991), breast cancer diagnosis (Richardson et al. 1992), prenatal care (Taggart and Mattson 1996; Zambrana, Dunkel-Schetter, and Scrimshaw 1991), and invasive cardiac procedures (Carlisle, Leake, and Shapiro 1995; Ell et al. 1995). Several works describe novel public health interventions among ethnic populations based on the growing belief that culturally relevant programs are needed to maximize diffusion of information (Flaskerud and Nyamathi 1990; Parker et al. 1996).

The only recent study that deals directly with some aspect of folk medicine in Los Angeles is Becerra and Iglehart's essay (1995) comparing the use of home remedies among African Americans, Mexican Americans, Chinese Americans, and non-Latino whites (see earlier works by Dwyer 1987 on Hmong; Edgerton, Karno, and Fernandez 1970 on Curanderismo; George 1980 on Santería; and Roeder 1988 on Latino traditions). The authors note the extensive use of folk medicine concurrently with biomedical care—contrary to long-standing assumptions that folk medicine is limited to rural settings or has nearly died out, and that the utilization of folk medicine and biomedicine is mutually exclusive.

Among the fourteen articles on the spiritual and herbal aspects of Latino health care listed on PubMed (the National Library of Medicine's internet bibliographical service of more than nine million entries), half a dozen based on research in other states relate to concerns in the present study.

Mikhail (1994) reports that 81 percent of Latinas relied on home remedies to manage their children's health problems and 17 percent sought help from a folk healer. According to Keegan (1996), nearly half of Mexican Americans responding to a questionnaire had used an alternative practitioner one or more times during the previous year—mostly herbal medicine and spiritual healing, including visits to a curandero or curandera—two-thirds of whom never reported these visits to their primary care provider. Zuckerman and others (1996) found Latinos far more likely than Anglos to self-medicate bowel problems with herbal teas and other folk remedies, the perception of health and bowel function in part determined by ethnicity. Suarez, Raffaelli, and O'Leary (1996) discovered through interviews that nearly two-thirds of their Latino subjects with AIDS engaged in folk healing, either Spiritism or Santería, and three-fourths believed in good and evil spirits, with nearly half stating that spirits had a causal role in their infection. Desired outcomes of folk healing included physical relief (44 percent), spiritual relief (40 percent), protection from evil (26 percent), and effecting a cure (23 percent). Zaldivar and Smolowitz (1994) surveyed the role of spiritual and folk medical beliefs in perceptions of diabetes and treatment choices and found that 78 percent of their Latino subjects believed they had diabetes because it was God's will and 17 percent reported using herbs to treat the disease.

These studies indicate that the health-related perceptions and behaviors of many Latinos are an integral part of cultural systems of religion and healing traditions (for African Americans, see Frankel 1977; Hyatt 1970–78; Jackson 1976; Kerr 1993; Mathews 1987; Snow 1974, 1977, 1979, 1993; Terrell 1990; and Weidman 1978). In regard to interventions, therefore, Stolley and Koenig (1997) posit that knowledge of the impact of spiritual beliefs among ethnic groups can help in designing culture-specific strategies for professional health care (see also Fishman et al. 1993; and O'Connor 1995, 1997). That ethnographic research and training based upon it are desperately needed is underscored by Brooks's findings (1992) at the Martin Luther King County General Hospital in Los Angeles: most personnel lack knowledge and understanding of the dominant Latino and African-American population treated at this facility, medical complaints from patients are inadequately communicated to health professionals, and instructions are not sufficiently related to the patients. While part of the problem is language competency, much of it is lack of cultural knowledge and sensitivity by health care workers. If the absence of insurance looms large as a barrier to accessing professional health care, additional obstacles result from the actions of providers themselves (Flores and Vega 1998). What other resources can ethnic populations avail themselves of, either instead of or (more commonly) in addition to biomedicine?

BOTÁNICAS AS SPIRITUAL AND HERBAL SHOPS

"Botánica" is a term first used in Cuba and later Puerto Rico by practitioners of the Afro-Cuban religions Santería, or Lucumí, and El Palo Mayombe (Stevens-Arroyo and Pérez y Mena 1995). Although immigrants from other parts of Latin America far outnumber those from the Caribbean in southern California, almost all of the spiritual-herbal centers bear the name botánica rather than *yerberia* (specializing in herbs) or *perfumería* (a source of candles, incense, and other sacramental objects) commonly found in Mexico (Trotter 1981). Botánicas recall the stalls in village or town markets in Mexico, Colombia, Guatemala, and other Latin American countries that sell herbs and sacramental items as well as those in African countries catering to the herbal requirements of traditional healers (in Nigeria called *kemwin-kemwin:* "anything and everything" shops; see Nevadomsky 1988). They also resemble African-American spiritual goods stores, occult stores (Winslow 1969), and "conjure shops." The latter is described in a 1930s account of a store in Jacksonville, Florida, "as just an ordinary store from the outside, but upon entering one is confronted by the exotic odor of soothing incense that evokes visions of foreign lands. Roots, herbs, oils, magic powers, charms, and spirit-chasing powders catch the eye among the thousands of labels on boxes and bottles arranged in neat rows on the long shelves" (McDonough 1993, 85). They have quickly proliferated throughout the Americas, for instance in Brazil, where they are known as *casas da umbanda*, and in Haiti among Vodou devotees returning from the U.S. As "omnibus stores" or "supermarkets" of religious and herbal goods, botánicas play a pivotal role, integrating multiple religious and healing traditions of their owners and clients through the varied ritual items, medical treatments, ceremonial preparations, and ecclesiastical instruction that they offer (Polk 1998). Among other shops in Los Angeles are those devoted to religious articles, "occult" stores (sometimes as part of store-front churches such as Winslow describes in Philadelphia [1969]), and the *centro espiritual* featuring readings and religious articles in the Spiritualist tradition associated with Allan Kardec.

The mere word botánica on a sign or window signals to the community that spiritual work is done here. Names like Botánica Obatala, Botánica el Negro Jose, Botánica Cristo Rey, Botánica el Milagro, and Botánica el Congo Manuel suggest different religious identities: Santería, or the preferred term Lucumí; Espiritismo, or Spiritism; Curanderismo; folk Catholicism; and El Palo Mayombe, respectively. All spiritual and herbal centers, however, offer assistance within a panoply of traditions. (Because these religions are embraced by hundreds of millions of people worldwide, we capitalize the names as is customary for Catholicism, Protestantism, Buddhism, et cetera, but use lower case when referring to religious functionaries such as priests, *paleras*, and *espiritistas*.)

Various sources place the number of these stores in Los Angeles from one hundred to one thousand or more (Quintanilla 1990; Sanchez 1997; Weightman 1993). Reasons for the disparity in estimates are that no one has systematically documented these centers, new ones spring up frequently, and some operate in homes rather than commercial shops, or they begin as storefronts, attract a clientele, and then move into the home. Their existence scarcely noticed by medical and cultural researchers, these religious-herbal centers appear to serve as community hubs and meeting places, "natural support systems" (Delgado and Humm-Delgado 1982), and sources of information, referrals, personal and family counseling, and medicinal plants and treatments. They are usually open from 9 A.M. to 6 P.M. Monday (the least busy day) through Saturday (the busiest day, in preparation for rituals and ceremonies).

Judging from published lists, Los Angeles seems to have the most botánicas. Some store owners or counselors and herbalists claim the identity of *curanderos* (male) or *curanderas* (female) in the Mexican tradition. Many others call themselves *espiritistas* or *spiritists* as they practice Espiritismo. Yet others are *santeros* or *santeras* indicating an affiliation with Afro-Cuban Santería, or Lucumí, or *paleros* or *paleras* associated with El Palo Mayombe. A number of them refer to themselves by several terms at once, depending on their familiarity with different religious systems and the needs of their clients. In a sampling of ten spiritual-herbal centers in downtown and east L.A., for instance, the man who operates one botánica is a santero and his wife a spiritist, the husband-wife owners of another are both a santero/a and a palero/a. One woman is a palera and santera as well as a spiritist while other healers practice only Santería or El Palo; some are also herbalists called *yerberos* or yerberes following the Curanderismo tradition or *osainistas* within Lucumí.

Inside a Botánica

The sidewalk in front of Botánica la Sagrada (pseudonym) is crowded and bustles with activity. As usual, street vendors have set up their small tables in front of the large, red brick building that houses the botánica and several other small shops. Carefully positioned in the narrow strip of shade that runs along the building's facade, they boisterously hawk candy, clothing, and a sundry of other goods to passersby. Behind them the bright glare of the sun fills the botánica's windows with reflections making it almost impossible to see the large, colorful statues of Catholic saints that announce the shop's trade in religious articles.

Like many other botánicas in southern California, the exterior of Botánica la Sagrada is relatively nondescript and easy to overlook. Nevertheless, a steady stream of people enter and exit the store. Upon entering this botánica, one is struck by how distant the interior seems from the din of traffic, the rush of curbside commerce, and the stifling vapors of automobile exhaust. Inside it is cool and quiet. The air is infused with enchanting aromas from the numerous perfumes, colognes, incense sticks, and scented oils filling the store. Each breath seems to bring a new sensation. Even the names of the products are captivating: Patchouli D'Amor, Secret Fruit Lotion, Ivory Elephant Spray, and Seven African Powers Incense.

The store's many shelves and display cases are packed to the ceiling with religious paraphernalia and, as you look around, your gaze is drawn to one icon, image, or statue after another, each seemingly more esoteric and fascinating than the last. The paneled wall behind the cash register is literally plastered with colorful chromolithographs of Jesus Christ, the Virgin Mary, and various Catholic saints. A shelf directly below these holds statues depicting saints in their respective poses of grace and divinity. Replicas of St. Anthony stare in wonder at the Baby Jesus resting in the saint's arms while those of the crippled and gaunt St. Lazarus remain steadfast and resolute despite obvious pain and misery. In the midst of these, and seemingly out of place, is a carefully arranged line of ceramic Native Americans. Some are on horseback while others stand with their arms outstretched and heads turned heavenwards as if frozen in the act of summoning the spirits of the sky. All around these, hanging from hooks on the shelves and walls, are a vast array of rosaries, wooden crucifixes, beaded necklaces, and attractive charms made from colored fabric and small images of Catholic saints.

At first glance, the botánica seems to be little more than a retail outlet for an incomprehensible jumble of religious icons, mystic symbols, and plastic bags of plants. In *Santería: An African Religion in America* (1988), Joseph Murphy addresses the confusingly complex accumulation of artifacts, sacramental objects, and herbs. He writes: "To the uninitiated, their merchandise must look mysterious indeed: candles and beads, herbs and oils, cauldrons and crockery, and plaster statues of Catholic saints. Yet, for those who know their meaning, each of these items has a part to play in santería" (39). The many disparate images and icons that are brought together in the botánica typify the process of artistic and ritual synthesis that is the hallmark of African and Afro-Caribbean religion.

A place of spiritual consultation as well as an outlet for ritual and sacramental objects, the botánica is best understood as a combination of community center, herbal shop, and religious supply house. Inside, a person encounters retail display cases bearing the amazingly wide variety of goods that are either used in ceremonies and rituals or utilized in the creation of altars and shrines. In addition to candles, statues, and so on, one shop in east Los Angeles owned by a Mexican woman in her fifties who is a santera (Lucumí) as well as a palera (El Palo Mayombe) displays the following items, whether herbs or products made from herbal oils and essences (quantities are approximate):

> 145 packaged herbs stored in covered plastic containers on shelves on two walls
> 50 loose herbs from an herbalist, stored in plastic containers above a counter on the back wall
> more than 100 plastic containers and boxes of herbal capsules
> 50 or more small bottles of different kinds of tincture
> at least 40 bars of herbal and perfumed soaps
> 25 or more containers of herbal lotions and bath oils
> 80 containers of powders

Almost all botánicas are divided into two sections, front and back, each having distinct ritual, aesthetic, and commercial qualities. The front is usually more spacious. The majority of the merchandise for sale is displayed here. Proprietors often use this space to erect a variety of public and semiprivate altars that clearly indicate the spiritual traditions to which they adhere and to which clients may look for help. For example, botánicas in which Lucumí is the principle religion will invariably have an altar for Eshu-Eleggua located near the front door.

The rear of the store is usually where the owner counsels clients who come for advice or ritual assistance. This area is customarily separated from the front by a door or curtain offering the owner and client confidentiality during consultations and demarcating public and private space. Chairs, stools, or small benches are placed near the entry to the back section and are often occupied by individuals awaiting their turn to see the owner or the friends and family members of those who have come for consultation. In some stores, the rear section takes on the appearance of a doctor's office, complete with waiting room, water coolers, and coffee tables stocked with popular magazines. Because the back is normally the place of consultation, this is usually where the altars dedicated to the spirits or divinities with whom the owner most frequently works are located. Walls are often adorned by chromolithographs, not only of saints but also Native Americans who are thought to be particularly knowledgeable about herbs and therefore powerful allies in health (eight large images of Indians adorn the walls of one small consultation room, either portraits in full headdress or men on horseback).

There are also several wholesalers. Customers often refer to one of them as "the supermarket of botánicas." Huge by standards of religious goods stores, they do indeed resemble supermarkets, down to the wheeled grocery carts. Goods include several hundred books in English and Spanish on religion, divinities, and herbs as well as tarot cards, bath crystals, bath salts, floor washes, soaps, herb baths, shampoos, candles of varied size and color, colognes, lotions, plants, herbal teas, incense (hundreds of different sticks, powder, and aerosol sprays), scented oils, perfumes and sachets, jewelry (talismans, good luck charms, apotropaic pendants), statues (Native Americans, Buddha, wizards), crucifixes, rosaries, chromolithographs of saints, holy water, empty containers with which to mix and store one's own preparations, and a wide variety of ritual implements from incense burners to Ouija boards. Some wholesalers specialize in herbs. Over the course of a year one shop carries more than three hundred different plants from both arid and tropical regions of North and Central America, freshly harvested and ready for resale or immediate use.

Services Provided by Spiritual-Herbal Shops

The demand for the services provided by botánicas and the sacramental objects and medicinal plants and products that they stock has increased dramatically in recent years. Although botánicas tend to be located in neighborhoods with large numbers of immigrants from throughout the Caribbean and Latin America, the full clientele of each shop reflects the broad ethnic diversity of the city where it is located as well as the specific demographics of its neighborhood. In Los Angeles, for example, Guatemalans and Mexicans constitute a significant percentage of botánica owners and customers (although there are Puerto Rican and Cuban owners as well). In New York and Miami, the presence of Haitians, Dominicans, and Puerto Ricans is more significant. (Now, however, Mexicans are New York City's third largest Latino group; see Alonso-Zaldivar 1999.) Botánicas in every city are also frequented by members of many other ethnic groups including Anglo-Americans, Armenians, Chinese Americans, and Filipinos.

People require the services provided by botánicas for two basic reasons. Some come in order to obtain materials that will help continue ongoing interactions with the divinities they worship. For instance, a Cuban man knows he must light a special candle on the day sacred to Afro-Cuban deity Ogun or a Guatemalan woman believes that she will be able to become pregnant if she obtains a statue of San Simon and places the appropriate offerings in front of it. Others enter botánicas with a specific goal in mind but do not know what path to take to achieve it. Is there an *oricha* (Lucumí deity) who can help me find a lover? To which saint should I pray in order to heal my sick child, and what herbal remedies should I administer? One woman's simple but eloquent words confirm this role: "I came to the botánica looking for a spirit to guide me." In short, people turn to these centers in order to obtain specific sacramental objects or to find solutions to troubling medical, social, and spiritual situations most often by way of divination or trance mediumship.

One santero who operates a botánica estimates that a fourth of client encounters are for advice in business and personal decision making. The following description of a divination session exemplifies both the context and process of the ritual prognostication he performs (see also Mason 1993): In October of 1996, Olivia (pseudonym), a regular client, was forced to make an extremely difficult personal decision, one she felt unable to make without spiritual guidance. Like many other immigrants from El Salvador who had come to Los Angeles in search of a better life, she and her husband had been unprepared for the realities of urban America. After years of struggling to secure a stable income and to establish a safe home environment, the couple came to the conclusion that they could no longer remain in the dangerous and impoverished neighborhood where they lived. They decided to return to their native country. Before finalizing their plans to relocate, however, Olivia insisted on consulting the santero to whom she had been going for many years.

Hoping to determine whether or not the decision to leave the United States was a prudent one, Olivia asked the santero to perform a "reading" using the Afro-Caribbean cowrie shell divination system known as *diloggun*. Should she and her husband go back home? Or should they stay in California? Based on the interpretation of patterns formed by sixteen cowrie shells (*caracoles*) when tossed onto a mat or tray by the diviner, diloggun is considered by Lucumí santeros to be one of the most direct means of obtaining sacred knowledge. In order to "read" the messages conveyed by the cowries, the diviner counts how many shells land open side up and how many land on the closed or "mouth" side when they are thrown—a simple binary system. Each of the sixteen possible configurations that can be formed by the shells is referred to as an *oddu*. Associated with each oddu is a proverbial expression and several mythological narratives (*pataki*) that will ultimately be used to solve the client's problem. As part of their training, diviners memorize the large corpus of sayings, myths, and legends associated with the oddu and must be able to recite and interpret these when they are indicated by the arrangement of the cowries (see Bascom 1969; Evanchuk 1996; Flores-Peña 1998; and Sandoval 1979; contrast with divination by an espiritista described by Garrison 1977).

Also associated with each oddu are a number of auxiliary divination tools (*igbo*) that are used in pairs. After the initial toss of the cowries, the diviner employs the igbo, each of which has a specific positive or negative connotation, to more accurately interpret the meaning of the oddu that has been cast. The primary igbo are a black stone (*otan*), a ball of chalk (*efun*), a seashell (*aye*), a piece of bone (*egun*), and a plastic doll's head (*ori agboram*). Once the oddu has been ascertained, the santero hands the appropriate igbo to the client and instructs her to shake them together and then separate them, holding one tightly clenched in each fist. The santero then picks up the sixteen cowries, touches each of the client's hands, asks a yes or no question of the oracle and tosses the cowries. As with the determination of the oddu, the pattern formed by the cowries signals whether the client's right hand or left hand should be opened to reveal an igbo that will provide either an affirmative or negative answer to the question posed by the diviner. If, for instance, the black stone (otan) is revealed, the answer is no. If the shell or white chalk is present then the response is positive. Using the cowries and igbo, santeros will generally work through a series of yes and no queries that clarify the meaning of the oddu and suggest the necessary course of action.

Upon arriving at the santero's botánica, Olivia was led to the consultation room where the priest performs the diloggun. He instructed her to sit down on a chair in front of his wooden desk. The divination instruments, cowries and igbo, were carefully arranged on the desktop. First the santero filled out the biographical data section of a blank client information sheet, making sure that his information was up to date. He then dipped his right middle finger into a small container of water and sprinkled a few drops on the floor as a purification rite. Next he recited a litany of prayers invoking both his ancestors and the orichas he worships. The first oricha entreated was Elegua, who facilitates interaction between humans and the supreme deity Olodumare, as his assistance is believed to be most critical in the process of divination. Following this, the santero picked up the cowrie shells in one hand and touched Olivia's forehead, hands, and knees in order to create a psychic connection between the client and the cowries. He then tossed the cowries to ascertain the oddu that would address Olivia's problem.

On the first cast, nine cowries landed mouth side up. This indicated that Olivia's oddu was *osu*—a configuration that warns of troubles or danger. The santero threw the cowries a second time in order to determine which pataki associated with the oddu should be recounted. Again nine cowries landed mouth side up. Acting accordingly, he recited a story about two friends whose argument over land brought ruin to both of them. He asked Olivia how she thought the events of the story applied to her situation. Using the igbo, he then tried to better determine the nature of the warning. Was it truly an ominous portent? He handed Olivia two igbo—the black stone and the chalk—and asked if the oddu signified good fortune (*ire*) or misfortune (*iku*) and then cast the shells. The resulting pattern designated the hand in which Olivia had concealed the black stone. The santero advised Olivia that the immediate implication was that the planned move could be disastrous, perhaps resulting in death. He suggested that she postpone the relocation at least until another reading of the oracle indicated that it would be safe to leave the U.S.

In order to find out if misfortune was unavoidable or if there was a way to elude it should she and her husband decide to leave the country in spite of the warning, the santero handed Olivia two other igbo, the bone and the shell, and then tossed the cowries. The resulting pattern pointed to the hand holding the shell igbo suggesting that the orichas could provide a solution (*ilesi ocha*) to Olivia's dilemma. Subsequent casts of the diloggun indicated that offerings (*ebo*) to two female spirits within the Santeria pantheon, Ochun and Yemaya, would prevent death or some other calamity from striking her.

Because the sacred narratives associated with each oddu contain explicit descriptions concerning the appropriate ebo that should be carried out by the diviner or his client, the santero immediately provided Olivia with a prescription of the necessary rites that should be performed. She was instructed to undergo two separate spiritual cleansings: one for three days using materials (herbs, oils, et cetera) sacred to Ochun and the other employing objects consecrated to Yemaya. Additionally, she was required to take an offering of food to the ocean, the domain of Yemaya. Two casts of the cowries were made in order to assure that the prescribed ebo would be accepted by Ochun and Yemaya. The answers were affirmative. Finally, the santero asked Eleggua if everything that could be done to help resolve Olivia's dilemma had, in fact, been determined. Again the answer from the oracle was yes. The santero performed a cleansing ceremony to Ochun with Olivia; later Olivia undertook her own cleansing with Ochun ("who knows the language of death," said the santero) using a sacrificed rooster and then made an offering at the beach of food for the angel of death so that death would not strike her. Her husband did none of these things. Olivia remained in Los Angeles. Her husband left for El Salvador. Two days later he was murdered.

This complicated example suggests the larger complexities of the system of divination as a whole. Specific remedies are associated with each of the sixteen oddu as are a large number of proverbs and stories that the santero must master. Santeros never ask clients to "tell me where it hurts," for it is up to the oracle to discover the nature of the problem and its possible solution. A divination is carried out whether the client seeks personal advice, family counseling, or treatment for a medical condition. A reading can last an hour and cost ten to fifty dollars depending on the stature and reputation of the santero.

Special ceremonies as well as herbal preparations and subsequent divinations might be required.

ETHNOMEDICAL AND RELIGIOUS SYSTEMS

Individuals seeking treatment may select from multiple and competing systems of healing. As Brodwin (1996, 13) notes in his study of medical pluralism in Haiti, "There are very few settings which offer only one way to conceive of the body and its suffering, or where people have recourse to only one brand of treatment." In Los Angeles, the botánica, best understood as a locus of coexisting and competing discourses on affliction and healing, provides health seekers with access to several ethnomedical systems or health care strategies. As a result botánicas provide a unique vantage point for the study of the ways these belief systems are shaping medical pluralism in contemporary, urban America.

In general, the religious and ethnomedical belief systems served by botánicas whether in Los Angeles or elsewhere can be said to share several fundamental precepts:

- The belief in supernatural beings who interact with humans
- The assumption that disease can be the result of natural causes, divine retribution, or sorcery
- The supposition that healers, many of whom admit to a divine calling, must be able to diagnose and treat illnesses brought on by either natural or supernatural causes
- The use of ceremonial and herbal therapies

To elaborate on the second point, each religious system postulates not only a supreme being but also spirits, whether the souls of the deceased or a pantheon of divinities. The body can fall ill on its own, requiring attention by a physician (the "material" world), but disease may also be provoked by sorcery. Moreover, spirits can mimic a disease or aggravate the condition; hence the notion of "traveling diseases" or sickness that moves around the body requiring the release of the spirit. As one santero said, "The spirits have fun with your disease." Aside from these basic similarities in beliefs, the mythologies, concepts of disease causation, procedures for diagnosis, and the ritual treatments of each belief system reflect the diverse cultural and historical contexts in which the traditions arose. In a multicultural context of dynamic interchange such as the botánica, however, distinctions blur. We pointed out earlier that stores carry accouterments for several religions, and ritual specialists often identify themselves with at least two or three different traditions at once. A health practitioner does not find, say, Catholicism, Espiritismo, and Lucumí mutually exclusive but rather complementary. Summarized below are a half dozen ethnomedical systems represented in botánicas by statues, chromolithographs, and other sacramental items, publications, materia medica, and diagnostic and treatment methods.

Santería and Lucumí

Practitioners of oricha worship—also known as Lucumí (a term used in Cuba to identify peoples of Yoruba ancestry) or Santería (the worship of saints)— posit one god, Olodumare (or Olorun or Olofi), who created spirits (orichas, santos) that function as intermediaries in ways somewhat similar to Catholic or Eastern Orthodox saints. Because humans cannot have direct contact with the supreme being, they must rely on orichas or santos in order to benefit from the spiritual energy (ache) of Olodumare. The Santería priest or priestess is responsible for opening paths to the orichas and thus, ultimately, to God. Initiation into the priesthood is seen as an important step toward the fulfillment of one's destiny and the attainment of harmony with the universe. Through sacrifice, divination, and spirit mediumship, the priest forges direct links to the divine that will benefit him and those on whose behalf he has petitioned the divinities. However, it is understood that si Dios no quiere, santos no pueden (if God does not wish, the santos won't be able to act); fortunately, most of the time changes are possible.

Adherents of the religion contend that health problems afflict people at any given time, and they recognize six main harmful forces (there are others) that may cause illness. In order of importance, these are iku (death), arun (sickness), ina (disaster), ofo (loss), fitibo (feeling overwhelmed), and araye (general struggle and strife). Opposing these are the ire or blessings: ire owo (money), ire omo (children), ire ichegun ota (defeating one's enemies), and ire ariku babawa (to become immortal). These elements (both positive and negative) are considered supernatural entities and can affect anyone. The negative forces can afflict a person because of a violation of a taboo, disobedience, and the breaking of a law (either human or divine). Lucumí belief holds that only two events in life cannot be altered: the day you are born and the day you will die. However, because of one's actions, death can come sooner than it normally would. Arun (sickness) may manifest via supernatural causes (curses, sorcery, divine punishments) or by natural causes (congenital and acquired conditions).

Divination determines the source of a patient's illness and suggests the best methods (both physical and supernatural) to treat the problem. If the cause is supernatural, an ebo or sacrifice is required. If the affliction is deemed to be a case requiring the attention of a medical doctor, the oracle will advise what needs to be done in order for the physician to more effectively treat the patient. Practitioners of Lucumí don't rule out the importance of doctors and pharmaceuticals, but they do use the oracle to supplement standard procedures. After a person has been treated by a medical doctor, he or she will consult a diviner in order to assure that all physical and spiritual problems have been resolved (see Brandon 1990, 1991, 1993; Cabrera [1940] 1975; Curtis 1982; Murphy 1988; Pasquali 1986, 1994; and Sandoval 1979, 1983).

El Palo Mayombe

Both Santería and El Palo Mayombe are New World religions that arose with European and African Creole society in Cuba during the era of slave trade. Lucumí, however, derives primarily from traditions of the Yoruba in southwestern Nigeria and Benin. El Palo Mayombe draws its impetus from the religious practices of the Kongo or BaKongo peoples of central Africa (Wetli and Martinez 1983).

El Palo Mayombe places emphasis on working with the spirits of the dead rather than on interaction with a pantheon of anthropomorphic deities as is the case with Santería. This is in keeping with the religion's central African heritage, for Kongo religious beliefs stipulate that communication with direct ancestors and the recently deceased are the best avenues by which humans can forge a relationship with the ultimate divinity, Nzambi Mpungu. Practitioners of El Palo Mayombe (paleros or paleras) create shrines (*ngangas*) dedicated to the spirits of specific deceased individuals and, through the maintenance of the shrines, are able to call upon these entities for assistance in a variety of spiritual matters.

In addition to postulating the existence of a creator deity, Nzambi, adherents to El Palo Mayombe recognize the existence of various lesser beings called *nkisi*. These include spirits of the dead, forces of nature (such as wind, lightning, the sea) and environmental elements (trees, plants, rocks, animals). Furthermore, each Palo practitioner has a personal spirit (*nfumbe*) who acts as a "guardian angel." Palo rituals center around the creation and utilization of a *nganga* or *prenda*: an iron pot or cauldron filled with dry branches (*palos*), vines, roots, animals, and objects that symbolize the forces of nature.

Palo accepts the influence of spirits and sorcery as the major sources of disease and interprets sickness as an attack on the body. Treatments involve chanting (*manbos*), therapeutic ritual designs (*firmas*), and, above all, the use of the nganga. The cauldron and its contents are said to be a microcosm of the natural, human, and spiritual realms in which the nfumbe and nkisi spirits, with whom paleros or paleras work, reside. Using the nganga and communicating with the spirits via mediumship and trance possession, the practitioner attempts to discover the causes of disease (natural or supernatural) and to channel the supernatural forces that will enable him or her to heal the affliction (Cabrera 1986; Montenegro 1994).

Espiritismo

Espiritismo (Spiritism) is also prevalent in botánicas. It derives from the European Spiritualist tradition of the early nineteenth century influenced by the French engineer and psychic investigator Hippolyte Rivail (1804–1869). Using the pseudonym Allan Kardec, he authored a series of books outlining a spiritual doctrine that emphasizes the importance of communication with the dead. According to Kardec, the spirits of deceased individuals are able to interact with the living, and when contacted through a medium, they can offer solutions to a variety of social, psychological, and medical problems. Spiritism diffused to the Caribbean where it syncretized with Native American and African religions. Spiritist altars usually display (in Spanish) Kardec's *The Gospel According to Spiritism* and *The Collection of Prayers*; the former often replaces the Bible.

Subscribers to the tradition contend that the spirit world is arranged in a hierarchy that places the Judeo-Christian God at one end of the spectrum and the restless, wandering souls of those who were unprepared for death at the other. Between the two is a series of categories representing benign "pure" beings such as angels and seraphim, Catholic saints and Afro-Cuban orichas, historical heroes and leaders, as well as the spirits of ordinary men and women. A spiritual seance is one of the primary means by which mediums (espiritistas) contact these ethereal beings on behalf of themselves and clients. In Los Angeles, types of spirits often encountered in ceremonies and also represented in the religious folk art of botánicas are African slaves, Native Americans, Latin American nationalist figures (for example, Pancho Villa), and ascended masters such as the Buddha.

Practitioners of Espiritismo believe that disease may result from a variety of physical and spiritual conditions, some of which may not be counteracted. Some afflictions are thought to have been ordained by God and, therefore, cannot be resolved by any means. Most illnesses, however, are recognized as physical or spiritual ailments that require treatment by medical doctors and spiritualists, usually in combination. Some maladies are diagnosed as manifestations of karmic conditions that were inherited by the soul upon incarnation. Even if these cannot be eliminated, they can be alleviated with rituals, prayers, and moral rectitude. Sorcery causes yet other medical problems.

The treatment of disease, physical or spiritual, may require herbs, rituals, other material remedies, and also the intervention of supernatural entities known as "spiritual protectors" and "spiritual guides." According to the doctrine of Espiritismo, these "guardian angels" know how to heal without interfering with the will of God. When patients consult an espiritisto or espiritista, they generally seek to ascertain not only the cause of their affliction but also the most effective means of treating it. Through the use of various divination implements and spirit mediumship, spiritists provide answers as to the source of a patient's problem and suggest courses of action. Depending on the nature of the problem, recommendations may include spiritual procedures at the botánica, herbal treatments self-administered at home, or referral to a mainstream health care practitioner (see Garrison 1977; Harwood 1977, 1981; and Koss-Chioino 1992).

Curanderismo

Curanderismo, the most common folk medical tradition practiced by Mexican Americans and Latino immigrants in the United States, integrates elements of popular Catholicism, Native American medicine, European magic and witchcraft beliefs, Spiritualist doctrines, and contemporary biomedicine. Healers who follow this tradition (curanderos or curanderas) believe that the ability to heal is God-given and often claim that they began their medical practice as a result of a divine calling. The healers generally work within a specific neighborhood or community and mainly tend to the needs of friends, relatives, and neighbors. Some practitioners, however, have become widely acclaimed for their healing abilities and, as is the case with the late Don Pedrito Jaramillo, may even achieve the status of folk saint (see *Spirit Doctors* 1997).

Curanderos or curanderas recognize illnesses of both natural and supernatural causes. The majority of the ailments seen are physical complaints such as headaches, gastrointestinal problems, or general pain. Folk illnesses brought on by improper eating habits (*empacho*) or traumatic experiences (*susto*) are also treated by these healers. Less commonly seen are supernatural afflictions *mal puesto* (a magical hex) and *mal ojo* (evil eye). Remedies for physical and spiritual problems require prayer, spirit mediumship, and the utilization of herbs, oils, holy water, and other sacred objects. A fundamental precept of Curanderismo is the idea that the patient must actively participate in his or her treatment for it to be effective. Acting as a medical and spiritual advisor, the practitioner helps the patient to harness the healing power of God (Clark 1959; *Eduardo the Healer* 1978; Graham 1976, 1985; Granger 1976; Kiev 1968; Madsen 1964; Roeder 1988; Rubel 1960, 1966).

Hoodoo (Conjure or Rootwork)

Understood fundamentally as a system of pharmacopedic practices and spiritual traditions developed and utilized by African Americans living in the South, Hoodoo offers individuals a means of transforming, revising, and reenvisioning reality. Largely comprising medicinal and ritual operations derived from African sources, the primary role of Hoodoo is to provide healing alternatives to those who are ill, to find love for the loveless, to secure work for the unemployed, and to offer empowerment within an often oppressive social environment. As with Curanderismo, the Hoodoo practices are normally family-based traditions that have been passed on from generation to generation. Although some individuals who practice Hoodoo have garnered reputations as powerful healers within their community, most people who utilize its remedies and rituals do so with anonymity. Hoodoo, as some practitioners say, is a "quiet" tradition; a system of healing that generally takes place in the home and is usually self-administered. There are, however, legendary practitioners such as Marie Laveau, Dr. Buzzard, and Dr. John with whom some modern conjurers claim association or inspiration. Hoodoo is the most pervasive of the African-based religions in American culture, known through allusion to "conjure" woman, "hoochie coochie man," "mojo" (bag or hand), "juju," "rootwork," and "voodoo"; and appearing in literary works by such authors as Zora Neal Hurston, Rudolph Fisher, Ishmael Reed, and Alice Walker; in music by bluesmen like Willie Dixon, Robert Johnson, and Sly Fox; and in art works from quilts and yard displays to easel paintings.

Much like El Palo Mayombe, the practice of Hoodoo, conjure, or rootwork centers around the use of animal, mineral, and vegetal materials as a means of affecting the spiritual force or vitality of an individual. Sickness can have natural or supernatural causes. Treatments for natural illnesses usually consist of herbal teas or other decoctions, poultices, and aromatic baths. Supernatural afflictions, generally thought to be caused by sorcery, are counteracted through the use of prayers, candles, cleansing rituals, and apotropaic devices. Supernatural illnesses imply that one's spirit has been "tied up" by someone working malign, conjure practices. In such cases the conjury must be broken and the spirit "released" (see Hurston 1935; Hyatt 1970–78; Jackson 1976; Lichstein 1992; Snow 1979; Maduro 1975; and Mathews 1987, 1992; for works on the related Vodou, see Brodwin 1992 and 1996; Cosentino 1995; Mena 1998; Metraux 1972; Polk 1997; and Straight 1983).

Biomedicine

Alternately called orthodox, official, professional, conventional, modern, or Western medicine, biomedicine is also a medical system. Some would contend that it is an *ethnomedical* system, for it too is part of a culture, embodies a worldview, expresses a set of values, and holds beliefs about health, healing, and the relationship of human beings to nature and the supernatural. While the other systems described above resemble one another in postulating a spiritual as well as material world and in assuming the interrelationship of mind, soul, and body, biomedicine differs on both counts.

Biomedicine separates mind from body, treating each with distinct methods, and both from the spirit or soul which is left to the clergy to deal with (if it is treated at all). It focuses on the biological or organic phenomenon of disease, thereby excluding the cultural, social, and psychological construction of illness by patient, friends, and family (Clark 1995). Biomedicine is quick to pathologize: the patient is diseased (rather than suffering an illness; see Eisenberg 1977), childbirth and menopause are not natural life-cycle events but pathologic conditions (Clark 1995; Davis-Floyd 1987, 1992), and ecstatic states and trances are neurotic or psychotic episodes. Its explanatory model dwells on the germ theory and on bodily deterioration, a wearing out of parts, which it treats in isolation from other factors using chemicals or surgery. While it can replace hip joints or remove malignant tumors, biomedicine can't explain why these problems befall us rather than other individuals (Hufford 1994). This medical system has much to offer (especially *inyecciones* or injections, which have become a cultural tradition for Latinos; see Gurza 1999 and Reza 1999). Many people need more, however, choosing treatments from other systems to complement biomedicine (Cassidy 1995).

A SANTERO AT WORK

Although the religious-medical systems differ owing to cultural and historical circumstances, they hold fundamental precepts in common. Already mentioned is the belief in supernatural beings who interact with humans and who can affect health. Most of the systems view health as a state of balance or equilibrium; should individuals fall into a state of imbalance, they become ill. Biomedicine's germ theory of disease may explain *how* people become sick but other systems explain *why* they do, particularly when other people remain well (Pasquali 1994). Restoration of health requires restoring equilibrium, accomplished through ceremonies and herbs (including baths and spiritual cleansings). Prevention of illness is a common concern. When sickness is attributed to supernatural forces, the way of protecting one's health is to neutralize the negative ones through moral action, deference or propitiation, and to cultivate the positive forces; in both instances, protective talismans, amulets, candles, incense, herbs, roots, and sometimes the ritual sacrifice of animals prove useful.

Another idea about health and illness fundamental to Curanderismo but also implicit in the Afro-Cuban religions and Espiritismo concerns "hot" and "cold" properties (having nothing to do with temperature) of the body, environment, illness, plants, and foods (see Anderson 1987; Harwood 1971). Some "hot" diseases or states are acid indigestion, diabetes, hypertension, pregnancy, susto, *ojo*, and *bilis*. Examples of "cold" diseases include menstrual cramps, pneumonia, colic, and empacho (however, ethnographic studies indicate that opinions differ from one community to another and even within communities as to which illnesses, and especially which plants and foods, are hot and which are cold). According to some Hispanics, a woman should avoid lemons, grapefruits, sauerkraut, pickles, vinegar, and tomatoes because they are cold or too acidic: "such things make the uterus very cold" and stop menstrual flow, congealing blood in the uterus to reappear later as cancer (Snow and Johnson 1978). The goal of treatment is to restore harmony and balance; for example, "cold" remedies like bananas and lemon juice as well as teas of passion flowers or linden are often used for hypertension. This system has elements in common with systems prevalent in Chinese and Ayurvedic tradition (Anderson 1987).

Each religious complex differentiates between the "material" and the "spiritual"; practitioners recommend that clients seek treatment by doctors for illnesses in the material realm (Garrison 1977), while they treat spiritual problems and also ailments of a material nature caused or aggravated by supernatural forces. All the ethnomedical systems have in common the use of herbal remedies (about one-fourth of the pharmacopeia of biomedicine is "green medicine," derived from plants, albeit in processed form). In Lucumí tradition, plants are sweet, strong, or neutral in one system; but in another system, baths and teas are composed of herbs "owned" by a particular oricha whose assistance is needed. Theories of health and illness, principles of disease causation, and therapeutic techniques become more apparent when interacting with a santero who is also an osainista or herbalist. The data that follow derive from interviews and observation (in October and December 1998, and February 1999) conducted jointly by Michael Owen Jones and Patrick A. Polk with a healer in the Los Angeles area introduced to them by Roberta J. Evanchuk. The analysis grows out of discussions among these three individuals as well as between them and Ysamur Flores-Peña, who specializes in African and European ethnomedical systems, and Donald J. Cosentino, who is an expert on Afro-Caribbean religious systems.

Biographical Background and Calling

Now middle-aged, Carmello Santiago (pseudonym) grew up in the Caribbean and moved to southern California in the 1980s. He opened a botánica within four years of his arrival and has since become a well-established member of the Lucumí community both locally and nationally. Carmello has long been involved with various religious systems. From the age of nine he has been a healer in the Espiritismo tradition (his father was a noted spiritist medium, his mother a healer). Like many folk practitioners he had the "calling" replete with visions, possession, and visitation by spirits (see *The New Believers* 1990; Espín 1996; Hand 1980; and Singer and García 1989). For three years in his teens he was a Jehovah's Witness. Then he considered entering the Jesuit seminary hoping to become a Catholic priest. "It was very hard soul searching," he said; "I didn't know what the hell I was looking for, but my basic question was, growing up as a spiritist, 'Is this it?' It's like you wonder if you're doing the right things, is this what you really want? I just got sick and tired of being a spiritist! I wanted something else. You have to realize, I'd been attending seances and dealing with people and healing people since I was nine years old, so by the time I was a teenager everyone was looking at me not as a regular teenager but just by what could I do for them. At nine years old I was already taking care of people. So you really get a sense like 'Oh my God, is there something else to life than this?' You really ask yourself those questions."

At eighteen Carmello suffered a severe injury that conventional biomedical treatment and other available therapies were unable to cure. As a last resort he visited a santero. With the help of this traditional priest and healer, Carmello employed offerings and prayers to the orichas as a supplement to his regular medical treatment and soon regained his health. Later, following his recovery, Carmello was initiated as a Lucumí priest. By the early 1990s Carmello had his own *ile* (house) or congregation for oricha worship and is now godfather to several score who joined the religion through him, some of whom he has initiated into the priesthood by means of a long, complex ceremony following theological instruction. As spiritist and santero, Carmello listens attentively to knowledgeable individuals around him, taking voluminous notes that he keeps on his bookshelf near his desk where he confers with clients. Of his adherence to the two spiritual traditions, Carmello states: "I have never left Spiritualism; both practices [Espiritismo and Lucumí] exist together. You use both. Spiritism is a tool and I never stopped being a Spiritist, because you never stop being that."

Carmello readily admits to having suffered some of the same ailments as his clients. For instance, he arrived in Los Angeles on a Thursday. His aunt in Whittier lent him her car to drive to downtown Los Angeles to locate the office where he was to report for work the following Monday. "So when I was exiting, when I took the five freeway south, I got absolutely overwhelmed by the sheer amount of cars and people and the sheer madness of it, and I just broke down, I just pulled over to the side, parked the car and started crying. I wanted to go back home!" Weeping hysterically, he couldn't move for more than an hour. He suffered susto, the folk-defined illness of fright (Kroesen 1994; Logan 1993). "That was my first experience with susto, and then I had certain ceremonies that I needed to do to put myself back together again." Managing to return to his aunt's home, he called friends in the Caribbean to send him by overnight delivery several fresh herbs (lantana, lemon grass, mint) that he used for a tea in conjunction with the necessary rituals to the orichas.

Preparation and Uses of Herbs

"When you're driving, you're always looking to see what herbs are around," said Carmello. As Brandon notes (1991), the Lucumí term for plants, herbs, and weeds is *egwe*. They help human beings through *ache* that makes them alive with divine power. All plants are thinking entities; all have personality and temperament, requiring rituals to entice them to give up their power. Some are frightened easily and withhold their powers by refusing to bloom. Others are shy and retiring. Yet others have explosive personalities, requiring great etiquette and respect before being picked. The powers of plants fluctuate over the course of the day, resting at night but enlivened by morning (Sandoval 1977). All must be gathered properly with prayers and token payment. Wild egwes possess the greatest power for healing.

Herbalists collect plants from the local mountains, river beds, and neighborhood sites such as empty, undeveloped, or untended plots of land. According to Carmello, abandoned homes with overgrown yards and weed-filled parking lots are often good sources of herbal materials. "Santeros work with weeds," he said. As we drove away from a wholesaler's store where he had just bought some fresh herbs imported from Latin America, Carmello noticed a certain type of plant growing on the fence surrounding a corner lot. He signaled us to stop, hopped out of the car, and enthusiastically began plucking portions of an orange-colored plant from the fence. It's known as "holy weed" he said, and can be used to soothe skin lesions and surgical wounds, reducing the scarring. He had assumed that the plant was no longer in season. Nonspecialists usually have to rely on botánicas in order to obtain the components of herbal remedies. However, some basic "home remedy" herbs are available at sidewalk plant or flower shops throughout east Los Angeles, such as lemon grass, rosemary, sweet basil, and "tree of life." Individuals often buy these plants as starter or home herbal kits.

Carmello is an osainista, defined by Brandon (1991, 60) as a priest or priestess "knowledgeable about the herbs, their prayers, personalities and temperaments, and able to collect them from the wild." Ritual uses of herbs include *osains* and *omieros*. The latter is the more powerful, not only for cleansing but also for empowering individuals and objects that are about to come in contact with the orichas (Brandon 1991). Ordinary herbal preparations may have up to nine ingredients, balancing strong and sweet qualities, said Carmello. Omieros (mixtures of plants associated with a particular oricha; see Cabrera [1940] 1975) are composed of up to 121 different egwes. "Strong" plants (like camphor) "increase the heat" and are used to "dislodge a situation," said Carmello; if the body is very hot (the condition of illness), then "sweet" herbs like basil, mint, and camomile reduce the heat through a bath, tea, or poultice. Generally speaking, in Lucumí one seeks to cool things down (in contrast to El Palo Mayombe). A knife (iron) is associated with the oricha Ogun. A client will consult the oracle to determine if surgery is truly necessary and will prove successful, and also to invoke the oricha's help to guide the surgeon's hand. After the operation ("hot"), the client will return to the santero for ceremonies, herbal baths (*despojos*), and perhaps ointments or poultices to "cool" the condition and aid recovery.

Carmello grows, dries, and stores many of his own herbs, collects them from abandoned lots and overgrown yards, purchases others from an importer, and also special orders fresh ones (unavailable or out of season in southern California) from Miami, Puerto Rico, and other sources in tropical climates. He not only utilizes the plants himself but also gives workshops on spiritual herbs and baths in which participants learn to identify the plants by traditional methods, perform correct procedures of herb collecting and drying, and prepare teas, soaps, tinctures, compresses, and bath salts using infusion, decoction, and maceration.

As a rule of thumb, "sweet" herbs include spearmint, mint, camomile, basil, lavender, and any other herb that is sweetly aromatic. "Strong" (or "loud") herbs taste bitter or smell pungent or harsh, such as rue, angel trumpet leaf, avocado, tree of life, and the leaves of most trees. Teas are made by infusion, that is, by pouring hot water over herbs that steep for ten minutes or more, releasing some of the oils and curative properties of the leaves. To make a decoction, Carmello recommends gently boiling water and herbs over a medium fire in a covered container, then letting it stand ten minutes or so to allow the steam to settle; this results in obtaining a higher amount of essential elements, but evaporation causes some loss. The most effective method is maceration: using a mortar or one's hands to crush the leaves to produce an aromatic liquid, dark green and full of the plant's essential elements as well as containing "personal vibrations."

Like other osainistas (Brandon 1991, 68), Carmello strongly advises against using commercial preparations, for one cannot be entirely sure of what they contain, and they are likely not to have been collected in the wild by a knowledgeable herbalist who, through proper rituals, maximizes their power. Some typical preparations consist of soaps, salts, poultices, and compresses. Carmello grates pure Castile soap, mixes it with herbs and other ingredients (honey, perfumes, oils), reshapes it, and allows it to dry. To prepare salts he combines an equal amount of table salt, baking soda, and Epsom salt and then adds perfumed oils, dried flowers, or leaves. A poultice consists of a moist, hot herb pack made by spreading a thick paste of crushed, fresh herbs over a clean cotton cloth and applied to the affected area for several hours. He makes a compress using a cloth soaked in a hot herbal preparation that is then wrung out and applied to the skin (he advises leaving both ends of the cloth out of the water for easier handling when applying it).

Carmello insists that most herbs be collected before 9 A.M., before the sun dissipates their oils. They should be picked by hand, starting at the top with the newest leaves, and then dried in a shady place on a ventilated object such as an old screen door, turned several times during the drying process, and stored in dark containers and in shade. The final product will be dark green and aromatic. When needed, the herbs are put in water, the purer the better. Traditional healers, he contends, never mix more than nine herbs in a single bath; a sweet herbal bath should follow a strong one. Each essence has its own therapeutic effect. For example, bergamot is refreshing and reduces irritability, anxiety, and depression; it also aids sleep. Calming and refreshing, camomile treats stress and depression. Frankincense relaxes and rejuvenates and also stimulates the mind. Lavender is balancing, normalizing, and tranquilizes the mind. Myrrh serves as a sedative and also rejuvenates the skin. Orange blossom soothes nerves. The soothing and relaxing rose helps resolve relationship problems. Spiritually enhancing, sandalwood treats impotency and frigidity. No matter the problem—whether social, emotional, or physiological—single essences and especially combinations of herbs, usually along with appropriate rituals and ceremonies, are often effective in alleviating it. Sometimes a ceremony alone will suffice.

Selected Cases

While other santeros and santeras generally keep records for a year, Carmello Santiago has three filing cabinet drawers filled with cases spanning the past thirteen years that he has been a practitioner in the U.S. One sheet for each problem notes the client's date of birth and ethnicity, the date that the client came to him, the divination, the "prescription"—the herbal preparations and ceremonies recommended by the oracle—and the ultimate outcome of therapy. Carmello has told us about a number of cases before, we have talked with several clients, and we have witnessed divinations as well as observed a ceremony conducted by his wife, Lilian (pseudonym), a santera and espiritista.

Recently we asked Carmello to pull some cases that he considers "representative" and to discuss them. These cases are, of course, self-selected. He selected nine from his files, three involving procedures carried out by Lilian. In each instance, the problem's nature, cause, and possible resolution were revealed through the oracle, in other words, complex Lucumí divination procedures as in the case described above involving Olivia.

Case 1.   The first case is an African-American male born in 1967. He was first seen 9 January 1990, last seen 28 February 1999. "He's been a continuous client of mine. One of the interesting things about this person—he was a healthy person, he was suffering a bad case of some kind of genital dysfunction, went to his company insurance, they couldn't find anything wrong with him. He's a person who played sports in school, he worked out, he's young, and he was having problems. . . . He wasn't able to conceive, was unable to even hold an erection, and he was having pain in the genital area." Through divination the oracle indicated that the problem was "a parasite, some kind of bug that lives in the body." He was given a combination of (strong) teas—in Spanish, *polao*—to drink three times a day. Alongside this he was told to drink a combination of juices that are a diuretic in a sense, which are cucumber, lettuce, and the like ("fresh" or sweet herbs that flush and refresh the system). After that there was a ritual performed on him with the oricha Ogun. The ritual included the use of a leaf called *vencedor*. Basically the translation is "to conquer." "It's a tree that has the tendency to grow up straight regardless of all the problems. Always shoots straight up."

"How did you determine the teas?"

"You ask the oracle. Basically on your knowledge of what the herbs do, you ask the oracle what combination of herbs is acceptable. So we did that with Ogun, and the man was supposed to wash the affected area with the leaves of the tree—meaning his groin. After that, the idea was to bring the bug out, whatever the bug was. Afterwards he went back to the doctor and was diagnosed, because the oracle advises you to go to the doctor. It's a medical problem, not a spiritual problem. And he was diagnosed with a severe case of genital herpes."

"And then how did you determine that it was rituals to be performed for Ogun?" (Ogun is the oricha of the forge and of war; see Flores-Peña and Evanchuk 1994.)

"Everything is to be asked of the oracle. You don't make a decision on your own. You have to ask the oracle if what you think, your particular choice, is acceptable." The teas (polao) had to be strong because Ogun is a hot deity. The symbolic significance of rubbing the genitals with vencedor—"the tree that grows erect"—is obvious. The man was treated by a doctor. He had first sought Carmello's aid in 1990, then he was initiated into the religion. By exact count of case notes, he has seen Carmello eighty times in nine years, mainly for help in personal decisions, social problems, and work-related matters.

Case 2.   Case 2 is a Mexican-American businessman, born in 1964, who came to Carmello for a single treatment on 3 November 1991. "He was discharged from the hospital after a month with inconclusive diagnosis—lack of strength, unable to stand, he needed to be held or carried in a wheelchair. Also he could not hold anything in his stomach. He was expectorating a lot even though he was not producing anything. Recently married at the time, and now he has two children the last I heard. He was diagnosed as being bewitched."

"Diagnosed by divination?"

"Yes. The divination established that something was put in his food. He was to have the equivalent of an exorcism with Osain [the oricha of herbalism, magic, and the power of nature] as a major cleansing: *rompemiento*, 'to break.' After that he was given a . . . it was suggested that he drink something to flush his kidneys because the oracle asserted that the problem was in the kidneys, not in his stomach. Contrary to what he was saying, that it was his stomach that hurt, it was the kidneys."

The man had been hospitalized for a month, and every conceivable test had been performed with no insights into his problem. "According to the oracle, what happened was that whatever spell was put on him was hindering the doctor's effort to see the disease." The ceremonial rompemiento was to break through that blockage. The man was required to sleep in old clothes in order to "pick up the humors of the body"; the clothes were then ripped ("broken"), and while he was naked Carmello and another priest cleansed him with herbs, a bath, coconuts, colored cloth, and cigar smoke. The clothes, candles, coconuts, and cigar smoke were wrapped together and sent to a cemetery for burial. Carmello gave him a tea of aloe vera gel and brazil bark to drink for fifteen days in order to flush the kidneys. The man was told to also drink a mixture of mint and warm milk before going to bed and on arising in the morning. Carmello instructed him to then return to the doctor; he was diagnosed with an early case of cirrhosis of the liver.

"See, usually the oracle distinguishes between different stages of the disease: the disease created by magic [sorcery], the disease created by punishment from divine forces, and the disease created by one's own actions. When the disease is created by physical conditions, [such] that it requires the intervention of the medical establishment, the oracle itself will acknowledge that. So the oracle becomes sort of like a triage, clarifying and clearing away what the doctors cannot see. Like my old teacher used to say, 'Machines cannot see spirits.'"

An individual can bring punishment upon himself or herself by violating a taboo or offending a divine force. Or sometimes "you did something that brought that disease to you. For example, in the middle of winter you walk out with no shirt and you get pneumonia. Well, you brought it upon yourself." One may also inherit genetic conditions or predispositions. "The diviner needs to ask if he can intervene to cure the whole thing with rituals and medicine [herbs], or if there's a need for the person to see a doctor. If the person needs to see a doctor, then the oracle will say you do this, and see a doctor; if the case is beyond [spiritual work], the diviner will just say forget it, go to a doctor, there's nothing I can do for you."

Finally, "some sicknesses cannot be cured and the oracle acknowledges that too. There's the case of a young Belizean woman. She came because of a diagnosis of cancer. And the oracle asserted that there was nothing to be done because it could not be stopped or cured, so basically the only thing you could do was alleviate it. So sometimes the oracle acknowledges that the body is already in such bad shape that it is impossible. All you can do is two things: alleviate the condition and prepare the person for death. There is cleansing, you talk to the person, there's all this preparation for death. The person receives ceremonies and rituals of Babalú Aye, the oricha of infectious diseases, and she receives beads of Babalú Aye. The cancer, like it often does, went dormant for about a year and a half, and then it came back again and she passed on. But she knew, we knew, everyone knew that what we were doing was basically getting things ready. Many times the oracle acknowledges that there is nothing to be done at all."

Case 3.   Case 3 is an African-American female born in 1959, last seen 25 February 1999. "This pertains to Lilian [the santero's wife, an espiritista]. Complaint: unable to conceive a child. Been through every fertilization technique and clinic there is, with no results. No other complaints, healthy, no addictions to anything. Two *santiguos* was the prescription. One with Ochun, the other [one month later] a santiguo espiritual" (see Evanchuk 1999). The first consists of songs, prayers, and incantations as well as the ritual massaging of the abdomen with a squash, gourd, or pumpkin; Lilian learned it from Carmello's mother. "The style of the second is completely different. It involves flowers, it involves certain perfumes, certain combinations of oils, that's directed by the spirit" and performed not in front of the orichas but in front of Lilian's spiritual altar. Seven days later the woman was to have a cleansing with Babalú Aye using a guinea hen sacrificed to this oricha concerned with disease. "According to Lilian, she had an inflammation that prevented the egg from doing what it was supposed to do. She did it [had the rituals], she got pregnant, and she had a kid. Lilian asserted that her ovulation was a mess, it was completely off rhythm. She was also supposed to receive a charm to carry with her and she did, a *niche*, just a charm for her protection. Lilian also thought that her desperation was preventing her from getting pregnant. Her own desperation of getting pregnant. And then the inflammation plus that, it was just a mess. So she did that [took part in the ceremonies], she's got a kid, she's thinking of having another one, she became initiated and became a worshiper." Lilian also had the woman drink (one time only) a combination of seven different oils. One was "egg oil" (in other words, a beaten egg yolk that has sat awhile) "as a purgative but also to bring down the inflammation." According to Carmello, "She has paid in excess of fifty thousand dollars getting pregnant. And she almost had a heart attack because she ended up spending here about three hundred dollars and she got pregnant." (Recently she conceived her second child.)

Case 4.   "Mexican female, two years of age. Diagnosis: susto. Constant crying, not eating, losing weight, not sleeping, always scared of everything. First of all she was taken in front of the orichas and she was cleansed with white flowers. The whole pantheon of orichas. Into the altar room [where the shrines are]. Then she was left standing there for a second—because you have to combat susto with susto—so when she was standing there, and when she's busy looking at everything, the person is supposed to grab the kid, throw it up, turn it around and bring it down."

After frightening the child to break the hold of susto, the santero prescribed a beverage containing orange blossom water and honey to be drunk for twenty-one days, and a bath at the same time consisting of white flowers and water that had been left outside to "pick up the dew." She had recovered the last time Carmello saw her in June 1997, when her parents brought her back for treatment of colic. "The prescription: change diet. Too much frijoles. She was developing gas, and that hurt, so drop the frijoles. Which is a problem because at the same time this is a family of very limited resources. So if you tell a family, don't give them frijoles, what are they going to feed her?" Other family members who had consulted Carmello about their own ailments include the mother, the father, the brother-in-law and the sister-in-law. "I was referred by the sister-in-law."

"Any idea what caused the susto?"

"Crossing the border! That will scare the wits out of anyone. The whole family is illegal."

"Is that a common source of susto that you treat?"

"Most of the susto cases that I treat, I don't even have to look at the oracle, I just can tell immediately that they probably just crossed the border. Male, female, kid, whatever, the ordeal of crossing the border, the ordeal of hiding and then adapting to this city. Even if they don't develop it when they cross the border, just living here in fear of being arrested and in fear of not being able to fulfill their obligations to pay the coyote and the whole thing is enough to give them susto."

Case 5.   "Another female kid, born 1990, Mexican, born in Los Angeles of illegal parents. She developed a rash, the skin will dry up and then break. Very painful, she was a living sore. It was all over, it was horrendous. You cannot pick up the kid, because whatever you did to her will hurt. She was kept basically naked, she could not wear clothes. Taken to the hospital, diagnosis inconclusive for fungus. The doctors did not know really if it was a fungus, a viral infection, nothing. Everything was inconclusive, they were just trying different treatments to see if one them will score."

The parents brought the child to Carmello. The oracle prescribed a treatment "with Babalú Aye [oricha of infectious diseases] and three baths, made with omiero. Omiero is a ritual preparation done with incantations and specific herbs to the oricha, with a minimum of seven herbs and then it is 'seasoned' with different things like roasted corn, palm oil, honey, rum, guinea pepper—it's a heavy preparation. Omiero means 'water that cools,' and it's used for consecration, usually, to consecrate sacred items. And also for medicine she was advised to take three baths in a seven-day period. She was supposed to take that and then make a mixture with aloe vera gel, palm oil and honey, and to smear the body to ease and prevent the skin from cracking. After that she was supposed to be cleansed with gun powder in front of Osain [the oricha of herbalism, magic, and medicine]. You blast the gun powder and when the smoke comes up you cleanse the person in the smoke of the gun powder. The kid got better, skin cleared, diagnosis from the laboratory inconclusive still. They don't know what she had, and to be honest with you, neither do I. In this case she didn't need to go back to the doctor, but I sent her back to the lab because we were curious about what the hell she had."

"The baths with omiero, what were the ingredients?"

"Seven different kinds of herbs. You have fern, *boton de oro*, sage, *romerillo,* tree of life, [unclear], the other one is angel trumpet, and that was it. It's a combination of both sweet and strong. The romerillo and the boton de oro are sweet but they're not taken because of that condition, but because it's a combination particular to the orichas. This is a preparation for the omiero and omiero doesn't go by sweet and strong category. The same plant that you might take in one place for sweet or cold or hot or strong doesn't feature in the omiero because the omiero goes by oricha. Whatever oricha owns the plant, that's what you use, not because of their qualities. If you're working with the plants on their own as plants and herbs, there's a set of rules that you follow. If you're dealing with them within the Lucumí tradition, or Palo, or any form of religion, there's another set of rules. And you don't mix both."

Case 6.   "Next case, Salvadoran male, born in 1967, came here on 7 October 1993, last time here was 6 January 1999. Working man, brought here by wife [whom Carmello had treated previously]; impotency. Prescription was a rum rompemiento, and also there was a cream made for him to apply to the affected area." The cream consisted of aloe vera, sage, honey, snake oil (the renderings from a fried snake). The prescription included a bath with Elegua omiero, in other words, herbs (plus appropriate "seasoning" in the form of honey, roasted corn and so on) that are owned by the divinity Elegua (also known as Eshu or Elegba), the oricha that stands at the cosmic crossroad between the human and the divine; his goodwill must be obtained for projects to succeed (Flores-Peña and Evanchuk 1994).

Because Elegua's number is three, the man was to bathe three times in the omiero consisting of a long list of herbs "seasoned and prepared according to the likes of the oricha." An oddu (a configuration of the sixteen cowries used in divination) indicated that he was to rub himself with a whole coconut that later was disposed of in a cemetery. "The idea is that the coconut will pick up whatever inflammation is in there to find out what was preventing the doctor from finding it." Because "the oracle said he had some kind of physical condition that was affecting everything," Carmello sent the man back to the urologist who then found a hernia high on the testicles that prevented the passage of sperm. "He's scheduled for surgery next month."

Case 7.   "Another case is a Salvadoran female, she was born in 1952, came here [recently] complaining of excessive bleeding, she was diagnosed by a doctor as having fibroids and scheduled for an operation: hysterectomy. Came for divination and was advised that two santiguos [seven days apart] be performed with Ochun [conducted by Lilian]. [After the second one] she had a hemorrhage— very, very heavy—taken back to the doctor, taken to the hospital, fibroids had dissolved, she was discharged, the surgery was canceled, she's fine."

Vivian Garrison (1977) describes the "spiritual working" on behalf of clients with organic gynecological disorders through the use of a *rogación* (petition) to Ochun (the oricha of love, fertility, and the beauty of life, she is a demanding lover and compassionate mother, the favorite daughter of Olodumare, the supreme being [see Flores-Peña and Evanchuk 1994]). It consists of a ceremony of songs, prayers, and incantations as well as the ritual massage of the abdomen with a squash or gourd (representing the abdomen and all of its internal organs). According to Garrison, as the squash rots, so too does the inflammation and sickness of the abdomen that has passed into the squash dissipate and disappear. Writes Vivian Garrison (1977, 146): "Most of the time, this ritual is a harmless procedure which serves to alleviate anxiety while the woman awaits her next menstrual period, visit to the doctor, or other, more decisive answer to questions about her gynecological condition. In the cases I know about the women continued to see a gynecologist as well, but the *santera* claimed a 'cure' effected by Ochún when the matter was resolved. In this way the *espiritistas* or *santeras* do claim to 'cure' infections and 'tumors' which purportedly 'the doctor could not cure,' and to prevent 'unnecessary operations.'" The author adds, however, that there are in fact frequent exploratory operations and unnecessary hysterectomies, a situation that promotes the search for alternative or complementary treatment.

Case 8.   "The daughter of this woman is the next case, Salvadoran female, born 1968. She had a miscarriage in an earlier pregnancy. Santiguo made, it was done, to help her womb get back into shape. She was advised to, by divination, not to get pregnant soon. Still she did. She was advised to come back for divination because the pregnancy was problematic, and the kid was probably not going to be healthy. Did not come back. Kid is ten months old, diagnosed with Down's syndrome. The oracle told her not to get pregnant, because it was too soon and if she got pregnant the kid was not going to be healthy. She just got pregnant and the kid was diagnosed with Down's syndrome. She came back to see if we could do something with the kid. But that was it. How can you reverse Down's syndrome?"

Case 9.   "Husband and wife, Mexican American. The female was born in 1975, diagnosed with a severe case of fibroids, scheduled for hysterectomy six months before her wedding. Lilian performed santiguo; the woman was also cleansed with two guinea hens and they were sacrificed to Babalú Aye, she was cleansed with an *awan*, which is a cleansing done with different kinds of dry grains like dry beans and vegetables and fruit and stuff and then there is bacon. And left there. She was advised to drink Elegua's omiero, half a cup in the morning, and she had to wear the beads of Babalú Aye. Everything done, the fibroids disappeared, no hysterectomy done, she's fine.

"Husband came, brought by wife [on a later occasion, after they were married], he was complaining of some sexual dysfunction. He was not able to hold an erection. He's Mexican American, about the same age. He was having trouble having sexual intercourse with his wife, pain, so we did rompemiento. Diagnosed with susto. I don't know what he saw. Something he saw. He was given three baths with sweet herbs, which means herbs of the likes of basil, mint, spearmint, castille rose, which is not an herb technically but is used as one, cinnamon stick, and jasmine flower. And he was cleansed with Osain, with gun powder. Lived happily every after. Okay? Those are the cases that I pulled for you."

Discussion

Many observations can be made about these cases. All were word-of-mouth referrals, whether from botánicas or other clients. None of the clients was a member of Carmello's ile (or congregation), although two (one man, one woman) later asked to be initiated into Lucumí; both have sought the help of the oracle on average once a month, usually for advice in social relations and work-related problems (such as finding, keeping, or changing jobs). Most clients are Latino or African American. They are from all age groups. Several are illegal aliens or their children are. Nearly all came to Carmello Santiago out of desperation when biomedical treatment proved unavailable, inadequate, or inappropriate. The illnesses include erectile dysfunction, infertility, sexually transmitted disease, hernia, general debility, sorcery, cirrhosis of the liver, an extreme rash, susto, colic, irregular periods, and fibroids. Treatment consisted of ceremony only (with prayers, songs, and incantations) or a combination of rituals (by Carmello, the patient, or both together) along with herbal baths, teas, ointments, and poultices or compresses. Carmello identifies the plants by common name, some in English, others in Spanish, and yet others in Lucumí. Several herbal preparations follow the system of sweet and strong while others have been recommended by the oracle because of their association with particular divinities that own them (the latter are omieros that both cleanse and empower, refreshing and preparing individuals and objects for contact with the orichas). The numbers three, seven, and nine, or combinations of them, occur frequently and have religious significance. A number of individuals, especially those who have become members of his ile or congregation, return regularly to consult the oracle in regard to personal decision making. For example, in case 1, the African-American male who first sought Carmello's help with erectile dysfunction has seen him eighty times in nine years; in case 3, the African-American female initially unable to conceive has also sought his help seventy to eighty times for other matters.

Carmello does not know how many cases he has seen, even those in the past thirteen years in California, for he has not counted all those in his files. Other priests call with difficult cases, some locally and others around the country, several of whom he schedules to see when in another city to perform lengthy and complex initiation rituals; these he does not record or keep on file. "I see about eight cases daily. I don't like to see more than that because if it's more than that I won't be able to give enough time to each case. Right now I'm working Mondays, Tuesdays, Fridays, and Saturdays. That doesn't include those cases where I go to Concord or San Francisco, or when I go to Chino, when I go to San Diego, when I go to New York. Now I'm just starting to open Texas. It really gets problematic! I work from 2:30 to 6:30, but that's not the end of my day. At seven I might be jumping in my van to go to some priest or priestess's house to keep working, and I'll be back around 11, 12 o'clock."

As far as the socioeconomic standing and education of clients are concerned (as suggested by the sample cases as well as other data), "I have people from all walks of life, and I think it balances itself out. I have everything, from illegal immigrants to the well-established movie producer that will come here. And of course these are the type of people that will come as needed, but I will have engineers, accountants, and people in the medical industry as well, for example, nurses. People who are very well read, very well educated. We deal with Hispanics, followed by African Americans, followed by Anglo-Americans, and then in the way, way back, Asians. We deal with people of lower income, medium, high income. The classic case of high income was this girl who was—I told you this story—she was chasing me and calling me desperately because she needed to make a huge decision, and she didn't know what to do, and she needed to see me. So finally I said well this will be important! So when she came she said she needed to ask Elegua; she had this big problem: her sales had been so good that she had this big surplus of money, and she had to decide whether to buy a Maserati or a Porsche. And that was a real big problem that she had! And I just look at her like, 'Is *that* your problem?' She said, 'Yeah, I need to know!' And she meant it. She was frantic. So a week later she went and bought a Porsche, and she brought the Porsche here to be blessed. I said, 'Do you realize that this is the type of problem that I hardly see here?'"

In commenting on the sample cases, Carmello often remarked on the desperation that each of the clients felt at the hands of professional health care providers. "They feel that they've been used as guinea pigs, that the doctor doesn't know what he or she is doing, so let's try this to see if it works. And in the meantime what they fear is that the remedy is going to be worse than the disease! So basically, when they come in [to me], they realize that they are sick, that something is not right, but the medical system is not able to understand their complaint. . . . The person is getting more frustrated, and that is when they decide to go and see someone. And at that time when they come to me, they're just on the edge of desperation. For example, the Salvadoran male that I gave you, the sixth case [impotency], when he came he was brought by his wife, and when I told him what was happening and what we should do, he told me something like, 'I'm glad you told me because if you couldn't help me I was going to shoot myself.' And he had a gun with him and he showed it to me."

Carmello emphasized a second point regarding the complementary role of his practice. "The idea is that this is a system that is not at war with the medical establishment. We don't have the slightest intention of proving we're better than the doctor. They have their job, we have ours. But we refer people to them even though they don't refer people to us, but that's okay." As Carmello sees it, "The person needs to clarify a situation. . . . We just map, we map the way to whatever is to be done, and that's what we do." The santero or santera will send the client to a doctor, for "we cannot prescribe medicines, and sometimes the person is just sick and he needs medicines and that's it!" He notes that many of his clients have already seen a doctor anyway, but often to no avail as most of the sample cases indicate.

One last point: when discussing instances of clients scheduled for surgery who come to him for a reading or the blessing of the orichas, Carmello said, "The power is that if the diviner tells a person, 'Don't get the surgery,' they won't! No matter how sick, they won't, because they understand that they're not going to come back alive. And if the diviner tells them, 'Yes, do get your surgery,' they will do it. And even if the doctor prescribes a surgery, they will come to us to find out if that surgery is needed. They will come and ask the oracle. This is the second opinion, and the heaviest one. In this community the second opinion comes from the oracle. So the power of this table is amazing. The person sitting doing the consultation has this very awesome power because he's speaking with the oracle, with divine force. . . . So when the doctor says, 'You need to have a surgery,' they say, 'Uuhhhh,' and they come here. *So the second opinion in Los Angeles usually is not a doctor, it is a diviner.*"

CONCLUSION AND IMPLICATIONS FOR HEALTH CARE DELIVERY

Latino and African-American communities have many sources of health care available to them, some more and others less visible. They range from self-treatment with home remedies and over-the-counter drugs to a variety of traditional healers to clinics and medical centers (Baer 1982; Mikhail 1994; Roeder 1988). A major source, rarely acknowledged much less described in the medical and ethnographic literature, is the spiritual-herbal center known generally by the Caribbean name botánica. This store dispenses sacramental objects as well as herbs and herbal products. It also serves as community hub and meeting place, a "natural support system," a referral center and, in the back room, an office for spiritual consultations, family counseling, psychotherapy, and treatment for various physical maladies.

Many reasons have been given for using home remedies or consulting traditional healers. Most are discussed by Beatrice Roeder in *Chicano Folk Medicine from Los Angeles* (1988). They range from necessity (no physician available) to economics (high cost of professional medicine and lack of health insurance), psychological factors (fear of doctors and hospitals; emotional support given through personal attention by the folk healer), culture (folk-defined illnesses, belief in witchcraft, integration of health and religion or custom as the path of least resistance), dissatisfaction with biomedicine (treatment failures, no known cure, not appropriate to nature or cause of illness, communication problems, modesty and embarrassment, lengthy wait in clinic, distance and transportation difficulties), education and attitudes of parents, gender (women are more likely to learn herbal remedies), confidence in the effectiveness of traditional medicine, continued contacts with influential believers and practitioners, ethnic pride (determination to maintain ethnic traditions versus the desire for acculturation), and the influence of the symbolic (for example, the impact on opinion and decision making by personal experience narratives told by others and by the drama of ritual and ceremonies entailed in some forms of traditional therapy such as Lucumí illustrated above).

What accounts for the apparent underutilization by Latinos of professional health services? By the 1980s a controversy raged over cultural versus socioeconomic and political factors (Roeder 1988), that is, whether Hispanics so often number fewer among those treated in hospitals and clinics because of a reliance on tradition and custom or owing to a structure of domination, exploitation, and inequality. Van Oss Marin and others (1983) cite the findings of a study of one hundred Mexican Americans in Los Angeles that the most important reasons mentioned by respondents for not seeking professional health care were "people don't have enough money" and "people don't have medical insurance," which implicates issues of equity. Other reasons include lack of proper documents and fear of deportation, problems arranging child care, inability to leave work, long waiting times, and difficulties with English (Van Oss Marin et al. 1983), too few community clinics, and a mind-set that doesn't assume entitlement to quality health care (Kim 1997). Along more cultural lines, going to a traditional healer is often less intimidating because

clients are seen in homes and stores, often at any time (Kim 1997); it is familiar and comforting, affordable, and the atmosphere of botánicas, with their
scent of incense, flickering candles, and statues of revered saints, remind many
customers of a church (Quintanilla 1990). Religious health care systems like
Lucumí put names on fears, explain why things go wrong, and offer specific
measures for people to regain control over their lives often through the mobi-
lization of beneficial supernatural forces, thus reducing stress and facilitating
decision making (Borrello and Mathias 1977, 67, 72; Fisch 1968, 380; Pasquali
1986, 15). Although some researchers contend that Latinos are less often served
by professional facilities because of their dependency on folk medicine, data
suggests a dual use with little competition between these two forms of health
care (Mayers 1989, 291; Mikhail 1994). Certainly the sample cases discussed by
Carmello Santiago indicate the use of both systems, sometimes because of
biomedicine's failures and other times as a complement because "machines
cannot see spirits."

A study of Curanderismo in urban Los Angeles thirty years ago posits
its diminished role in the future (Edgerton, Karno, and Fernandez 1970), a
prediction that has not been borne out (see Alvarez 1997; Mozingo 1998;
Quintanilla 1990; and Sanchez 1997). The authors' anticipation of the demise
of tradition coincided with notions at the time that folk medicine will decline
with acculturation, less interest among the young as well as greater accessibility to formal health care. However, traditional knowledge is durable
(Bhopal 1986, 105; Hufford 1992, 1994) and barriers to health care persist, such
as lack of health insurance and regular sources of care along with obstacles
resulting from the actions of providers (Flores and Vega 1998; Snow 1974;
Stekert 1970). New waves of immigrants and migrants along with trips back
and forth from the U.S. to the home country and extensive travel by highly
sought-after ritual leaders and noted herbalists like Carmello Santiago reinforce traditional patterns of behavior (Borrello and Mathias 1977). Moreover,
recent years have witnessed a revival of interest in alternative medicine as
well as the proliferation of internet sites enabling practitioners to exchange
information and helping healers and patients to make contact. Santería has
become known to many through Latin jazz and other popular music by Tito
Puente, La India, Eddie Palmieri, Conrad Herwig, David Byrne, Milton
Cardona, Celia Cruz, Francisco Aguabella, and even Paul Simon, whose
musical "The Capeman," in which santeros were cast to sing and drum their
prayers to the orichas, opened on Broadway in 1997 (he has also released an
album titled *Rhythm of the Saints*; and in the 1950s when Desi Arnaz as Ricky
Ricardo sang "Babalu" on the *I Love Lucy* show, he was referring to Babalú
Aye, the oricha that presides over disease). The result of all this is a rapid

increase in the number of botánicas whose spiritual and herbal therapies appeal to a diverse clientele.

This is not to suggest that all instances of folk healing and alternative medicine are efficacious, that every healer can always differentiate successfully between illnesses in the spiritual and material realms, or that each folk practitioner unfailingly insists that clients seek professional health care for ailments of a material nature. Nor do we contend that all traditional healers are conscientious and well intentioned. All four of the authors have utilized different forms of alternative and complementary medicine to varying degrees and three have been treated by folk practitioners (including healers representing traditions in this study); regardless of sympathy toward some forms of alternative medicine, we are aware that exploitation and harm may occur within any medical practice. A product sometimes sold in botánicas for ritual use can result in mercury poisoning (Zayas and Ozuah 1996). Questions have been raised about whether the use of herbal remedies delays treatment by professional practitioners and whether the use of plant medicines in conjunction with pharmaceuticals might compromise the latter's efficacy. Obviously there is a need for more qualitative research on traditional healing systems and health practices.

Assuming, however, that much alternative medicine is effective or at least is not harmful, then the question remains as to what uses studies of folk medicine can be put. How might traditional healers and their methods participate more fully, and with greater understanding and respect, within a medically pluralistic system?

Frequent suggestions from the late 1970s to early 1990s included informing professional medical personnel of typical beliefs and practices of ethnic populations that would interfere with patient compliance, and instructing the physician on how to elicit home remedies that the patient is using with a view toward eliminating harmful practices while leaving the harmless ones in the treatment plan. The notion that compliance is the goal has been challenged in recent years, especially by folklorists such as Hufford (1994). Ascertaining what is harmful or harmless is difficult at best, and ignores practices that may be beneficial because of suggestion or the placebo effect, psychotherapeutic results or, in the case of herbs, pharmacological properties (or a combination of all three). These approaches stereotype patients (O'Connor 1997) and promulgate a "deficit model" rather than identify and utilize cultural strengths (Delgado and Humm-Delgado 1982, 88). On the other hand, more recent proposals to "integrate" traditional medical practices within the biomedical system run the risk of co-opting the former, weakening the very concept of pluralist medical systems whose advantage is the gamut of "cultural adaptive strategies necessary for survival and the management of disease and illness" (Pedersen and Baruffati 1989, 494).

We suggest four applications, three of which have been recommended by others to varying degrees. One is to document more extensively the plants utilized in herbal preparations, including those for ceremonial purposes (which sometimes are also drunk, inhaled, or applied to the body in some fashion; see Brandon 1991). The search for potentially new drugs to prevent, treat, or cure illnesses can benefit from folk medical knowledge as a mode of screening, which is certainly superior to random experimentation (Spjut and Perdue 1976), although it raises potential ethical issues regarding exploitation of traditional healers and a country's ecosystem (Barton 1994; Houghton 1995; King and Tempesta 1994). A number of articles in the *Journal of Ethnopharmacology* report efforts to identify plants used in traditional medical systems (Laguerre 1987, 89; see, for example, Appelt 1985; Kelley, Appelt, and Appelt 1988; and Trotter 1981), but rarely does such documentation occur in the U.S. or within the religious-health traditions considered in the present essay (for methods in ethnobotanical and ethnopharmacological fieldwork, see Croom 1983; Etkin 1993; Lipp 1989; and Young 1983). In her article on Hispanic mothers' practices regarding children's health problems, for instance, Blanche I. Mikhail notes that herbs commonly used by the study sample have known pharmacologically active ingredients: camomile has an antiseptic, anti-inflammatory, antispasmodic, and carminative effect; mint has carminative, antispasmodic, and cholagogic consequences; cinnamon has astringent, stimulant, and carminative properties; and eucalyptus has antiseptic, expectorant, and astringent qualities (1994, 635). But many other plants have not been studied (for possible models for field research, see Browner 1985 and Halberstein 1997). The research needs to pay careful attention to which parts of the plant are used in particular preparations and for which ailments, how and when the plants are harvested, whether they are used fresh or dried, how they are stored, and precisely how a remedy is prepared and administered.

A second application, often remarked upon in the literature, falls into the area of education and sensitivity training, based on the assumptions that folk medicine is engaged in by most of us anyway (from home remedies to religious interventions) and that it may be as effective as some forms of biomedical care (Applewhite 1995). Knowledge about traditional practices helps professionals in the medical system better understand the orientation toward health and illness that may be held by patients (DeSantis and Thomas 1990; Laguerre 1987). But knowledge must be accompanied by a degree of empathy and respect (Pasquali 1986; O'Connor 1995; Scott 1974), lest health care workers generate fear, distrust, or rejection of their services (Krajewski-Jaime 1991;

Pasquali 1994). The santero Carmello Santiago emphasizes this very issue: clients came to him out of desperation, distrustful of the medical establishment, and displeased by their treatment; for many in southern California, the second opinion comes from a diviner, not a doctor.

One Lucumí priest remarked, "If a person comes and sits down and says, 'I'm feeling sick, and the doctor orders a battery of tests and they all come back negative, they'll say, 'Look, you have nothing. Go home.' Or worse, they'll say, 'Go see a psychologist,' which in Spanish culture is like a real bad thing to do, because that tells everybody you're 'nuts.'" Religious health care systems involving mediumship or possession—such as Curanderismo (Kiev 1968), Hoodoo (Maduro 1975), Espiritismo (Garrison 1977; Harwood 1977; Koss 1975; Koss-Chioino 1992), and Santería (Sandoval 1979) have often been interpreted as forms of psychotherapy. Garrison goes so far as to contend that "people do not seek the help of the spiritist with organic disorders" and "the mediums studied do not treat [organic] disorders," only mood and feeling states associated with diagnosed organic disorders or psychophysiological conditions and intrapsychic and interpersonal disorders (1977, 71), an observation not borne out by our own study in which it appears that a santero treats not only emotional states and processes but also some organic disorders as well as performing a type of "triage" in which patients are assessed by divination as to whether they have spiritual (and hence to an extent, emotional) or material (organic) problems, or a combination of the two.

The third application, therefore, involves the folk practitioner actively engaged in a patient's emotional recovery. Since medical practitioners have "first chance" at the treatment of spiritist clients, writes Garrison (1977, 164), "I would place the onus upon physicians to make it as clear as possible to patients when there are organic or psychological explanations for complaints presented. And I would weigh against the possible detrimental effects of *Espiritismo*, the role that spiritists play in treating the psychological component of illness *and encouraging clients to receive necessary medical care*" (emphasis in the original). Garrison (165) notes that spiritists already participate significantly in the professional health and mental health care delivery system whether or not this is recognized by professionals, an observation borne out by our study as well. "Therefore, it would seem clear that some strategy for bringing the general medical services, the mental health services, and the spiritists into closer integration would clearly benefit the Puerto Rican community." As an example, she took three healers "to make presentations to professional audiences, to 'consult' to clinicians regarding patients, and to participate in clinical team case conferences regarding specific patients who were also deeply involved in Espiritism or Santería" (166; see also Weclew 1975, 153).

She warns, however, that such participation must be done in a way that prevents the folk healers from being co-opted to the professional system, discrediting their own distinct specialty (see also Koss 1980, who describes a therapist spiritist training project in Puerto Rico as an experiment to relate the traditional healing system to the public health system).

In an article on "natural support systems" in the Hispanic community, Delgado and Humm-Delgado (1982, 88) write that "outreach could be done at *bodegas* [grocery stores], *botanicas*, and churches." The santero Carmello Santiago contends, "We don't want to antagonize, we can be a great asset to them [professional health care workers] and it would cost them nothing. When they were doing the vaccination of the kids [measles epidemic, late 1980s], I got calls here. People don't trust the system. And whatever new technique comes in, they feel that it's not proven so they're going to use it even if it kills, it's just one less Mexican. They tell me that!" Because of the authority and trust so often accorded the traditional healer, a fourth application involves the practitioner and botánica as intermediary between the medical establishment and the public, providing information and referrals as well as urging action regarding health care issues (for example, the need for inoculations and screening for cancer, cholesterol, hypertension, and sexually transmitted diseases).

We end this essay with a modest example of how the fourth application involving botánicas and healers might serve an intermediary role. About one-quarter of California's residents lack health insurance, a disproportionate number of whom are Latinos. Children have the poorest health status and highest health risks as well as least access to desirable prevention and health promotion programs. On 1 July 1998 the state initiated a five hundred million dollar Healthy Families program offering low-cost health benefits to more than four hundred thousand children whose working parents are too impoverished to buy insurance but not poor enough to receive welfare benefits. The state has a twenty-one million dollar education and outreach campaign promoting the program that includes billboards, radio, and TV spots. A local assemblyman in the Southland organized an educational forum in El Monte where three-fourths of the population of 106,209 is Latino; it is also home to numerous botánicas and traditional healers such as curanderas, paleras, santeras, and espiritistas. "After two hours, most chairs in the auditorium [still] sat empty. The formal presentation was scrapped" (Marquis and Ellis 1998, A24). The sparse attendance indicates that many families did not know of the program, including the santero Carmello Santiago. Recognizing the potential value of the enterprise, he insists, he would have urged qualifying clients to attend if he had been informed about it, and further, other practitioners and owners of botánicas would have done likewise. To most agencies and researchers outside the community, however, these spiritual-herbal centers are invisible; yet every day their waiting rooms are filled with clients seeking care.

REFERENCES

Alonso-Zaldivar, Ricardo. 1999. Big Apple takes on a flavor of Mexico. *Los Angeles Times*, 19 February, A1, A20–21.

Alvarez, Lizette. 1997. Santería: A once-hidden faith leaps into the open. *New York Times*, 27 January, B1.

Anderson, E. N., Jr. 1987. Why is humoral medicine so popular? *Social Science of Medicine* 25: 331–37.

Appelt, Glenn D. 1985. Pharmacological aspects of selected herbs employed in Hispanic folk medicine in the San Luis Valley of Colorado, USA: I. *Lingusticum porteri* (osha) and *Matricaria chamomilla* (manzanilla). *Journal of Ethnopharmacology* 13: 51–55.

Applewhite, Steven Lozano. 1995. Curanderismo: Demystifying the health beliefs and practices of elderly Mexican Americans. *Health and Social Work* 20: 247–53.

Baer, Hans A. 1982. Toward a typology of black folk healers. *Phylon* 43: 327–43.

Barton, J. H. 1994. Ethnobotany and intellectual property rights in ethnobotany and the search for new drugs. In *CIBA foundation symposium 185: Ethnobotany and the search for new drugs*, 214–28. Chichester, U.K.: Wiley.

Bascom, William. 1969. *Sixteen cowries: Yoruba divination from Africa to the New World*. Bloomington: Indiana University Press.

Bastani, R., C. P. Kaplan, A. E. Maxwell, R. Nisenbaum, J. Pearce, and A. C. Marcus. 1995. Initial and repeat mammography screening in a low income multi-ethnic population in Los Angeles. *Cancer Epidemiology Biomarkers Preview* 4:161–67.

Becerra, R. M., and A. P. Iglehart. 1995. Folk medicine use: Diverse populations in a metropolitan area. *Social Work Health Care* 21 (4): 37–58.

Bhopal, Rajinder Singh. 1986. The inter-relationship of folk, traditional and Western medicine within an Asian community in Britain. *Social Science of Medicine* 22: 99–105.

Borrello, Mary Ann, and Elizabeth Mathias. 1977. Botanicas: Puerto Rican folk pharmacies. *Natural History* 86, no. 7 (August–September): 64–72, 116–17.

Brandon, George. 1990. Sacrificial practices in Santeria, an African-Cuban religion in the United States. In *Africanisms in American culture*, ed. Joseph E. Holloway, 119–47. Bloomington: Indiana University Press.

———. 1991. The uses of plants in healing in an Afro-Cuban religion, Santeria. *Journal of Black Studies* 22: 55–76.

———. 1993. *The dead sell memories: Santeria from Africa to the New World*. Bloomington: Indiana University Press.

Brekke, J. S., and C. Barrio. 1997. Cross-ethnic symptom differences in schizophrenia: The influence of culture and minority status. *Schizophrenia Bulletin* 23 (2): 305–16.

Brodwin, Paul. 1992. Guardian angels and dirty spirits: The moral basis of healing power in rural Haiti. In *Anthropological approaches to the study of ethnomedicine*, ed. M. Nichter, 57–74. Philadelphia: Gordon and Breach.

———. 1996. *Medicine and morality in Haiti: The contest for healing power.* New York: Cambridge University Press.

Brooks, T. R. 1992. Pitfalls in communication with Hispanic and African-American patients: Do translators help or harm? *Journal of the National Medical Association* 84: 941–47.

Browner, Carole H. 1985. Criteria for selecting herbal remedies. *Ethnology* 24: 13–32.

Cabrera, Lydia. [1940] 1975. *El monte: Notas sobre las religiones, la mágia, las supersticiones y el folklore de pueblo de Cuba.* Reprint, Miami: Ediciones Universal.

———. 1986. *Reglas de Congo: Mayombe Palo Monte.* Miami: Ediciones Universal.

Carlisle, D. M., B. D. Leake, and M. F. Shapiro. 1995. Racial and ethnic differences in the use of invasive cardiac procedures among cardiac patients in Los Angeles County, 1986 through 1988. *American Journal of Public Health* 85: 352–56.

———. 1997. Racial and ethnic disparities in the use of cardiovascular procedures: Associations with type of health insurance. *American Journal of Public Health* 87: 263–67.

Cassidy, Claire M. 1995. Social science theory and methods in the study of alternative and complementary medicine. *Journal of Alternative and Complementary Medicine* 1: 19–40.

Clark, Margaret. 1959. *Health in the Mexican American culture: A community study.* Berkeley: University of California Press.

Clark, Marta. 1995. Biomedicine, meet ethnomedicine. *Healthcare Forum Journal,* May/June, 1–9 (published through www.thfnet.org).

Cosentino, Donald J., ed. 1995. *The sacred arts of Haitian vodou.* Fowler Museum of Cultural History, University of California, Los Angeles.

Croom, E. M. 1983. Documenting and evaluating herbal remedies. *Economic Botany* 37: 13–27.

Curtis, James R. 1982. Santeria: Persistence and change in an Afrocuban cult religion. In *Objects of special devotion: Fetishism in popular culture,* ed. Ray Browne, 336–51. Bowling Green, Ohio: Bowling Green Popular Press.

Davis-Floyd, Robbie E. 1987. The technological model of birth. *Journal of American Folklore* 100: 479–95.

———. 1992. *Birth as an American rite of passage.* Berkeley and Los Angeles: University of California Press.

Delgado, Melvin, and Denise Humm-Delgado. 1982. Natural support systems: A source of strength in Hispanic communities. *Social Work* 27: 83–89.

DeSantis, Lydia, and Janice T. Thomas. 1990. The immigrant Haitian mother: Transcultural nursing perspective on preventive health care for children. *Journal of Transcultural Nursing* 2: 2–15.

Dwyer, Philip. 1987. Herbalism and ritual: Folk medical practices among Asian immigrants in southern California. Ph.D. diss., University of California, Los Angeles.

Edelman, Marian Wrights, Wendy Lazarus, and Lois Salisbury. 1998. A first step to providing health care for all kids. *Los Angeles Times*, 30 June, B7.

Edgerton, Robert B., Marvin Karno, and Irma Fernandez. 1970. Curanderismo in the metropolis: The diminishing role of folk psychiatry among Los Angeles Mexican Americans. *American Journal of Psychotherapy* 24 (1): 124–34.

Eduardo the healer. 1978. Produced by Richard Cowan and Douglas C. Sharon. 55 min. Distributed by Penn State Public Broadcasting. Videocassette.

Eisenberg, Leon. 1977. Disease and illness: Distinctions between professional and popular ideas of sickness. *Culture, Medicine and Psychiatry* 1: 9–23.

Ell, K., L. J. Haywood, M. deGuzman, E. Sobel, S. Norris, D. Blumfield, J. P. Ning, and E. Butts. 1995. Differential perceptions, behaviors, and motivations among African Americans, Latinos, and whites suspected of heart attacks in two hospital populations. *Journal of the Association for Academic Minority Physicians* 6 (2): 60–69.

Espín, Olivia. 1996. *Latina healers.* Encino, California: Floricanto Press.

Etkin, Nina L. 1993. Anthropological methods in ethnopharmacology. *Journal of Ethnopharmacology* 38: 93–104.

Evanchuk, Roberta J. 1996. When the curtain goes up, the gods come down: Aspects of performance in public ceremonies of orisha worship. Ph.D. diss., University of California, Los Angeles.

———. 1999. "Bring me a pumpkin": A healing ceremony in orisha worship for women of all ages. *Southern Folklore* 56 (3): 209–21.

Fisch, Stanley. 1968. Botanicas and spiritualism in a metropolis. *Milbank Memorial Fund Quarterly* 46: 377–88.

Fishman, B. M., L. Bobo, K. Kosub, and R. J. Womeodu. 1993. Cultural issues in serving minority populations: Emphasis on Mexican Americans and African Americans. *American Journal of Medical Science* 306: 160–66.

Flaskerud, J. H., and L. T. Hu. 1992. Relationship of ethnicity to psychiatric diagnosis. *Journal of Nerve and Mental Disorders* 180(5): 296–303.

Flaskerud, J. H., and A. M. Nyamathi. 1990. Effects of an AIDS education program on the knowledge, attitudes and practices of low income black and Latina women. *Journal of Community Health* 15 (6): 343–55.

Flores, Glenn, and Luis R. Vega. 1998. Barriers to health care access for Latino children: A review. *Family Medicine* 30: 196–205.

Flores-Peña, Ysamur. 1998. "The tongue is the whip of the body": Identity and appropriation through narrative in Lucumí religious culture. Ph.D. diss., University of California, Los Angeles.

Flores-Peña, Ysamur, and Roberta J. Evanchuk. 1994. *Santería garments and altars.* Jackson: University Press of Mississippi.

Frankel, Barbara. 1977. *Childbirth in the ghetto: Folk beliefs of Negro women in a north Philadelphia hospital ward.* San Francisco: R and E Research.

Garrison, Vivian. 1977. Doctor, espiritista, or psychiatrist? Health-seeking behavior in a Puerto Rican neighborhood in New York City. *Medical Anthropology* 1: 65–191.

———. 1982. Folk healing systems as elements in the community. In *Therapeutic intervention: Healing strategies for human systems*, ed. Uri Rueveni, Ross V. Speck, and Joan L. Specks, 58–95. New York: Human Sciences Press.

George, Victoria. 1980. Santeria cult and its healers: Beliefs and traditions preserved in Los Angeles. Master's thesis, University of California, Los Angeles.

Graham, Joe S. 1976. The role of the *curandero* in the Mexican American folk medicine system in west Texas. In *American folk medicine: A symposium*, ed. W. D. Hand, 175–89. Berkeley and Los Angeles: University of California Press.

———. 1985. Folk medicine and intracultural diversity among west Texas Mexican Americans. *Western Folklore* 44: 168–93.

Granger, Byrd Howell. 1976. Some aspects of folk medicine among Spanish-speaking people in southern Arizona. In *American folk medicine: A symposium*, ed. Wayland D. Hand, 191–202. Berkeley and Los Angeles: University of California Press.

Gurza, Agustin. 1999. A dangerous cultural tradition. *Los Angeles Times* 27 February, A18.

Halberstein, R. A. 1997. Traditional botanical remedies on a small Caribbean island: Middle (Grand) Caicos, West Indies. *Journal of Alternative and Complementary Medicine* 3: 227–39.

Hand, Wayland D. 1980. *Magical medicine: The folkloric component of medicine in the folk belief, custom, and ritual of the peoples of Europe and America. Selected essays of Wayland D. Hand.* Berkeley and Los Angeles: University of California Press.

Harwood, Alan. 1971. The hot-cold theory of disease: Implications for treatment of Puerto Rican patients. *Journal of the American Medical Association* 216: 1153–58.

———. 1977. *Rx: Spiritist as needed: A study of Puerto Rican community mental health resources.* New York: Wiley.

———. 1981. Mainland Puerto Ricans. In *Ethnicity and medical care*, ed. Alan Harwood, 397–481. Cambridge: Harvard University Press.

Houghton, Peter J. 1995. The role of plants in traditional medicine and current therapy. *Journal of Alternative and Complementary Medicine* 1: 131–43.

Hufford, David J. 1992. Folk medicine in contemporary America. In *Herbal and magical medicine: Traditional healing today*, ed. James Kirkland, Holly F. Mathews, C. W. Sullivan III, and Karen Baldwin, 14–32. Durham, North Carolina: Duke University Press.

———. 1994. Folklore and medicine. In *Putting folklore to use*, ed. Michael Owen Jones, 117–35. Lexington: University Press of Kentucky.

Hurston, Zora Neale. 1931. Hoodoo in America. *Journal of American Folklore* 44: 317–417.

———. 1935. *Mules and men.* New York: J. B. Lippincott.

Hyatt, Harry Middleton. 1970–78. *Hoodoo, conjuration, witchcraft, rootwork.* 5 vols. New York and Quincy, Illinois: Memoirs of the Alma Egan Hyatt Foundation.

Jackson, Bruce. 1976. The other kind of doctor: Conjure and magic in black American folk medicine. In *American folk medicine: A symposium,* ed. Wayland D. Hand, 261–72. Berkeley and Los Angeles: University of California Press.

Keegan L. 1996. Use of alternative therapies among Mexican Americans in the Texas Rio Grande Valley. *Journal of Holistic Nursing* 14 (4): 277–94.

Kelley, B. D., G. D. Appelt, and J. M. Appelt. 1988. Pharmacological aspects of selected herbs employed in Hispanic folk medicine in the San Luis Valley of Colorado, USA: II. *Asclepias asperula* (inmortal) and *Achillea lanulosa* (plumajillo). *Journal of Ethnopharmacology* 22: 1–9.

Kerr, H. D. 1993. White liver: A cultural disorder resembling AIDS. *Social Science of Medicine* 36: 609–14.

Kiev, Ari. 1968. *Curanderismo: Mexican-American folk psychiatry.* New York: Free Press.

Kim, Myung Oak. 1997. Folk healers still practice across city: Immigrants combine traditional ways (with our modern medicine). *Philadelphia Daily News* (www3.phillynews.com/packages/immigration/immi30.asp.).

King, S., and M. S. Tempesta. 1994. From shaman to human clinical trials: The role of industry in ethnobotany, conservation and community reciprocity in ethnobotany and the search for new drugs. In *CIBA foundation symposium 185: Ethnobotany and the search for new drugs,* 197–213. Chichester, U.K.: Wiley.

Koss, Joan D. 1975. Therapeutic aspects of Puerto Rican cult practices. *Psychiatry* 38: 160–71.

———. 1980. The therapist spiritist training project in Puerto Rico: An experiment to relate the traditional healing system to the public health system. *Social Science and Medicine* 14B: 255–66.

Koss-Chioino, Joan. 1992. *Women as healers, women as patients: Mental health care and traditional healing in Puerto Rico.* Boulder, Colorado: Westview Press.

Krajewski-Jaime, Elvia R. 1991. Folk-healing among Mexican-American families as a consideration in the delivery of child welfare and child health care services. *Child Welfare* 70: 157–67.

Kroesen, Kendall W. 1994. Politics, affect, and culture in illness etiology: *Susto* and *coraje* in Mexico. Paper presented at the American Anthropological Association meeting (http://weber.ucsd.edu/~kkroesen/aaapaper.htm.).

Laguerre, M. S. 1987. *Afro-Caribbean folk medicine.* South Hadley, Massachusetts: Bergin and Garvey.

LeVine, E. S., and A. M. Padilla. 1980. *Crossing cultures in therapy.* Monterey, California: Brooks Cole.

Lichstein, P. R. 1992. Rootwork from the clinician's perspective. In *Herbal and magical medicine: Traditional healing today,* ed. James Kirkland, Holly F. Mathews, C. W. Sullivan III, and Karen Baldwin, 99–117. Durham, North Carolina: Duke University Press.

Lipp, F. J. 1989. Methods for ethnopharmacological field work. *Journal of Ethnopharmacology* 25(2): 139–50.

Logan, Michael H. 1993. New lines of inquiry on the illness of susto. *Medical Anthropology* 15: 189–200.

Madsen, William. 1964. *The Mexican-Americans of south Texas*. New York: Holt, Rinehart, and Winston.

Maduro, Renaldo J. 1975. Hoodoo possession in San Francisco: Notes on therapeutic aspects of regression. *Ethos* 3: 425–47.

Marquis, Julie, and Virginia Ellis. 1998. Health plan for needy children launched. *Los Angeles Times*, 1 July, A3, A24.

Mason, Michael Atwood. 1993. "The blood that runs through the veins": The creation of identity and a client's experience of Cuban-American Santeria dilogun divination. *Drama Review* 37 (2): 119.

Mathews, Holly F. 1987. Rootwork: Description of an ethnomedical system in the American South. *Southern Medical Journal* 1980: 885–91.

———. 1992. Doctors and root doctors: Patients who use both. In *Herbal and magical medicine: Traditional healing today*, ed. James Kirkland, Holly F. Mathews, C. W. Sullivan III, and Karen Baldwin, 68–98. Durham, North Carolina: Duke University Press.

Maugh, Thomas H., II. 1998. Insurance unaffordable for millions, study says. *Los Angeles Times*, 22 June, E4, S6.

Mayers, Raymond Sanchez. 1989. Use of folk medicine by elderly Mexican-American women. *The Journal of Drug Issues* 19: 283–95

McDonough, Gary W., ed. 1993. *The Florida Negro: A federal writers' project legacy*. Jackson: University of Mississippi Press.

Mena, Aipy. 1998. Cuban Santeria, Haitian vodun, Puerto Rican spiritualism: A multiculturalist inquiry into syncretism. *Journal for the Scientific Study of Religion* 37: 15–27.

Metraux, A. 1972. *Voodoo in Haiti*. New York: Schocken Books.

Mikhail, Blanche I. 1994. Hispanic mothers' beliefs and practices regarding selected children's health problems. *Western Journal of Nursing Research* 16: 623–38.

Montenegro, Carlos. 1994. *Palo Mayombe: The dark side of Santería*. Bronx, New York: Original Pubs.

Mozingo, Joe. 1998. Latin American faith healing draws many adherents in L.A. *Los Angeles Times*, 8 March, B1–2.

Murphy, Joseph M. 1988. *Santería: An African religion in America*. Boston: Beacon Press.

Nevadomsky, Joseph. 1988. Kemwin-kemwin: The apothecary shop in Benin City. *African Arts* 22, no. 1 (November): 72–83, 100.

The new believers. 1990. Produced by Tom Corboy. 28 mins. Distributed by Extension Media Center, University of California, Berkeley. Videocassette.

Newell, G. R., and P. K. Mills. 1986. Low cancer rates in Hispanic women related to social and economic factors. *Women and Health* 11 (3–4): 23–35.

Norris, S. L., M. deGuzman, E. Sobel, S. Brooks, and L. J. Haywood. 1993. Risk factors and mortality among black, Caucasian, and Latina women with acute myocardial infarction. *American Heart Journal* 126 (6): 1312–19.

O'Connor, Bonnie Blair. 1995. *Healing traditions: Alternative medicine and the health professions.* Philadelphia: University of Pennsylvania Press.

———. 1997. Applying folklore in medical education. *Southern Folklore* 54: 67–77.

Parker, V. C., S. Sussman, D. L. Crippens, D. Scholl, and P. Elder. 1996. Qualitative development of smoking prevention programming for minority youth. *Addictive Behavior* 21: 521–25.

Pasquali, E. A. 1986. Santeria: A religion that is a health care system for Long Island Cuban-Americans. *Journal of the New York State Nurses Association* 17: 12–15.

———. 1994. Santeria. *Journal of Holistic Nursing* 12: 380–90.

Pedersen, Duncan, and Veronica Baruffati. 1989. Healers, deities, saints, and doctors: Elements for the analysis of medical systems. *Social Science and Medicine* 29: 487–96.

Polk, Patrick A. 1993. African religion and Christianity in Grenada. *Caribbean Quarterly* 39: 74–81.

———. 1995. Sacred banners and the divine cavalry charge. In *The sacred arts of Haitian vodou,* ed. Donald J. Cosentino, 325–47. Fowler Museum of Cultural History, University of California, Los Angeles.

———. 1997. *Haitian vodou flags.* Jackson: University Press of Mississippi.

———, ed. 1998. *Botánica: Art and spirit in Los Angeles.* Folk Art Group, University of California, Los Angeles.

Pyle, Amy. 1999. Many Latinas lack health insurance, study finds. *Los Angeles Times,* 28 January, B1, B3.

Quintanilla, Michael. 1990. Dreams in bottles. *Los Angeles Times,* 14 December, E1, E10–12.

Reza, H. G. 1999. Sale, misuse of smuggled drugs spread. *Los Angeles Times,* 27 February, A1, A18.

Richardson, J. L., B. Langholz, L. Bernstein, C. Burciaga, K. Danley, and R. K. Ross. 1992. Stage and delay in breast cancer diagnosis by race, socioeconomic status, age and year. *British Journal of Cancer* 65: 922–26.

Roeder, Beatrice. 1988. *Chicano folk medicine from Los Angeles.* Berkeley and Los Angeles: University of California Press.

Rubel, Arthur J. 1960. Concepts of disease in Mexican-American culture. *American Anthropologist* 62: 795–814.

———. 1964. The epidemiology of a folk illness: Susto in Hispanic America. *Ethnology* 3: 268–83.

———. 1966. *Across the tracks: Mexican Americans in a Texas city.* Austin: University of Texas Press.

Sanchez, Kimberly. 1997. Encyclopedia botanica. *Los Angeles Times,* 4 April, D2, D5.

Sandoval, Mercedes C. 1977. Afrocuban concepts of disease and its treatment in Miami. *Journal of Operational Psychiatry* 8: 52–63.

————. 1979. Santería as a mental health care system: An historical overview. *Social Science and Medicine* 13B: 137–51.

————. 1983. Santería. *Journal of the Florida Medical Association* 70: 620–28.

Scott, C. 1974. Health and healing practices among five ethnic groups in Miami, Florida. *Public Health Reports* 89: 524–53.

Shrout, P. E., G. J. Canino, H. R. Bird, M. Rubio-Stipec, M. Bravo, and M. A. Burnam. 1992. Mental health status among Puerto Ricans, Mexican Americans, and non-Hispanic whites. *American Journal of Community Psychology* 20: 729–52.

Singer, M., and R. García. 1989. Becoming a Puerto Rican espiritista: Life history of a female healer. In *Women as healers: Cross-cultural perspectives*, ed. C. S. McClain, 157–85. New Brunswick, New Jersey: Rutgers University Press.

Snow, Loudell F. 1974. Folk medical beliefs and their implications for care of patients: A review based on studies among black Americans. *Annals of Internal Medicine* 81: 82–96.

————. 1977. Popular medicine in a black neighborhood. In *Ethnic medicine in the Southwest*, ed. E. H. Spicer, 19–85. Tucson: University of Arizona Press.

————. 1979. Voodoo illness in the black population. In *Culture, curers, and contagion*, ed. N. Klein, 179–84. Novato, California: Chandler and Sharp.

————. 1993. *Walkin' over medicine*. Boulder, Colorado: Westview Press.

Snow, Loudell F., S. M. Johnson, and H. E. Mayhew. 1978. The behavioral implications of some old wives' tales. *Obstetrics and Gynecology* 51: 727–32.

Spirit doctors: Three Latina healers. 1997. Produced by Monica Delgado and Michael Van Wagenen. 28 min. Distributed by Filmmaker's Library, New York. Videocassette.

Spjut, R. W., and R. E. Perdue, Jr. 1976. Plant folklore: A tool for predicting sources of antihumor activity? *Cancer Treatment Reports* 60: 979–85.

Stekert, Ellen J. 1970. Focus for conflict: Southern mountain medical beliefs in Detroit. *Journal of American Folklore* 83: 115–56.

Stevens-Arroyo, Anthony M., and Andres I. Pérez y Mena, eds. 1995. *Enigmatic powers: Syncretism with African and indigenous peoples' religions among Latinos*. New York: Bildner Center for Western Hemisphere Studies.

Stolley, J. M., and H. Koenig. 1997. Religion/spirituality and health among elderly African Americans and Hispanics. *Journal of Psychosocial Nursing and Mental Health Services* 35 (11): 32–38.

Straight, William M. 1983. Throw downs, fixin, rooting and hexing. *Journal of the Florida Medical Association* 70: 635–41.

Suarez, M., M. Raffaelli, and A. O'Leary. 1996. Use of fold healing practices by HIV-infected Hispanics living in the United States. *AIDS Care* 8(6): 683–90.

Suro, Frederico. 1991. Shopping for witches' brew. *Américas* 43 (5–6): 84–88.

Taggart, L., and S. Mattson. 1996. Delay in prenatal care as a result of battering in pregnancy: Cross-cultural implications. *Health Care for Women International* 17: 25–34.

Terrell, S. J. 1990. *This other kind of doctors: Traditional medical systems in black neighborhoods in Austin, Texas.* New York: AMD Press.

Trotter, R. T., II. 1981. Folk remedies as indicators of common illnesses: Examples from the United States-Mexico border. *Journal of Ethnopharmacology* 4: 207–21.

Van Oss Marin, B., G. Marin, A. Padilla, and C. de la Rocha. 1983. Utilization of traditional and non-traditional sources of health care among Hispanics. *Hispanic Journal of Behavioral Sciences* 5: 65–80.

Vega, W. A., B. Kolody, S. Aguilar-Gaxiola, E. Alderete, R. Catalano, and J. Caraveo-Anduaga. 1998. Lifetime prevalence of DSM-III-R psychiatric disorders among urban and rural Mexican Americans in California. *Archive of General Psychiatry* 55: 771–78.

Weclew, Robert V. 1975. The nature, prevalence, and level of awareness of "Curanderismo" and some of its implications for community mental health. *Community Mental Health Journal* 11: 145–54.

Weidman, H. 1978. Southern black health profile. Offprint, Miami Health Ecology Project, University of Miami.

Weightman, Barbara A. 1993. Changing religious landscapes in Los Angeles. *Journal of Cultural Geography* 14: 1–20.

Wetli, Charles V., and Rafael Martinez. 1983. Brujeria: Manifestations of Palo Mayombe in south Florida. *Journal of the Florida Medical Association* 70: 629–34.

Winslow, David J. 1969. Bishop E. E. Everett and some aspects of occultism and folk religion in Negro Philadelphia. *Keystone Folklore Quarterly* 14: 59–80.

Young, Kathleen L. 1983. Ethnobotany: A methodology for folklorists. Master's thesis, Western Kentucky University.

Zaldivar, A., and J. Smolowitz. 1994. Perceptions of the importance placed on religion and folk medicine by non-Mexican-American Hispanic adults with diabetes. *Diabetes Education* 20 (4): 303–6.

Zambrana, R. E., and S. C. Scrimshaw. 1997. Maternal psychosocial factors associated with substance use in Mexican-origin and African American low-income pregnant women. *Pediatric Nursing* 23 (3): 253–59.

Zambrana, R. E., C. Dunkel-Schetter, and S. Scrimshaw. 1991. Factors which influence use of prenatal care in low-income racial-ethnic women in Los Angeles County. *Journal of Community Health* 16 (5): 283–95.

Zayas, L. H., and P. O. Ozuah. 1996. Mercury use in espiritismo: A survey of botanicas. *American Journal of Public Health* 86(1): 111–12

Zuckerman, M. J., L. G. Guerra, D. A. Drossman, J. A. Foland, and G. G. Gregory. 1996. Health-care-seeking behaviors related to bowel complaints: Hispanics versus non-Hispanic whites. *Digestive Diseases and Sciences* 41: 77–82.

4

The Poor Man's Medicine Bag:
THE EMPIRICAL FOLK REMEDIES OF
TILLMAN WAGGONER

RICHARD BLAUSTEIN, ANTHONY CAVENDER,
AND JACKIE SLUDER,
WITH COMMENTS BY TILLMAN WAGGONER

PART I: BECOMING AN HERB DOCTOR

As the old saying goes, Tillman (Tim) Waggoner of Knoxville, Tennessee, is a "man of many parts." Born in 1940 and raised in the Marble City community in the formerly rural Third Creek section of west Knoxville, at various points in his life Tim Waggoner has been a moonshiner (very briefly), soldier, Missionary Baptist preacher and radio evangelist, folk healer, blue-collar laborer, folk festival performer, university guest lecturer, and also author and publisher of several collections of local folktales, recipes, and home remedies, including *The Poor Man's Medicine Bag* (1984). Tim Waggoner wrote *The Poor Man's Medicine Bag* "to help people who couldn't afford to go to the doctor" and to preserve some of the traditional knowledge of southern Appalachian folk medicine still current during his childhood. Realizing that he "just got in on the last of this great thing" (meaning traditional Appalachian folk medicine), Tim took on the role of native folklorist, interviewing approximately one hundred of his friends and neighbors concerning herbs and home remedies. *The Poor Man's Medicine Bag*, however, is much more than simply a compendium of Appalachian folk remedies; it represents the confluence of diverse streams of medical tradition, old and new, local and exotic, distilled from popular literature as well as oral tradition, all of which Tim considers to be empirical therapeutic alternatives.

Tim Waggoner still lives in the Third Creek section of Knoxville where he was born and raised. His parents, Tillman Hollis Waggoner and Lillian Omeda Waggoner, were hardworking east Tennessee country people who moved to Knoxville from small rural communities in Union and Sevier Counties, respectively, in the late 1930s. The third of seven children, Tim nostalgically remembers his formative years as a time when a genuine sense of community still prevailed, an era when neighbors helped out in time of need. Following the old pioneer adage of "make do or do without," Tim recalls that his family and their neighbors made extensive use of botanicals and other traditional materia medica. However, medical knowledge in the Marble City community was not exclusively passed along via oral transmission, contrary to prevalent romantic stereotypes of southern Appalachian folk culture. Some of the Waggoner family's herbal knowledge came from official rather than folk sources: Tim's mother (actually his aunt: see afterword) often referred to a U.S. Department of Agriculture monograph dealing with the collection, preservation, and medicinal uses of botanicals. Practical in all aspects of their lives, Tim's family and neighbors were by no means opposed to official medicine, as long as they could afford to pay for it. Tim notes that he was hospitalized twice during his childhood, at the age of two for diphtheria and again at five for spinal meningitis. Two of Tim's sisters are now practicing nurses.

During his teenage years, Tim became acquainted with two older men, Doc Harris and Dewey Lincus, who sparked his budding interest in herbs and their medical uses. Not a licensed physician, Doc Harris was a self-taught herbalist who sold his botanical concoctions on Market Street in downtown Knoxville. According to Tim, Dewey Lincus was "an old mountain man from Rogersville" (the county seat of Hawkins County, Tennessee), who was well known around south Knoxville as an especially adept herb doctor. Lincus made the greatest impression on the young Tim Waggoner. He recalls that Doc Harris was somewhat secretive and unwilling to reveal the ingredients of his herbal preparations, which he prepared and sold commercially like so many other old-fashioned herbalists and medicine-show men. Dewey Lincus, however, was a generous and amiable old soul who was glad to have the young Waggoner accompany him on his forays into the nearby Great Smoky Mountains to gather herbs. Tim spent countless hours on the front porch of Lincus's shack soaking in the older man's knowledge of herbs and home remedies. Seemingly a reclusive folk mystic, Lincus was "close to nature" and could communicate with animals, bringing to mind St. Francis of Assisi, who could allegedly talk with birds. Tim Waggoner insists that "Dewey talked to animals like I talk to you . . . I have sat down on his porch with him and they would come in to be healed" (1995a).

Shortly after graduating from high school in 1958, Tim joined the U.S. Army. Returning home from the service, he married Joyce Ann Boles and began working for a grocery chain and later took a job with TRW Plastics, where he worked for thirty-three years. A few years after his marriage, Tillman Waggoner received a spiritual call to preach the gospel and was subsequently ordained as a Missionary Baptist minister. From early childhood, he was intensely religious and a regular churchgoer, even though his own parents were not always so inclined. He has ministered to a small congregation in the Marble City neighborhood for many years and at one time had a religious program on a Knoxville AM radio station. Though profoundly religious in orientation, Tim's philosophy of medicine (described in detail in part II) is both highly eclectic and pragmatic. Rather than relying solely on faith healing as do adherents of radical fundamentalist sects, who are actually only a small if highly sensationalized segment of the southern Appalachian population, Tim's predominantly naturalistic and empirical medical beliefs and practices are arguably closer to the Appalachian norm and the American cultural mainstream in general.

Tim Waggoner is hardly typical in any other respect, however. Few ordinary people could have mustered the energy required to work a regular industrial job, minister to a small church, conduct his own radio program, help raise a family of three children, and still find time to read about herbs and healing. Tim began frequenting an area health food store in the late 1970s, where he acquired books, monographs, and pamphlets dealing with herbs and nutrition. *Prevention* magazine remains one of his most valued sources of alternative health care information. Three popular health books particularly influenced Tim's ideas about health and natural diet: John Lust's *The Herb Book* (1974), Jethro Kloss's *Back to Eden* ([1939] 1970), and D. C. Jarvis's *Folk Medicine* (1958).

The Herb Book introduced Tim to a wider range of medicinal herbs than those customarily used in southern Appalachian folk medicine. Written by a Vermont physician, D. C. Jarvis's national best seller *Folk Medicine* extolled the salubrious health benefits of honey and vinegar. Though popularized by a Vermont Yankee, the honey and vinegar regimen was quickly incorporated into contemporary southern folk medicine, not only by Tim Waggoner in *The Poor Man's Medicine Bag* but also by an Alabama entrepreneur who promotes a commercial honey-vinegar health drink called "Jogging in a Jug." (Recent TV ads repeat the statement that honey and vinegar have no official proven health benefits, strongly suggesting that the FDA may have warned the makers of "Jogging in a Jug" to tone down their advertised health claims.) However, Jethro Kloss's *Back to Eden* had the greatest influence upon Tim Waggoner's personal philosophy of health and healing, highly consonant with Kloss's contention that "the fundamental principle of true healing consists of a return to natural habits of living" ([1939] 1970, iv). The return to natural habits of living has been a recurrent theme of health reform movements in the United States and elsewhere at least since the early nineteenth century. Early health care reformers such as Sylvester Graham and authors of popular home health guides like Wooster Beach and John C. Gunn espoused what would now be termed a "holistic" approach to preventive health care, largely based upon diet (primarily or exclusively vegetarian), rest, exercise, and stress management. Some early health care reformers were purely naturalistic and rationalistic; others, like the founders of the Seventh Day Adventist Church and the Latter-day Saints, equated return to natural diet with spirituality and the rejection of worldly corruption, artificiality, and impurity. *Back to Eden* by Jethro Kloss is a twentieth-century expression of this ongoing tradition of American religious health care reform. Health reform is defined in religious terms. According to Kloss, "natural habits of living" were established by God to enjoy a life free from illnesses which stem from the rejection of divine wisdom. If humans would only follow the principles Kloss terms "simple laws of health," including pure food, pure water, fresh air, sunshine, rest, nature's remedies, herbs, etc."([1939] 1970, ii), then natural good health can be restored.

Kloss's influence on Waggoner is evident in this excerpt from a taped interview Jackie Sluder recorded with Tim:

> You see, a lot of people don't understand this but everything comes from God. Every disease, they don't come from the devil. The devil didn't create anything; they come from God. Of course, Satan uses the law of nature to let you catch them. (1995b)

Tim's statement echoes Kloss's theories concerning the divine nature of healing clearly expressed in the following excerpt from *Back to Eden:*

> God has provided a remedy for every disease that might afflict us. Satan cannot afflict anyone with any disease for which God has not provided a remedy. Our Creator foresaw the wretched condition of mankind in these days, and made provision in Nature for all the ills of man. Many who violate the laws of health are ignorant of the laws of living (eating, drinking, and working) to their health. Until they have some kind of sickness or illness, they do not realize that their condition is caused by the laws of nature and health. ([1939] 1970, ii–iii).

Waggoner elaborates on his view of some of the basic tenets of the law of Nature in his preface to *The Poor Man's Medicine Bag:*

First, let me say that I believe in doctors and the medical profession. Now, let me say that I want to go to heaven as bad as anyone else, but I will take every pill that I can take to help me stay longer. This is the will to survive that God has placed in man. Without it, a person would not want to overcome the second death either. It would be stupid to say that there is no divine healing, just as it would be stupid to say that there is not natural healing which includes the aid of doctors and the medical profession. Go to a hospital and see for yourself. It happens everyday. It doesn't matter whether it is divine healing with God's intervention, or whether it is natural healing with the aid of doctors. God does all the healing. He made our bodies and it would be stupid to say that He cannot heal them. The world in which we live is ruled by the law of nature. This is God's law in which he lets nature take its course except where He would intervene. Nothing can break the law of Nature except God. (1984, 2)

Tim promoted his philosophy of health on his radio programs, encouraging listeners to acknowledge and conform to the divine law of Nature while dispensing practical advice concerning the health benefits of herbs, fresh air, exercise, proper nutrition, and the like. Occasionally, he advertised some of his herbal preparations (tonics and liniments) on his radio show. Seeking to expand his audience, Tim also became a regular contributor on health advice to the editorial pages of Knoxville's two daily newspapers.

By the 1970s, Tim began taking what he calls his "traveling herb wagon" to local fairs, flea markets, and community festivals in and around Knoxville. He assembled a portable table display including herbs, tonics, liniments, and—after its publication in 1984—*The Poor Man's Medicine Bag*, and offered advice concerning healing through following God's law of Nature. Tim finally gave up traveling around with his herb wagon around 1985, but not before he had attracted the attention of folklorists who first recruited him as a participant in the Stokeley Folklife Festival at the Knoxville World's Fair in 1982, which in turn led to his selection as a member of the Tennessee contingent at the Smithsonian Festival of American Folklife in Washington, D.C., in 1986. Today, Tim looks back at his traveling herb wagon as an effort to educate the public concerning the law of Nature. Following the example of his old mentor Doc Harris, Tim's herb wagon and his radio advertisements for tonics and liniments represent a continuation of an old entrepreneurial medicine show tradition which still survives here and there throughout the southern United States, despite the advances of modern medicine and the regulatory efforts of the Food and Drug Administration. While making the circuit with his traveling herb wagon, Tim came to know and learn from other vernacular healers. He particularly respected and admired Chief Two Trees, a Native American healer from Old Fort, North Carolina, who claimed success in treating various forms of cancers. Waggoner attended several seminars by Chief Two Trees and was so impressed by him that he referred several friends and acquaintances to him for treatment. Though Chief Two Trees eventually succumbed to prostate cancer, this did not diminish Tim's confidence in him. As he told Jackie Sluder, "He could have probably cured himself. Knowing him, he smoked, he ate what he wanted, he lived like he wanted, and he died like he wanted" (1995c).

Though Tim began receiving a degree of official validation for his herbal work in the mid-1980s, not only appearing at major folk festivals but also giving guest lectures on herbalism at the University of Tennessee in Knoxville on several occasions, he actually quit taking his traveling herb wagon to area gatherings by 1985. Holding down a full-time job while promoting natural healing on the side was becoming too stressful; besides, Tim's herb business was never profitable enough for him to support his family. Nonetheless, people kept seeking him out for advice on herbs and healing, and he would not turn away anyone in need. *The Poor Man's Medicine Bag* became his primary instrument for educating people about the law of Nature and common-sense, God-given knowledge about maintaining health.

Though Tim says that he believes in doctors and official medicine, his attitude towards official medicine, like that of many other unorthodox healers (see Gevitz 1978, 18–21), is highly critical. Basically, Tim's attitude to official medicine is in accord with the adjuration to Christians to "render unto Caesar what is Caesar's." While he does accept the value and efficacy of conventional medicine in coping with critical life-threatening ailments, particularly sexually transmitted diseases, he believes along with Jethro Kloss that healing ultimately comes from conformity to God's law of Nature, not from human cleverness or ingenuity. In Tim's estimation, official medicine is fundamentally misdirected; its technological achievements have had the unfortunate consequence, he believes, of further alienating humankind from the law of Nature. Like many Americans, he considers professional medicine corrupt, motivated by monetary gain rather than the desire to ease human suffering. Doctors are less interested in curing people than in making them drug-free. In Tim's opinion, the United States is "a nation of drug addicts." Hospitals are "slaughterhouses" where much unnecessary surgery is performed. Doctors would not be needed if people would only follow the law of Nature. Like Jethro Kloss, Tim Waggoner firmly believes that medical science ought to devote itself to understanding the therapeutic powers of God's law of Nature, which is the basis of healthful living.

Part II. Analyzing the Contents of *The Poor Man's Medicine Bag*

Published in 1984, two years after Tim presented his program on herbs and natural healing at the Stokeley Folklife Festival at the Knoxville World's Fair, *The Poor Man's Medicine Bag* includes a variety of remedies, recipes, useful advice, and homespun philosophy leavened with Tim's tongue-in-cheek humor. Part I of *The Poor Man's Medicine Bag* is devoted to remedies; part II includes recipes for food and wines, also advice on planting by the signs of the zodiac, bringing to mind *The Old Farmer's Almanac* and that longtime southern favorite, *Moore's Almanac*. Waggoner includes a few astrological heath care tips as well. When is it best to break bad habits such as smoking, drinking, or overeating? "When the signs come down out of the bowels, quit the next day. It will be easier than you think" (1984, 74).

Similarly, Tim recommends puncturing a burn or blister after sundown to promote healing. This is analogous to healing by signs of the zodiac, based upon belief that there is a natural rhythm and order pervading all of God's creation. Following the natural order leads to healing and increase; disorderly living leads to sickness and decay. Possibly the principle of sympathetic magic links the setting of the sun and the dwindling of the burn or blister, which is congruent with a literal belief that to everything there is a season, including the correct time of day or month to undertake the sowing of a field or the healing of a wound.

Though Tim does not use the term, his approach to health and healing can be characterized as holistic. This is particularly evident in his discussion of alcoholism and alternative treatments for it. Tim recognizes that alcoholism is a complex condition, entailing psychological and social factors as well as chemical dependency. He recommends that the alcoholic needs to be kept busy, but also suggests that goldenseal tea, eating apples, and drinking apple cider vinegar, or an infusion of Virginia creeper leaves, can also help kill the craving for strong drink.

Reading like a nineteenth-century domestic medical book, *The Poor Man's Medicine Bag* is a compendium of homely knowledge derived from a variety of sources, including oral tradition and popular publications. One indication of Tim's wide-ranging reading of health care literature is his use of exotic medicinal plants such as archangel root and palmetto berries, not typically associated with southern Appalachian folk medicine. Use of exotic botanicals by southern Appalachian herbalists is not necessarily a recent development. In the nineteenth century, domestic medical books typically included sets of botanical illustrations and descriptions of the curative properties of various plants. One of the oldest established commercial botanical companies in the United States, the Indiana Herb Company (established in 1910 and now known as Indiana Botanical Gardens), not only bought medicinal roots and herbs in bulk from pickers in various parts of the U.S., but its founder and proprietor Joseph E. Meyer (1878–1950) even published his own pocket-sized herb-picking guide, *The Herbalist*, first published in 1918 and reprinted as recently as 1960, which doubled as a mail-order catalogue, including advertisements for exotic medicinal botanicals and also magical roots and aphrodisiacs. Here again, it is important that scholars concerned with nonofficial medicine recognize the importance of various forms of vernacular (nonprofessional) literature in addition to oral transmission in the continuing evolution of pluralistic health care belief systems like those converging in *The Poor Man's Medicine Bag*.

Some of the popular health theories Tim advocates include finger acupuncture (1984, 7), reflexology for headache (7), and color therapy to calm emotional distress (24 and 75). While some proponents of official medicine might be tempted to laugh off some of the medical theories Tim espouses, at various points Tim appears to have picked up a few ideas through his reading in health care literature which have since been validated by systematic scientific research, especially his advice to drink red wine daily to lower high blood pressure.

An exhaustive item-by-item survey of 650 remedies listed in part I (see appendix) reveals the pluralistic character of Tim Waggoner's empirical health care options, summarized below:

- herbal: 276
- home remedy (nonherbal): 246
- over the counter: 42
- diet: 18
- consult professional: 16
- inhalation (steam, vapors): 9
- conventional first aid: 7
- conventional medicine: 7
- magical: 6
- massage: 4
- fumigation: 3
- popular health theories: 3
- cold therapy (ice packs, et cetera): 3
- warnings against traditional remedy: 3
- avoid strenuous exercise: 2
- mind, body, and health: 2
- old folk remedies or medical history: 2
- environment: 2

- warning regarding dosage: 1
- warning against popular remedy: 1
- emetics: 1
- enemas: 1
- exercise: 1
- heat therapy (heating pads, et cetera): 1
- prayer or faith healing (recite Ezekiel 16:6 or blood stopping): 1

Discussion of Results

Our analysis of these items listed in part I of *The Poor Man's Medicine Bag* shows that the ten leading types of remedies advocated by Tim Waggoner fall into four major categories:

A. *Noncritical naturalistic*
  1. Herbalism
  2. Home remedies
  3. Over-the-counter remedies
  4. Diet
  5. Massage or physical therapy
  6. Popular health theories
B. *Critical naturalistic*
  7. Conventional medicine
  8. Conventional first aid
C. *Noncritical supernatural*
  9. Magical remedies
D. *Critical supernatural*
  10. Prayer or faith healing

Tim believes people ought to use their God-given intelligence and common sense to take care of their ailments and infirmities. For the most part, *The Poor Man's Medicine Bag* provides naturalistic remedies for noncritical health care problems. Herbal remedies are the leading category, closely followed by nonherbal home remedies making use of items normally used for cooking or other domestic purposes or generic nonprescription materia medica such as castor oil, Epsom salts, and mineral oil. In accord with his eclectic, empirical approach, Tim also recommends over-the-counter remedies he believes to be effective as convenient alternatives to herbal preparations or nonherbal home remedies. Over-the-counter medications Tim particularly advocates include Pepto-Bismol and Save the Baby, a patented expectorant he discussed at considerable length in a taped interview with Jackie Sluder. Tim consistently advises his readers to seek professional attention and to use conventional first aid techniques in critical situations.

Despite the predominantly naturalistic orientation of *The Poor Man's Medicine Bag*, Tim does advocate a few magical cures, though he is well aware that many people dismiss them as superstitious nonsense. He prefaces these magical remedies by saying, "Now some people may laugh at this . . ." before proceeding to give well-known cures for warts, including rubbing warts with sliced potato and tying knots in wool, rubbing nine times on each wart, and then burying the wool, a form of sympathetic magic.

Having a seventh son or an orphan blow into an infant's mouth to cure thrush is also another well-documented Appalachian folk remedy. Tim's eclecticism is clearly evident in the various alternatives he offers as cures for this condition: "Thrash is a yeast infection which causes small white blisters in the mouth. For a cure have a seventh son of a seventh son to blow in the mouth, or someone who has never seen their parents, then use over-the-counter gentian violet or purple medicine" (1984, 74). Tim also gives these alternative cures for the same condition: "Drink water from a shoe, or go to a doctor" (74). Tim seemingly makes fun of belief in the inherent magical healing power of seventh sons in his humorous parody of a well-known traditional folk remedy: "For headache, have the seventh son of a seventh son blow in ear and then take two aspirin" (7).

From the folklorist's point of view, it is ironic that Tim describes vernacular medical practices he considers bizarre and outmoded as "old folks remedies," such as putting warm urine in the ear to ease earache, or cutting off a black chicken's head and smearing its blood on the affected skin to cure shingles. Variations upon the motif of killing or drawing blood from a black animal (generally a hen or cat) and using its blood to cure shingles can be found throughout the South (Hand 1980, 192; Waller and Killion 1972, 87; Clark 1970, 78). Waggoner finds these medical curiosities amusing, but he does not recommend them to his readers; they are not effective therapeutic alternatives in his view.

Surveying the individual items included in Tim's remedies reveals the open-ended eclecticism of his approach to healing. Honey plays an important therapeutic role as an ointment and for other healing properties. Honey appears twenty-four times, in six cases mixed with vinegar following the practice of D. C. Jarvis. Vinegar appears twenty-eight times, used for a wide variety of purposes. Sassafras is mentioned five times, once with the warning that some doctors believe it may cause cancer. Ginseng is mentioned twice, as a remedy for impotence and also rheumatism. Kerosene occurs three times, as a mosquito repellent, applied as a poultice for croup, and once with the warning *not* to apply it to cuts or wounds as an antiseptic but to use hydrogen peroxide instead. Tim advises against the medicinal use of kerosene, once a common southern folk practice, along with turpentine. The burning, astringent properties of kerosene and turpentine are of positive value according to the antiquated medical doctrine known as counter-irritant theory. Like the use of purgatives to which it is historically and conceptually related, counterirritant theory is quite literally the medical expression of the idea of fighting fire with fire, sometimes by deliberately raising blisters and creating irritations believed to draw out the noxious humors causing various diseases, particularly congestion of the lungs, which is remedied by the application of poultices. Regarding the empirical therapeutic validity of counterirritant theory, it is worth noting the increasing use of capsicum oleoresin found in chili peppers as an active ingredient in over-the-counter liniments and rubs, which creates a mild topical irritation stimulating the production of pain-relieving endorphins.

Red clover is recommended for use as a healing ointment and as blood purifier. Waggoner also advocates drinking a gallon of red clover tea daily for a year to cure cancer (1984, 80), a treatment he likely acquired from Kloss.

Some other items recommended in *The Poor Man's Medicine Bag* and their respective frequencies include:

- castor oil: 8
- plantain leaves or sap: 8
- baking soda: 5
- sage: 9
- slippery elm: 9
- goldenseal: 2
- vitamins: 2
- aspirin: 3
- foxglove (digitalis) tea (for heart condition, with warning regarding overdosage: 1
- WD-40 lubricant spray (to relieve arthritis): 1

Though Tim advocates WD-40 for arthritis pain in *The Poor Man's Medicine Bag*, he later disavowed it on the grounds that the lubricant spray intended for use on mechanical joints contained harmful substances which go into the bloodstream. Researchers have recorded use of WD-40 as an arthritis remedy in southern Appalachia. (Lang et al. 1988; Cavender and Beck 1995). The most common herbal remedy for arthritis and rheumatism in the southern Appalachians is to drink pokeberry tea or wine (see Waggoner 1984, 69).

Summary and Conclusion

This brief overview of the healing knowledge contained in *The Poor Man's Medicine Bag* illustrates the diversity of Tim's materia medica, his consistent ethical concern for the welfare of readers making use of these remedies, and his critical evaluation of traditional home remedies. Tim points out ill-founded or harmful traditional remedies and consistently warns his readers against common practices such as putting butter on burns or daubing insect stings with moist tobacco. Though his remedies are largely naturalistic, Tim advocates prayer as the last resort in case of severe bleeding. This set of remedies from *The Poor Man's Medicine Bag* graphically illustrates Tim's fundamental hierarchy of beliefs:

1. Stop bleeding: apply instant tea to wound
2. Stop bleeding: in dire cases, apply spider web to wound
3. Stop bleeding (serious wounds): apply tourniquet
4. Stop bleeding: as last resort, recite Ezekiel 16:6, inserting the name of the victim as directed. (1984, 17)

Tim Waggoner believes that critical health problems call for professional care and conventional first aid techniques, or if all else fails, prayer. Noncritical health problems can be treated with inexpensive home remedies, herbal infusions, or commercial over-the-counter preparations. A few magical remedies are effective; some traditional naturalistic remedies are harmful and should be avoided. Proper diet, stressing fresh fruits and vegetables as well as vitamin and mineral supplements, is also essential to good health.

Like modern people in general, many people in the southern Appalachians today probably share a largely but not exclusively naturalistic attitude towards health care. Cavender and Beck's recent systematic survey of remembered and current health care beliefs and practices of a rural community in Scott County, Virginia (the home of country music's original Carter family), strongly indicates that these longtime residents of southern Appalachia are quite pragmatic concerning their health and consistently seek out the most effective care they can afford (1995). Though most older community members were well acquainted with herbs and home remedies like those described in *The Poor Man's Medicine Bag*, few still relied upon them, nor would very many hesitate to avail themselves of official medicine if they felt they needed it, regardless of romantic, misinformed stereotypes of Appalachian antimodernism and fatalism.

Tim Waggoner is definitely not fatalistic, nor is he necessarily antimodern, though he, like many modern Americans, is critical of official medicine. However, as our analysis of *The Poor Man's Medicine Bag* shows, Tim is also critical of ill-founded and dangerous folk or popular remedies which are not empirically beneficial and effective. Rather than being fatalistic and antimodern, Tim Waggoner's medical beliefs and practices are actually both pluralistic and dynamic, deriving from a diversity of cultural traditions and sources and open to innovations with demonstrable therapeutic value. In this regard,

Tim Waggoner is like many other Americans for whom official medicine is neither their first nor their last therapeutic option but rather only one of a range of alternatives (see Blaustein 1992). Waggoner's eclectic and empirical approach to healing is shared by other notable folk herbalists in the region, including the late A. L. Tommie Bass of northern Alabama (Crellin and Philpott 1990) and Clarence "Catfish" Grey of West Virginia (Green 1978). Earlier we described Tim Waggoner as a man of many parts. A close reading of *The Poor Man's Medicine Bag* reveals its author to be a true populist educator, a man of the people without advanced formal education who has nonetheless become a self-taught scholar whose mission it is to bring beneficial knowledge to the community he serves. Interpreting Tim Waggoner's ideas and practice within the broader history of the American health care reform movement and the particular context of the Christian naturalist movement in the United States helps us to better appreciate the pluralistic and dynamic character of unofficial medical beliefs and practices in the modern world in general.

AFTERWORD: A CONVERSATION WITH TIM WAGGONNER

We thought it would be valuable to invite Tim Waggonner to read our essay and comment upon our interpretation and presentation of his medical theories and practices. Happily for us, Tim also thought this was a worthwhile idea. On Friday, 15 May 1998, we visited Tim at his home in Knoxville where we taped our conversation with him. Tim had anticipated our questions by preparing the following written notes:

> 1. The main reason I quit seeing people medically—people will not do what you tell them. I still lecture.
> 2. One of the main reasons for my driving effort for knowledge is that I am a poor man, and I hate to pay someone to do something I can do myself. People today have become lazy. There are over 5 million people who weigh over 500 pounds. Don't take me wrong, because being a few pounds overweight can be healthier than being underweight, but people are getting so lazy that they cannot function. Others will not work simply because it takes less energy to steal. This I blame on John F. Kennedy who put millions on welfare instead of requiring people to work. A person will not let himself starve. He will work if he is made to.
> My driving force which has caused me to work has been a Bible verse which says that a man who will not provide for his family is worse than an infidel. I'm here to tell you. I have made many blisters.
> My approach to medicine is God. God made this world, and he has told us in the Bible what we should & should not eat to make us healthy.

He has also told us to work. I believe in exercise, but I believe in it in the form of work. Put your energy to good use, and something gets accomplished. You may not like this, but if you don't ever accomplish anything, there is really no need for you to be in this world. You are a disease carrier of a different kind.

Many people only get in tune with God when they need something, such as a miracle. They throw the ball into God's court, and many people have died praying for a miracle, but it was not God's will that they should receive it. Probably due in part to broken promises, etc. However, this is not the approach I take. I let God throw the ball into my court, which he has done. God has said, "My grace is sufficient to overcome all things." I let the church pray for a miracle, mainly because I feel unworthy of one but since I have the ball instead of God having it, I play the game to test God's grace. Read and study about the ailment. Quit eating things that are bad for it, and start eating things that help cure it, etc.

In his taped conversation with us, Tim elaborated on these key principles of his medical beliefs and practices for nearly an hour. Edited excerpts of this transcribed conversation follow below:

[TW=Tim Waggoner; TC=Tony Cavender; RB=Richard Blaustein]

RB: . . . for the sake of the record, Tony [Cavender] and I have gone ahead and written this piece about your work and have sent you a copy in the mail. You've been very charitable with us: it looks like we have a few typos and a few spelling mistakes that you also helped us identify. Otherwise I would be very interested to know what you think of how we have described you, how we have described your approach to medicine and such things.

TW: Well, my approach hasn't changed a whole lot. It's still religiously based, which needs some more clarification: I think God made the world, I think he created the body, and I think it's up to him to cure it. Now, I talk to you in the book about the law of Nature, which is God's law, and nothing can stop the law of Nature except, of course, God. And when he stops it and reaches down and heals the body, it's a miracle. That's what we call a miracle.

Now there are people dying every day—they do nothing but pray for a miracle. Seemingly the doctors cannot help them, and they die praying for a miracle. And you wonder why that happens: well, personally, I don't feel worthy of a miracle. I don't think I'm going to look for one when there's something medically wrong with me.

I take God's other approach. Rather than dying begging God to perform a miracle, I take the approach that God's grace is sufficient to help me overcome all things. And I believe that. In other words, when you pray for a blessing—I mean a miracle—you throw the ball in God's court. When you believe that God's grace is sufficient to help you overcome all things, the ball's in your court. You see what I am saying? The thing for you to do is not give up praying for a miracle, get the church to do that. And start reading and studying and learning what's wrong with you. I'm not one of these people that . . . I believe that anything can be cured.

My great-great grandfather looked out at nature, and he said, "There's a cure there for everything." If I'm going to waste my time, I'm going to waste it hunting a cure for what's wrong with me, see what I'm saying. I'm going to read, study, take other people's opinions . . . I'll take every pill I can take to stay in this world. I want to see the Lord as much as anybody else, but I ain't in no hurry.

But there are things in the Bible that lead me to believe . . . well, flat out, God said to let your medicine be herbs, and flat out he said you can shorten your days or you can lengthen them. And I read and study these things. You're not going to live forever. Something's going to take you out of this world. But, if we can try and do live longer, we've left this world a better place, because it'll help the next fellow that's got it, you know. But I just don't see us a-layin' and a-prayin' for a miracle, 'cause first of all, I'd be the first to admit that I'm not worthy of no miracle. And I guess ninety percent of the people feel the way I do.

TC: But yet some people are worthy of a miracle, but the miracle doesn't come.

TW: That's right. Like the law of Nature, God's got two or three wills. It's not his will in the first place for you to be sick, but he permits it, according to the law of Nature, you see. He permits you to be sick. He's got a will, and a permissive will. And if it's his will to give you a miracle, and if it's his will that you be healed, it'll be there. But if it's his permissive will to let you die, that's just following the law of Nature. So the only thing you can do is ease your pain till your time to go.

TW: There are several reasons I quit seeing people. I've not completely quit; I still tell folks things, you know. But I used to have them come here, you know, and I'd see 'em.

Two main reasons—I'm a poor man. The reason I got interested in this in the first place: I don't believe in paying anybody for anything I can do myself. And if you look at the medical profession, it's expensive, and a poor man cannot afford it. Now, that's the reason I got into it.

Now the reason I quit seeing people, there's two reasons. They will not do what you tell them to do. When I tell you what to do, I want it done exactly like I tell you [laughs]. And I'll give you an example, my own mother, she wanted a laxative—gentle, soothing laxative. She couldn't get one from the doctor; nothing she tried worked. So I told her, "Yeah, I can help you." I took some out; I preached to her for fifteen minutes. I said, "Momma, *one* teaspoon." When it come time to take it: "Ah, I feel so bad I'll take two teaspoons." Well, she was using the vacuum and the pain hit her, and she just had to throw it down and run. It nearly turned her inside out.

TC: What kind of laxative was it?

TW: It was already premixed; you can buy 'em at the health food store. But another thing, like my son, he was getting married and they wanted me to make a gallon of my sex tea to take on their honeymoon. Well, at the time all I had was a quart jar. My recipe called for a gallon. I set him down and . . . another fifteen minutes, "Make this into a gallon!" So I made it into a quart and told him all he had to do was add water to make a gallon. They got on their honeymoon: "Well, we'll just drink it like it is!" Well, you can overdose on herbs. That's what happened to him: he overdosed. She was smokin' like a cheap cigar; he was sick for [*laughs*] . . . three or four days, you know. But the list goes on and on and on. And if you're not willing to do what I tell you, I don't want to see you. I don't want to harm you [*laughs*] . . . or make you worse.

But you've got to do what your doctor says, regardless of who it is, you know. If they won't take my word for it, they'll just have to learn by experience.

TC: So that was the main reason, people not complying with you . . .

TW: Yeah, going back to what I was telling you, the reason I got into this— this is an interesting theory, too—way back when I got into it, there were few doctors making house calls, not many. Like I said, I was always a person that if I could do it myself, I wouldn't pay for it. That's the way the old-timers used to be. My daddy could do anything to a house or a car or anything else, you know. He was a walking book of knowledge, the smartest man I ever knew. All the men of that day were; they knew how to do *everything*. And they didn't pay for anything they could do for themselves. People have gotten away from that.

TC: We've become specialists.

TW: We've become fat and lazy. There's over five million people over five hundred pounds in this country because of it. Got the wrong mental outlook, they're not willing to work . . . course, I blame John F. Kennedy for that.

TC: Why's that?

TW: Put 'em all on welfare. He's the one who started all that stuff. Now they're too lazy to work. But that's my opinion, you know [*laughs*] . . . political. I'll give you a good comment to go with that: if you're not willing to work and make this world a better place, then we don't need you in this world. You're a disease carrier of a different kind. You know what I'm talking about. And the only remedy I get for that is just to get a job.

Now if you want to know what I have accomplished that I am real proud of, I have read all the books by the Bible scholars, highly educated, and none of them seen the truth. And as a dumb hillbilly, I'm going to be able to show 'em [*laughs*]. I've about got my book finished; I lack about four or five paragraphs. It cannot be denied.

RB: What is the title of this book?

TW: *Looking for a City,* I believe it is. I've changed it so many times; I've wrote it four or five times; didn't like it.

TC: You've been working on this for several years?

TW: Oh yeah. They've not been able to see it, and for a dumb hillbilly to show scholars, you know, to me, that's an accomplishment. But that's what's wrong with the world today. We've got disease; men are not willing to make the world a better place for the people. Course, that goes back to environment and everything else. . . . That goes right back to the Bible. The devil, he wants everything concrete, he wants it to be pavement. He wants buildings sitting on it so you can't see the handiworks of God. He's no fool; got to give the devil a little credit. Yeah, he's shrewd. People can't see it.

What scares me, though, the Bible says over in Revelations, I forget the chapter, but the reason he is coming—talking about Christ—to destroy them that destroy the earth. And it's in there in black and white.

I don't even like to dig in the earth. We've dug in the earth. The earth has given us and given us and given us, and we've given nothing back. Keep on raping and plundering. But it's sad. In the process, we're destroying the very things that can cure us. There's so many species of animals, species of wildlife that are disappearing every day. Somewhere out there, we're just destroying the very things it's going to take to cure us. I like things natural, not synthetic.

The body gets sick naturally. If you eat the wrong things, you're going to be sick. And that's what's happening in America: we've got a sweet tooth, and ninety percent of what we eat is sugar. Or it's salt or pepper. Now, red pepper is good for you, but black pepper is not.

And they worry about cigarettes. More people are going to die of diabetes than have tobacco cancer. Course, when I was a young man—talking about tobacco—you never seen people dying of cancers; very rare. But they put all this junk in cigarettes today: ammonia, make it go to your brain faster. If they went back to just smoking tobacco just like it was, you know, they wouldn't have much of a problem. Tobacco companies are killing themselves.

In fact, some forms of tobacco, Life Everlasting, what they call "rabbit tobacco," has been smoked for centuries for asthma. But we're too involved in politics to see straight of anything, really, in this country. We just can't stand to see a bunch of woods or a field; got to build something on it. It irks me no end for every tree I see cut. God put 'em there for a reason. Course, now we're finding out why he put 'em there! Look at the Bible . . . all the fruit-bearing trees, eat the fruit thereof. And you're talking about the fruits and the vegetables and the medicines, things, you know, berries. We'd be healthy as a horse if we left alone what God says. Pork! We're finding out everything he said to eat is good for us, and everything he said not to eat will kill us. I can't match wits with God. I've got to figure out what I can, you know.

TC: It sounds like your philosophy of healing that we wrote about in that paper hasn't changed . . .

TW: . . . just refined . . .

TC: You still adhere to the basic tenets you talked about in your interviews with Jackie Sluder and that you elaborate on so eloquently in your book, *The Poor Man's Medicine Bag.* Is there anything about *The Poor Man's Medicine Bag* you would change if you were to do it again?

TW: Probably . . .

TC: What would that be?

TW: Well, I've a vast knowledge accumulated. Started writing another book. There's so much in my mind, it'd be that thick.

TC: What would you add?

TW: Well, like . . . cancer scares us to death, you know. You mentioned one, red clover tea a gallon every day for a year. Well, my increase in knowledge would add other things to it, you see. Stuff like that.

TC: So, basically adding and refining additional bits of information.

TW: Yeah.

TC: You've always been an avid reader . . .

TW: Still, gold's where you find it. We get information from other people, we get it from reading, and by trial and error. So I guess that your vast knowledge that you can call a concrete foundation is trial and error. I like to know whether it works or not before I comment on it.

Now, I'll give you a little piece of information. You're getting older. I've tried everything . . . your ears begin to itch as you get older. Take you a Q-Tip, dip it down in brown vinegar, shake it off. Bacteria can't live where vinegar is. Ear infection, the whole works; just one minute. Now, that I'd like to put in *The Poor Man's Medicine Bag*. I've got a million of them! They have now come out with a solution that you put in your ears, but you can't beat straight vinegar.

TC: So those are the kind of things you would add to it. But your underlying philosophy of healing has remained intact.

TW: Oh yeah.

TC: Like the laws of Nature: our responsibility to Nature, our connectedness to God.

TW: Well, let's face it: the Bible says he's got us on a string. We're like puppets, and he puts the fuel in us to make us move. We're a machine. He makes us move, but he's still got it in his hands. He can cut it anytime he wants to. Well, that's a clear picture of the Bible. To me, he's God, and he rules the world. There've been a lot of fools didn't think so, but they found out when he cut the rope. That's an interesting theory; I don't know if you ever thought about that or not. But he's got us each individually from the heart on a string.

We're individuals. When he cuts that string, just one person dies, the one that's on that string. So each person's got a string, and he moves us around in this world the way he wants us to go—usually. He always gives us some freedom of choice. We choose to stay around people we get along with, but we need the other people. We cluster for sex and survival and whatever. I don't know if you ever saw it that way or not, but really that's the way it is in the Bible. When you see that, and you're reading and studying the Bible, everything begins to make sense to you . . . . But there is a cure for everything, if we just take time to find it. But we got to learn which direction to look.

RB: How do we recognize these things, how do we know these cures, how do we sort out the good ones from the bad ones, the effective ones from the ones that aren't effective?

TW: Yeah, all of that's got to be found under what I call the law of Nature. Sometimes you can make a little scratch, my dog's got me pretty good, and you just leave it alone. They'll heal theirselves—most of the time. Sometimes they get infected. A little scratch has caused people to lose their arm, even their life, you know. Sometimes it turns sour. Under the law of Nature, we've got to find a cure. Outside of the law of Nature, of course, that's a miracle.

RB: What you seem to be stressing in *The Poor Man's Medicine Bag* is mostly naturalistic cures . . .

TW: . . . Definitely!

RB: Except for the one cure for the blood stopping, they all seem to be natural cures [*aside from six noncritical magical folk remedies*]. Why is that?

TW: Well, I think the body eats natural things. I found out through the years that you can cure practically anything by what you eat, or you can prevent it, you know. So, to me, science is way out on a limb. Instead of looking at the natural things that we do everyday, it's got to be in the natural.

RB: I guess what I was thinking was there are some people who would put more emphasis on prayer than you would seem to in this book. I'm just curious about that . . . it's not that you're not religious, because you are very religious, but why do some people put so much emphasis on healing through prayer while you seem to be emphasizing common sense?

TW: Well, we know that we need to pray, but we also should know. . . . Reason . . . there are a lot of religious fanatics that do not believe in going to the doctor but we need to reach these people. If they won't go to the doctor, at least they need to know a few fundamentals about healing themselves, you know what I'm saying? But to be frank with ye, I think God helps them that helps themselves.

RB: Yeah, that's what you seem to be saying in this book.

TC: One of my acquaintances up in Scott County, Virginia, said God wants you to do everything that's possible when you're ill, and that would include learning all you can about yourself, your body, medicines to use, as well as going to the doctor if necessary. She said a person should do all they can that's possible and let God take care of the impossible.

RB: That's well put.

TC: She's a Methodist. She said, "God doesn't like a lazy Christian." God doesn't want you to sit back and let God do all the work. God put a brain in your skull . . .

TW: That's basically what I believe.

TC: And you would say God laid out the laws of Nature, and it's up to you to get out there and learn what those laws are.

TW: You can't stop 'em; you just have to learn to live with them. And to learn to live with them, sometimes we have to . . . See, we're not all perfect. We make mistakes. We eat things and we do things in our lives that we shouldn't do, and we're going to pay for them, sure as we see another day coming around to us; that's how positive that it is you're going to pay for it.

TC: Can you think of any other comments you would like to make about our paper?

TW: My momma, you mentioned her; she used a lot of home remedies. My interest in home remedies came from her. [*Tim dedicated* The Poor Man's

Medicine Bag *to his mother*]. Now her aunt is the one who read about the herbs and all. She was . . . oh gosh, what's the word . . . delivered babies . . .

RB and TC: Midwife!

TW: Midwife. She was a midwife and everything else. They said it was amazing what she could do with colds and flus. Read an interesting article: they've about got the flu conquered. They've got it conquered in mice. But every flu they tried it on, it worked. I don't know what they made it out of, natural or anything else. But thank God for miracles! They work the other way, too . . .

RB: I don't know if I've got any more questions if you're reasonably satisfied with what you've seen. That really was the main concern: do you feel that this is reasonably accurate?

TW: Sounds good to me! You heard me . . .

TC: . . . We wanted to make sure that we were representing you fairly and accurately. . . .

TW: I love your wording. It's down-to-earth; I can read it.

RB: This makes me feel very good, Tim, because seriously, the two of us are very conscious about trying not to fall into that trap . . . [excessive use of academic jargon which cannot be understood by nonspecialists] [*laughter*].

TW: I'm a self-educated man, and a lot of that stuff I haven't gotten to yet! I enjoyed it. Everything I corrected [*referring to misspellings and typos*], except the one I just told you about my aunt. Mom, she was into home remedies. She really wasn't into herbs; maybe one every once in a while. Now, she could tell you the home remedies, my mom. Everything from constipation. They had a big old water bag, you know, for enemas. All sorts of stuff.

But I've helped a lot of people. An old man came to me one time. He had emphysema, couldn't walk across the street. I had him walking all over the neighborhood with just a simple little remedy: get out in the front yard . . .

RB: We just wanted to make sure you're represented accurately and honestly.

TW: Hey, that's one of the best ones I've seen. It's down-to-earth where I can comprehend it.

RB: Then we've succeeded . . . [in presenting Tim Waggoner's beliefs and ideas in terms that make sense to him].

TW: My head is full of knowledge, but it's not "above my raising," you know. I'm still on that level; I always will be. I spent years trying to grasp knowledge of a different sort. Some people spend their lives trying to get the big words and all that: all I want is the knowledge. I could care less about the big words.

APPENDIX

Types of Remedies Listed in part I of *The Poor Man's Medicine Bag:*

hair
herbal: 8
home remedy: (nonherbal): 7
environmental factors: 2
over-the-counter remedies: 1
diet: 1

head
diet: 3
massage: 3
home remedy (nonherbal): 2
herbal: 2
over-the-counter remedies: 1
humorous: 2
other: 3

face
home remedy (nonherbal): 4
herbal: 2
diet: 2

skin and impediments
home remedy: 22
herbal: 19
over-the-counter remedies: 6
diet: 3
environment: 2
consult physician: 2
magical: 2
hygiene: 1

wounds, cuts, burns, et cetera
herbal: 27
home remedy: 17
over-the-counter remedies: 3
fumigation (blowing smoke on
    wounds): 2
drawing out heat from wound with heat
    (heat therapy): 1
consult physician: 1
warning against traditional remedy: 1

blood
herbal: 19
diet: 11

conventional first aid (tourniquet): 1
consult physician: 1
prayer or faith healing (Ezekiel 16:6): 1
other: 2

insect and serpent bites
home remedy: 14
herbal: 9
consult physican: 2
conventional first aid: 2
over-the-counter remedies: 1
warning against traditional remedy: 1
cauterization: 1

eyes
home remedies: 8
herbal: 5
popular health theories: 3
diet: 3
over-the-counter: 2
conventional medicine: 2
consult physician: 1

nose
herbal: 5
home remedy: 4
diet: 2
magical: 2
over-the-counter: 1
humorous: 1

mouth
home remedy: 27
herbal: 16
over-the-counter: 6
humorous: 3
diet: 1
consult professional: 1
conventional first aid: 1
behavior modification: 1

ears
home remedy: 6
conventional medicine: 4
fumigation: 3

herbal: 2
over-the-counter: 2
humorous: 2
old folk remedy or medical history: 2
consult physician: 1
diet: 1
warning against traditional remedy: 1

neck and throat
herbal: 30
home remedy: 9
conventional first aid: 3
consult professional: 1
over-the-counter: 1
diet: 1

chest, lungs, and heart
herbal: 16
home remedy: 7
diet: 3
over-the-counter: 2
conventional medicine: 1
warning regarding dosage: 1

colds, flus, fevers, et cetera
herbal: 48
home remedy: 37
over-the-counter: 7
diet: 7
consult physician: 5
magical: 3
conventional medicine: 1

hands, arms, shoulders, and back
home remedy: 11
heat therapy: 4
herbal: 4
over-the-counter: 2
consult physician: 2
environment: 2
conventional medicine: 1
diet: 1
exercise: 1
massage: 1
warning against popular remedy: 1
magical: 1
humorous: 1

fumigation: 1

stomach, liver, kidneys, and gall bladder
herbal: 64
home remedy: 28
diet: 20
over-the-counter: 6
consult physician: 3
conventional first aid: 1
cold therapy: 3
heat therapy: 1
emetics: 1
enemas: 1
mind, body, and health: 1
warning against traditional remedy: 1

sexual information
herbal: 14
home remedy: 9
over-the-counter: 3
consult physician: 1
diet: 5
heat therapy: 1
mind, body, and health: 1
popular health theories: 1
warning against conventional
    remedy: 1
behavior modification: 1
avoid strenuous exercise: 1

rectum
herbal: 10
home remedy: 4
behavior modification: 2
avoid strenuous exercise: 1
over-the-counter: 1
consult physician: 1
enema: 1

feet and legs
herbal: 23
home remedy: 22
over-the-counter: 8
conventional medicine: 3
consult physician: 1
fumigation: 1
old folk remedy: 1

NOTES

Support for this study was provided by the Center for Appalachian Studies and Services. The authors wish to thank James Kirkland, Paul Bergner, and John Crellin for suggestions and research assistance. For further information concerning Waggoner and *The Poor Man's Medicine Bag*, write to Tim Waggoner, 3447 Reagan Avenue, Knoxville, Tennessee, 37919.

REFERENCES

Blaustein, Richard. 1992. Traditional medicine today: Moving beyond stereotypes. In *Herbal and magical medicine: Traditional healing today*, ed. James Kirkland, Holly F. Mathews, C. W. Sullivan III, and Karen Baldwin, 32–40. Durham, North Carolina: Duke University Press.

Cavender, Anthony, and Scott Beck. 1995. Generational change, folk medicine, and medical self-care in rural Appalachian community. *Human Organization* 54 (2): 129–42.

Clark, Joseph D. 1970. North Carolina popular beliefs and superstitions. *North Carolina Folklore* 18–19: 6–67.

Farr, T. J. 1935. Folk remedies. *Tennessee Folklore Society Bulletin*, 1 (2): 4–16.

Gevitz, Norman. 1988. Three perspectives on unorthodox medicine. In *Other healers: Unorthodox medicine in America*, ed. Norman Gevitz, 1–28. Baltimore: Johns Hopkins University Press.

Green, Edward E. 1980. A modern Appalachian folk healer. *Appalachian Journal* 6: 2–15.

Hand, Wayland D. 1980. *Magical medicine: The folkloric component of medicine in the folk belief, custom, and ritual of the peoples of Europe and America. Selected essays of Wayland D. Hand.* Berkeley and Los Angeles: University of California Press.

Jarvis, D. C. 1958. *Folk medicine: A Vermont doctor's guide to good health.* New York: Henry Holt and Company.

Kloss, Jethro. [1939] 1970. *Back to Eden.* Reprint, Coalmont, Tennessee: Longview Publishing House.

Lang, Forrest, Dana Thompson, Brock Summers, Wesley Hanson, and Michael Hood. 1988. A profile of health beliefs and practices in a rural Tennessee community. *Journal of the Tennessee Medical Association* 81: 229–33.

Lust, John D. 1974. *The herb book.* New York: Benedict Lust.

Meyer, Joseph E. [1918] 1960. *The herbalist.* Reprint, Glenwood, Illinois: Meyerbooks.

Sluder, Jackie L. 1996. Folk healers in Appalachia: A case study. Master's thesis, East Tennessee State University, Johnson City.

Waggoner, Tim. 1984. *The poor man's medicine bag.* Knoxville: Kingdom Press.

————. 1995a. Tape-recorded interview with Jackie Sluder, Knoxville, Tennessee, 3 February.

————. 1995b. Tape-recorded interview with Jackie Sluder, Knoxville, Tennessee, 10 March.

————. 1995c. Tape-recorded interview with Jackie Sluder, Knoxville, Tennessee, 23 March.

Waller, Tom, and Gene Killion. 1972. Georgia folk medicine. *Southern Folklore* 36: 71–92.

communication and the interplay of systems

5

Integrating Personal Health Belief Systems: Patient-Practitioner Communication

Shelley R. Adler

As students of folk medicine are well aware, the uneasy coexistence of diverse health belief systems in the United States is nothing new. Popular interest in these various healing systems seems to have increased with the development of patient empowerment and medical consumerism, as well as recent changes in the organization of health care delivery, particularly managed care (Adler, McGraw, and McKinlay 1998). Despite this widespread public interest, researchers noted in 1992 that "most physicians are unaware of [alternative medicine's] popularity, much less that many of their own patients are also being cared for by practitioners of alternative medicine" (Murray and Rubel 1992). Only one year later, many physicians became aware of the "invisible mainstream in the U.S. healthcare system" (Eisenberg 1997) with the publication of Eisenberg and others' seminal article on the prevalence and cost of complementary and alternative medicine (1993). The rate of usage and amount spent on complementary and alternative medicine, although surprisingly high to many biomedical scientists, were not the only significant findings—the investigators revealed that "72 percent of the respondents who used unconventional therapies did not inform their medical doctor that they had done so" (1993, 246). Four subsequent studies (including Eisenberg et al. 1998 as a follow-up) confirmed the high rates of patient nondisclosure (Keegan 1996; Begbie, Kerestes, and Bell 1996; Elder, Gillcrist, and Minz 1997; Eisenberg et al. 1998), but until now very little has been known about patients' own reasons for sharing or withholding information about their own alternative treatment use.

CONTEMPORARY COMPLEMENTARY AND ALTERNATIVE MEDICINE USE

Health belief systems have been explored by scholars from diverse academic backgrounds, including folklore, medical anthropology, sociology, history of medicine, public health, nursing, and biomedicine. This diversity of theoretical and methodological orientations is evidenced by the myriad disciplinary terms that are presently used—for example, folk medicine, ethnomedicine, traditional medicine, unorthodox medicine, and unproven remedies, to name a few. My own training and research in folkloristics and medical anthropology results in my being most comfortable with terms and definitions that are appropriate to healing systems and practices in any location and at any point in time. The definition developed by a multidisciplinary panel convened by the National Institutes of Health Office of Alternative Medicine (recently reconfigured as the National Center for Complementary and Alternative Medicine) comes closest to doing justice to this large, diverse, and dynamic field of research: "Complementary and alternative medicine (CAM) is a broad domain of healing resources that encompasses all health systems, modalities, and practices and their accompanying theories and beliefs, other than those intrinsic to the politically dominant health system of a particular society or culture in a given historical period" (Panel on Definition and Description 1997).[1] I have selected this definition of CAM to inform my ongoing study of women's treatment choices for breast cancer. For the purposes of this research, therefore, all nonbiomedical healing strategies used in the contemporary United States will be referred to as CAM. I conceptualize folk medicine as a subset of CAM, distinguished by its dependence on oral transmission, informal structure, and lack of commercialism (Hufford 1997).

The extensive use of CAM in the United States has been documented by a number of studies. Estimates of the percentage of adults using CAM cancer treatments in a variety of populations have ranged from 9 percent (Lerner and Kennedy 1992) to 50 percent (Cassileth et al. 1984).[2] My own research, based on face-to-face interviews with women with breast cancer, indicates that 72 percent use at least one CAM treatment in the first few months after diagnosis (Adler 1999).

The notion that the majority of patients a doctor sees are engaging in CAM usage on a regular basis has caused concern on the part of many physicians. Although it is always beneficial for doctors to be alert to their patients' health-related beliefs and practices, many argue that the importance of this awareness is elevated in the context of CAM usage: "The medical literature expresses a number of primary concerns about alternative therapies: that they are incorrect and unfounded; that they will cause direct harm; that they will delay or replace use of conventional medicine, thus causing indirect harm; and that they are perpetrated by quacks and frauds motivated by profiteering impulses" (O'Connor 1995; see Guzley 1992 for a representative example of this type of thinking). A more neutral portrayal of the reasons for physicians to stay aware of patients' use of different treatments is that "certain CAM therapies have demonstrable beneficial effects; some can be harmful under certain conditions; and others may interact with pharmacologic therapies in clinically significant ways (Lazar and O'Connor 1997).

The overwhelming majority of users of CAM also use biomedicine, either concurrently or serially. This is a remarkable situation, in which vast numbers of patients consistently participate in complementary and alternative healing practices outside of their physician's purview—and usually without his or her knowledge.

PREVIOUS APPROACHES TO CAM USE

For purposes of expedience (Sharma 1993), most researchers have selected CAM cancer treatments to study based on two criteria: the treatments have been limited to a specific number of therapies derived from the literature, from pilot studies, or intuitively (Eidinger and Schapira 1984; Eisenberg et al. 1993; Faw et al. 1977; Harris, Louis, and Associates 1987; Yates et al. 1993); and the selected treatments tend to be those with the greatest structural similarity to biomedicine (practitioner-dependent and clinic-oriented). Investigators' catalogs of CAM treatments most often reveal an exclusively etic perspective, with no evidence of informants' actual knowledge or usage. Many of the same problems that plagued earlier folk medical studies have been present in CAM research, with the result that patients' behavior is made to appear foolish, risky, and illogical. Historically, folk medical research in the United States has been conducted among marginal or peripheral communities, to the exclusion of more mainstream groups. The long-standing scientific misconception of the distribution of nonbiomedical practices is in large part a result of earlier notions of where populations of users of folk medicine could be found for study. From at least as early as the beginning of the present century, the belief has been widespread—in both the health professions and much of nonmedical academia—that folk and popular healing systems were in the process of gradually dying out with the advent of modern, Western medicine. An evolutionary model of the development of health systems has been to a large extent responsible for the perception of the waning popularity of nonbiomedical health practices. "Progress" implicitly defined as "increasing similarity to the culture of the scholar" (Hufford 1983, 307) was viewed as a natural and inevitable process. Discarded, obsolete ideas drifted down and were preserved in the sediment of the lower layers of culture—*gesunkenes Kulturgut* (Hufford 1988, 228; Hultkrantz 1960, 158–59).

The legacy of nineteenth-century social theories, which incorporated positivist assumptions of the unilinear evolutionary process of human thought, remains remarkably influential today. In this context, the persistent fascination with recent reports of the high prevalence of CAM usage (Eisenberg et al. 1998) and the "conventional" and "mainstream" characteristics of CAM users (Cassileth et al. 1984; Eisenberg et al. 1993; McGuire 1988) becomes clear: research findings challenge the still-prevalent view of the marginalized user of nonbiomedical therapies.

Evolutionist and survivalist assumptions have sustained a series of stereotypes of participants in nonbiomedical health systems as being socially marginal. The stereotypes of marginality typically include one or more of the following features: geographic remoteness or isolation (the image of rural Appalachia is frequently invoked); recent immigration or minimal acculturation to core American culture; ethnic minority membership or strong ethnic self-identification or group affiliation; poverty or low socioeconomic status; low formal educational attainment; mental or emotional imbalance; or desperation induced by grave illness or poor outcomes of conventional therapeutic efforts (O'Connor 1995, 17). I add three characteristics to this list of common stereotypes: being a woman, being elderly, and being gullible (see Pepper 1984 for classic examples of belief in these stereotypes). I think that this view of marginality has contributed to the fact that many physicians feel that their patients' use of CAM is intentionally enveloped in secrecy (Gray et al. 1997). In the medical literature, patients have been portrayed as willfully withholding information about their health beliefs because they are "afraid to 'confess' to the general practitioner their contacts with non-medical practitioners" (Guzley 1992, 523).

Scientific research has also contributed to the stereotype of the CAM user by focusing on nonrepresentative groups of people (Brown 1975; Ingelfinger 1976; Durant 1991). Convenience sampling has resulted in study populations that are poorly differentiated in terms of ethnicity and age. Prevalence studies have included people who use CAM for a variety of different conditions—from short-term discomforts to chronic or life-threatening illness—thus confounding the informants' reasons for and satisfaction with the choice of CAM treatments. Additionally, clinic-based samples, which continue to comprise the most common study populations, can introduce recruitment bias in terms of the types of patients that physicians allow researchers to approach ("compliant" patients). Finally, there is also a "context bias" that can arise when informants are interviewed in a clinic or hospital, locations at which "an adherent is least likely to feel at ease discussing beliefs and practices deemed 'deviant' by the larger society" (McGuire 1988).

Another problem in CAM research has been the difficulty of ascertaining accurate prevalence estimates. The broad range of reported prevalence rates (from 7 to 50 percent in the U.S.) appears to be directly related to each project's chosen methodology. The continuum of research findings from low to high rates of usage is paralleled by a methodological continuum ranging from quantitative telephone survey research to qualitative, face-to-face interviews. Also, not surprisingly, studies that rely on narrow definitions of CAM culled from the biomedical literature report lower prevalence of usage than investigations that utilize broader, emically derived definitions. Problems due to unclear definitions, nonrepresentative study populations, and underestimated prevalence rates have hindered progress toward a better understanding of the nature of people's use of CAM.

The Women's Breast Cancer Treatment Choices Study

The findings discussed in this chapter are based on two cycles of interviews from an ongoing five-year qualitative study of treatment decision-making on the part of women with breast cancer. In order to interview a representative group of women as soon as possible after their breast cancer diagnosis, participants were recruited using a unique population-based rapid case finding method. A team of case finders from the Northern California Cancer Center was sent to the medical records offices of each hospital in San Francisco County biweekly for thirteen months. The team assembled a list of all new cases by reading pathology reports, supplemented by hospital records. After patients' physicians were contacted, the women were sent introductory letters, followed by a recruitment telephone call.

Eligibility requirements for study participants included the following: ages 35–49 and 60–74, inclusive; residents of San Francisco, California, at the time of diagnosis; ability to be interviewed in English, Spanish, or Chinese (Cantonese or Mandarin); histological diagnosis of breast cancer (in situ or invasive); diagnosed at a hospital within San Francisco County; and diagnosed during the thirteen-month period of case ascertainment (May 1995–May 1996). Exclusion criteria included recurrent breast cancer and patients whose physicians refused to grant permission for them to be contacted. A total of eighty-six women were enrolled (87 percent of those known eligible).

Data is being collected through a series of four in-depth, face-to-face interviews. Informants are initially interviewed within a few months of diagnosis (two to four months average) and again after six months, eighteen months, and thirty months. The interviews take place in participants' homes or at private locations of their choosing. The study utilizes a semistructured interview guide that is specifically adapted for each of the four interview cycles. The open-ended questions are designed to encourage informants to articulate their personal understandings of their beliefs and practices regarding health and illness. The domains of questions asked during the initial and first follow-up interviews include: (a) conceptualizations of health and illness; (b) the process of discovery and confirmation of the breast cancer; (c) the individual's views on the cause, nature, and extent of her illness; (d) biomedical and/or CAM cancer treatments utilized to date; (e) experiences with and attitudes toward physicians and alternative practitioners; and (f) interactions regarding CAM and biomedical treatment use with physicians and alternative practitioners, respectively. In order to elicit answers with unbiased questions, informants were asked to describe all aspects of their health beliefs in their own words: potentially etic terms or concepts, such as cancer or alternative medicine, were not used by the interviewer unless introduced by the informant.

All interviews were audiotaped and transcribed verbatim. Cantonese, Mandarin, and Spanish interviews were translated by the interviewers and then transcribed. Concurrent qualitative text-based analysis is conducted with the use of QSR NUD*IST software. The data related to patients' disclosures of treatment use and interactions with physicians and alternative practitioners were analyzed separately. Transcripts were reviewed and coded by two persons who did not conduct the interview. After the identification of topics and themes that repeatedly appeared in the data, codes were developed, and subsequently assigned to the transcribed interviews. The data set was then analyzed and interpreted in terms of linkages between the derived concepts and recontextualized data.

Logics of Disclosure

Of the patients simultaneously being treated by an alternative practitioner, 54 percent discussed their CAM use with their physicians.[3] Conversely, 94 percent of the participants seeing alternative practitioners discussed details of their biomedical treatments with these providers. These quantitative rates of disclosure, however, can be misleading. In the vast majority of cases, patients who are using self-treatment are much less likely to initiate discussions of CAM use with their doctors than those who are seeing a practitioner. Also, even among those patients who actively seek to initiate discussion, many do not achieve their goal of prompting an interaction or receiving feedback.

Therefore, even more significant than the number of patients who disclose CAM use to their physicians is the nature and quality of any subsequent discussion. In the biomedical encounter, this interaction was frequently brief and superficial, while discussions with alternative practitioners were quite comprehensive, often including a review of biomedical data, such as laboratory tests and pathology reports.

Patients' disclosure of CAM usage was cautiously modulated and carefully adapted, even by those who would welcome an open discussion with their physicians. Informants who chose not to reveal their CAM practices gave one or more of the following reasons for their decision (listed in decreasing order of participant emphasis): the impression of physician disinterest; the anticipation of a negative response; the conviction that the physician is unwilling or unable to contribute useful information; the perception that the CAM therapies used are irrelevant to the biomedical treatment course; and the patients' views regarding the appropriate coordination of disparate healing strategies. Although a few participants implicated insufficient time as a barrier to disclosure, it was considered a relatively minor impediment. An abbreviated appointment was seen as contributing to the problem of poor communication, but was not viewed as a primary or determining factor.

The reason for lack of disclosure most frequently cited by informants was the feeling that the physician was simply not interested in a patient's use of CAM: "He'd think it was frivolous . . . I think he wouldn't take it very seriously." Even when patients did attempt to initiate discussion, their efforts were frequently not reciprocated: "The oncologist knows . . . but she's never asked me for details" and "Yeah, I told him—I don't know if he remembers or not." Unresponsiveness was taken as a clear message that the physician did not want to hear more about the patient's practices: "I don't feel that they're interested . . . I did tell the oncologist . . . and he didn't say, 'Good,' or 'Not good,' or 'Okay,' or anything. It's kinda like, 'We're looking at the platelets here, and the white count—let's not get too far afield! [laughs]." The impression of physicians' disinterest—even on the part of women who had initially volunteered information—often prevented further discussions.

Patients are aware of the persistent ambivalence and occasional hostility of some biomedical practitioners towards CAM (Lazar and O'Connor 1997; Adler and Fosket 1999): "When I said to my oncologist, 'I've used shark cartilage,' he almost laughed me out of the office." Because patients sometimes fear a negative response from their physicians, they carefully assess the potential receptivity before disclosing information about their practices: "My Chinese-American doctor is very against qi gong . . . He told me that qi gong is really just full of it—that it is really a scam. I think that's somewhat biased, so I didn't talk to him about my practicing of the qi gong—that I went back to China to learn more—'cause I don't want him to make me feel bad." The same participant, however, did disclose her CAM use in another context: "My radiation oncologist—he's a white person, but he knew something about qi gong. He seemed to be a lot more open." A physician's indiscriminate disapproval can be viewed as having a broader scope than merely discouraging the use of a specific CAM treatment: "When I raised the subject of alternative medicine, my oncologist would really pooh-pooh it. It isn't that I need him to believe in it—I just don't want someone to dismiss it all . . . and thereby, in some ways, be disrespectful to me." Informants' perceptions of physician disinterest and ambivalence echo findings from a preliminary study of physicians' attitudes toward patient use of CAM. Among the physicians interviewed, "there was little interest in initiating communication about unconventional therapies, with most seeing such discussions as a poor use of their time" (Gray et al. 1997, 14).

Another common reason for withholding details about personal CAM use was patients' conviction that disclosure would not yield any benefit. Whether the physician was felt to be unable to help because of inadequate training or unwilling to help due to a bias against alternative health systems, the unlikelihood of a useful outcome was a sufficient deterrent to pursuing further discussion. As one participant recounted, "When I started taking these herbs, I gave my primary care doctor a description of what was in them and what they were supposed to do—and she never said, 'I think it's good' or 'I think it's bad.' She looked at them and just goes, 'I don't see anything in here that's harmful.' . . . My Chinese herbalist requested that I get copies of my [lab] tests, which I did. My medical doctor gave me copies, but, again, without any comment or questions—indicating to me a sort of unwillingness to work with this alternative doctor."

Patients may feel that their use of CAM is not germane to the process of medical decision making. Some participants believed that the CAM therapy they used was not directed at the same target as concurrent biomedical treatments and therefore could not cause a harmful interaction: "I'm just using it to strengthen my antibodies" or "I really just took [the herbs] to control the spread of the tumor before my surgery. It really wasn't for treating my cancer." One participant who felt it unnecessary to inform her oncologist of her CAM usage, however, was concerned enough about potential cross-reactions to keep her herbalist informed about her biomedical treatment: "Just in case when the Chinese herbalist gives me herbs they might have some side effect on the Western medical treatment that I'm receiving. You know, you don't want to be mixing Chinese herbs and Western medicine, because the combination of the two could be pretty lethal. You can't just combine them."

Participants also based disclosure decisions on their understanding of the proper roles for the various practitioners in their therapeutic encounters. For women who thought of their CAM use as a personal healing strategy— "Just something positive that I'm doing for myself"—there was a sense of protectiveness regarding their treatment choices. Other participants distinguished between the realms of knowledge and authority of physicians and alternative practitioners: "I didn't bring it up with the surgeon . . . I don't feel like that's why I go to her. That's not really her job." Perhaps most interesting, though, are the cases in which patients perceive the value of integrating and coordinating their care, but choose to focus their efforts entirely on the alternative practitioner: "I send my acupuncturist my pathology reports" and "When you do surgery, of course you listen to your Western doctor—but I also went to my Chinese herbalist. I actually took my pathology report to him, and he looked at it, and felt that it's a good idea to have a surgery."

Not unexpectedly, the preliminary data available on doctors' attitudes toward CAM usage presents an entirely different picture of the context of disclosure. In discussing barriers to communication, the majority "identified the problem as being with the patients" (Gray et al. 1997, 17): "[patients'] unrealistic expectations of their physicians, inability to tolerate reality, hostility or denial in the face of bad news, disorganization in seeking information, and secretiveness about use of unconventional therapies" (18). Some doctors identified systemic communication problems associated with an overloaded health care system, such as limits on time. In general, "learning about, or having access to information, seemed to be much more important to physicians than actually discussing [CAM] issues with or passing the information on to patients" (18).

Finally, in order to understand better patients' disclosure decisions, it is helpful to consider the factors that promote discussion. When study participants did choose to reveal details about CAM treatment use it was because they perceived their physician to be respectful, open-minded, and willing to listen. Patients found it easier to discuss their alternative treatments when they believed that their physician expected them to be using some form of CAM. Participants also were particularly impressed by the few instances in which physicians opened a dialog with patients' alternative practitioners (most frequently by recommending or trading journal articles).

Participants mentioned different reasons for discussing their use of biomedical treatments with their alternative practitioners: concerns about biomedical/CAM treatment cross-reactions; the desire to target specific biomedical treatment side effects; and the view that alternative practitioners are relatively more "open-minded" and more adept at integrating diverse strategies than physicians are: "[My acupuncturist] always asks me—she writes down in her chart when my next [medical] visit is. When I go to see her the next time . . . that's one of the first questions she asks me. So, she's really up on what other people tell me or what I've done. And in any other area, she's really good at wanting to know about it, what I've been told." The nature of the interaction after a patient describes her biomedical treatment use to her alternative practitioner is thus often qualitatively different than in the medical encounter.

Personal Integrated Health Belief Systems and Virtual Collaborators

Interest in CAM use may be prompted by a wide range of factors, from the desire to avoid the invasiveness of a biomedical procedure to the fact that a particular healing modality is a part of a patient's cultural heritage (Lazar and O'Connor 1997; Hufford 1992; O'Connor 1995). The significance of a patient's use of CAM, therefore, is not limited to the impact of the discrete treatment itself; it usually indicates (concurrent) belief in at least one nonbiomedical explanatory health model (like the influence of the mind on the body, the importance of holistic healing, or the role of spirituality in medicine). A physician's indiscriminate criticism of alternative treatment use has broad implications for the medical encounter, as well as patient outlook and hope. Respectful discussion of CAM, however, "sheds light on patients' worldviews, values, explanatory models, lifestyles, health beliefs, and goals for care—all of which are clinically relevant and contribute to the ongoing development of effective and mutually rewarding doctor-patient relationships" (Lazar and O'Connor 1997). The interviews emphasized patients' spontaneous, that is, unsolicited, disclosures of CAM use. It is likely that some women would have overcome their hesitation to discuss CAM if their physician had asked them a direct question. It is telling, however, that, even in a part of the country with a reputation for open-mindedness regarding health care diversity, physicians rarely initiated discussion of CAM use.

The emic perspective that the informants provide reveals that an intricate framework of logic underlies their health behavior. A patient's integration of biomedical and various CAM therapies is, of course, not desperately haphazard, as sometimes portrayed in the medical literature: patients' integrative healing systems involve deliberate and complex strategizing. A helpful construct for the study of complementary and alternative medicine is personal integrated health belief systems, in which individuals combine disparate elements—from what may appear to be mutually exclusive health traditions—into a syncretic whole. In order to understand better the intricacies of these unique syncretic healing systems, the individual's own health beliefs must be studied as the locus for integration. As is often the case, the different biomedical and alternative health traditions may only appear to be irreconcilable— their apparent inconsistencies are either not viewed as such or are deemed insignificant from the individual's perspective.

The interviews with women with breast cancer revealed that accurate models of patient decision making regarding breast cancer treatments, even exclusively biomedical therapies, must take into account the role of alternative practitioners. The conventional view of the dyadic patient-physician relationship only reveals one side of a potential triangle of patient and practitioners. In actuality, the majority of physicians are engaged in a virtual collaboration with patients' alternative practitioners. Although the "partnership" is frequently invisible, its effects are not.

FOLKLORISTICS AND CAM RESEARCH

To conclude, I would like to emphasize that folkloristics is ideally situated to investigate the wide variety of CAM systems, including modalities, practices, theories, and beliefs. As Claire Cassidy explains, qualitative research methodologies display a high degree of "model fit"; that is, they comprise "research design and techniques [that] fit the explanatory model/s of the study population/s" (Cassidy 1995, 35). By sharing what amounts to a common perspective with many CAM systems, folkloristic inquiry avoids many of the problems that can arise with mismatched methodological techniques.

Another strength of folkloristics is its "populist" orientation (Hufford 1992)—an approach that links well with the patient consumerism that is so influential in the phenomenon of complementary and alternative medicine. Folklorists emphasize—or, more accurately, insist on—taking into account the emic perspective. As David Hufford observed, "ordinary people tend to be underestimated and . . . their knowledge tends to be discredited by authorities" (1992). By promoting participants' views and understandings, folklorists and other qualitative researchers can interpret CAM phenomena in terms of the meanings that people bring to them. Through the use of unstructured or semi-structured interviews, informants are given the opportunity and encouraged to describe their beliefs and practices using their own logic and terminology.

The holistic nature of qualitative inquiry blends well with the holistic model of many CAM healing systems (Cassidy 1995). Just as many CAM systems do not involve the traditional biomedical hierarchy of doctor and patient, for example, in qualitative inquiry the researcher-participant dyad is constructed to promote a more egalitarian relationship. Perhaps the most important contribution a folkloristic approach can make to CAM studies is the valuing of participants' "subjective" views as expert and the integration of informants' conceptualizations and models into research design and analysis.

NOTES

This research has been supported by joint funding from the National Cancer Institute and the National Institute on Aging (CA64634) and a grant from the University of California, San Francisco, Academic Senate Committee on Research. Cancer incidence data used in this research have been collected by the Northern California Cancer Center under contract No1–CN–05224/25482 with the Division of Cancer Prevention and Control, National Cancer Institute, National Institutes of Health, Department of Health and Human Services, and under subcontract 0501–8701/8708–S0207 with the California Public Health Foundation. I am grateful to the women with breast cancer who are generously sharing their thoughts and experiences by participating in this project: their altruism makes this research possible.

1. "Complementary and alternative medicine" is defined as "all health care resources to which people have recourse other than those intrinsic to biomedicine and the specific theoretical and practice models of biomedicine" (Panel on Definition and Description 1997).
2. Studies of patients in a variety of populations outside the U.S. have shown that between 9 percent and 75 percent of adult patients with cancer use CAM (Lerner and Kennedy 1992; Gray et al. 1997; Eisenberg 1997; La Valley and Verhoef 1995; Hufford 1997; Clinical Oncology Group 1987; Downer et al. 1994; Eidinger and Schapira 1984; Himmel, Schulte, and Kochen 1993; Millar 1997).
3. Overall disclosure for women using CAM generally was 33 percent, similar to reported findings in the general population.

REFERENCES

Adler, Shelley R. 1999. Complementary and alternative medicine use among women with breast cancer. *Medical Anthropology Quarterly* 13 (2): 214–22.

Adler, Shelley R., and J. Fosket. 1999. Disclosing complementary and alternative medicine use in the medical encounter: A qualitative study in women with breast cancer. *Journal of Family Practice* 48 (6): 453–58.

Adler, Shelley R., Sarah A. McGraw, and John B. McKinlay. 1998. Patient assertiveness in ethnically diverse older women with breast cancer: Challenging stereotypes of the elderly. *Journal of Aging Studies* 12 (4): 331–50.

Begbie, S. D., Z. L. Kerestes, and D. R. Bell. 1996. Patterns of alternative medicine use by cancer patients. *Medical Journal of Australia* 165: 545–48.

Brown, Helene. 1975. Cancer quackery: What can you do about it? *Nursing* 5 (5): 24–26.

Cassidy, Claire M. 1995. Social science theory and methods in the study of alternative and complementary medicine. *Journal of Complementary and Alternative Medicine* 1 (1): 19–40.

Cassileth, R. Barrie, Edward J. Lusk, Thomas B. Strouse, and Brenda J. Bodenheimer. 1984. Contemporary unorthodox treatments in cancer medicine: A study of patients, treatments, and practitioners. *Annals of Internal Medicine* 101: 105–12.

Clinical Oncology Group. 1987. New Zealand cancer patients and alternative medicine. *New Zealand Medical Journal* 100: 110–13.

Downer, S. M., M. M. Cody, P. McCluskey, P. D. Wilson, S. J. Arnott, T. A. Lister, and M. L. Slerin. 1994. Pursuit and practice of complementary therapies by cancer patients receiving conventional treatment. *BMJ Clinical Research Ed* 309: 86–89.

Durant, John R. 1991. If it quacks. . . . *Cancer* 67: 2225–26.

Eidinger, Richard N., and David V. Schapira. 1984. Cancer patients' insight into their treatment, prognosis, and unconventional therapies. *Cancer* 53: 2736–40.

Eisenberg, David M. 1997. Advising patients who seek alternative medical therapies. *Annals of Internal Medicine* 127: 61–69.

Eisenberg, David M., R. B. Davis, S. L. Ettner, S. Appel, S. Wilkey, M. Van Rompay, and R. L. Kessler. 1998. Trends in alternative medicine use in the United States, 1990–97. *Journal of the American Medical Association* 280: 1569–75.

Eisenberg, David M., Ronald C. Kessler, Cindy Foster, Frances E. Norlock, David R. Calkins, and Thomas L. Delbanco. 1993. Unconventional medicine in the United States: Prevalence, costs, and patterns of use. *New England Journal of Medicine* 328 (4): 246–52.

Elder, N. C., A. Gillcrist, and R. Minz. 1997. Use of alternative health care by family practice patients. *Archives of Family Medicine* 7: 181–84.

Faw, Cathy, Ron Ballentine, Lois Ballentine, and Jan van Eys. 1977. Unproved cancer remedies: A survey of use in pediatric outpatients. *Journal of the American Medical Association* 238: 1536–38.

Gray, R. E., M. Fitch, M. Greenberg, P. Voros, M. S. Douglas, M. Labrecque, and P. Llart. 1997. Physician perspectives on unconventional cancer therapies. *Journal of Palliative Care* 13: 14–21.

Guzley, Gregory J. 1992. Alternative cancer treatments: Impact of unorthodox therapy on the patient with cancer. *Southern Medical Journal* 85 (5): 519–23.

Harris, Louis, and Associates. 1987. Health information and the use of questionable treatments: A study of the American public. Washington, D.C.: U.S. Department of Health and Human Services.

Himmel, W., M. Schulte, and M. M. Kochen. 1993. Complementary medicine: Are patients' expectations being met by their general practitioners? *British Journal of General Practice* 43: 232–35.

Hufford, David J. 1983. Folk healers. In *Handbook of American folklore*, ed. Richard M. Dorson, 306–13. Bloomington: Indiana University Press.

———. 1988. Contemporary folk medicine. In *Other healers: Unorthodox medicine in America*, ed. Norman Gevitz. Baltimore and London: Johns Hopkins University Press.

———. 1992. Folk medicine in contemporary America. In *Herbal and magical medicine: Traditional healing today*. Durham, North Carolina: Duke University Press.

———. 1997. Folk medicine and health culture in contemporary society. In *Primary Care: Clinics in Office Practice* 24 (4): 723–42.

Hultkrantz, Ake, ed. 1960. *International dictionary of regional European ethnology and folklore*. Vol. 1. Copenhagen: Rosenkilde and Bagger.

Ingelfinger, F. J. 1976. Quenchless quest for questionable cure. *New England Journal of Medicine* 295 (15): 838–39.

Keegan, L. 1996. Use of alternative therapies among Mexican Americans in the Texas Rio Grande Valley. *Journal of Holistic Nursing* 14: 277–94.

La Valley, J. W., and M. J. Verhoef. 1995. Integrating complementary medicine and health care services into practice. *Canadian Medical Association Journal* 153: 45–49.

Lazar, J. S., and Bonnie Blair O'Connor. 1997. Talking with patients about their use of alternative therapies. *Primary Care: Clinics in Office Practice* 24: 699–714.

Lerner, Irving J., and B. J. Kennedy. 1992. *CA: A Cancer Journal for Clinicians* 42 (3): 181–91.

McGuire, Meredith B. 1988. *Ritual healing in suburban America*. New Brunswick, New Jersey: Rutgers University Press.

Millar, W. J. 1997. Use of alternative health care practitioners by Canadians. *Canadian Journal of Public Health* (Revue Canadienne de Sante Publique) 88: 154–58.

Murray, Raymond H., and Arthur J. Rubel. 1992. Physicians and healers: Unwitting partners in health care. *New England Journal of Medicine* 326 (1): 61–64.

O'Connor, Bonnie Blair. 1995. *Healing traditions: Alternative medicine and the health professions*. Philadelphia: University of Pennsylvania Press.

Panel on Definition and Description, CAM Research Methodology Conference, April 1995. 1997. Defining and describing complementary and alternative medicine. *Alternative Therapies in Health and Medicine* 3: 49–57.

Pepper, C. 1984. Quackery: A $10 billion scandal—A report by the chairman of the subcommittee on health and long-term care. Washington, D.C.: U.S. Government Printing Office.

Sharma, Ursula. 1993. Contextualizing alternative medicine: The exotic, the marginal, and the perfectly mundane. *Anthropology Today* 9 (4): 15–18.

Yates, P. M., G. Beadle, A. Clavarino, et al. 1993. Patients with terminal cancer who use alternative therapies: Their beliefs and practices. *Sociology of Health and Illness* 15: 199–216.

6

COMPETING LOGICS AND THE
CONSTRUCTION OF RISK

DIANE E. GOLDSTEIN

"Risk" is a word we hear a lot these days, whether it be in academic discussions of "risk assessment," "risk analysis," or "risk perception" or in discrete areas of life such as "environmental risks," "financial risks," or "public health risks." AIDS literature uses the word "risk" perhaps more than any other term and, in fact, a significant moment in the epidemiological understanding of AIDS is marked by the change in reference from "risk groups" to "risk activities." The notion of "risk groups" (such as Haitians, homosexuals, and intravenous drug users) rather than "risk activities" (such as sharing needles or sex without a condom) was seen in the mid-1980s to stigmatize specific groups while simultaneously allowing individuals to disassociate themselves from perceived vulnerability by disavowing memberships in identified risk groups. The logic of this change in usage is clear, shifting the focus from groups to specific behaviors. The shift in reference and in thinking would seem to be both a public health and a human rights victory. And indeed, it was.

Still, the stigmatizing nature of "risk" theory did not simply disappear. While "risk groups" were no longer in academic discourse, "risk activities" were, and the popular association of specific behaviors with specific groups remained. Sharing needles, for example (or even access to used needles), generally occurs in certain contexts; contexts require participants, and participants make up groups. Cindy Patton observes, for example:

> Despite efforts among activists to shift the terminology from risk *groups* to risk *behaviors*, AIDS education information concerning risk *reduction*

was directed almost exclusively toward gay men, and soon (though much less consistently and effectively) toward injecting drug users. (1994, 14)

But other issues exist in relation to the fragile attempts at disassociation of risk activities from groups. As Mary Douglas notes in her book *Risk and Blame: Essays in Cultural Theory*, the word "risk" has been removed from its older connotation involving choice to a generalized notion of danger. Douglas notes:

> "Risk" is the probability of an event combined with the magnitude of the losses and gains that it will entail. However, our political discourse debases the word. From a complex attempt to reduce uncertainty it has become a decorative flourish on the word "danger." (1992, 40)

This association of danger with the sense of risk distanced the notion from issues of cultural understanding involved in weighing of gains and losses used in personal risk assessments. Risk activities (translated in Douglas's terms as danger) tend to be seen in institutional terms as generalized, predetermined, and unquestionable. Richard Stoffle et al., in writing about environmental risks, discuss this institutional imposition of risk estimation. They note:

> Often, the specialists who conduct these assessments believe their estimates reflect the "real risks" of a technology or project because the estimates derive from scientific calculations. These "real risks" typically are presented through formal processes, such as public meetings, in which information flows one way, from risk communicator to the public with little or no exchange of information between these two groups. (1991, 612)

The emphasis on "real risk activities" as predetermined areas of danger framed risk assessment in etic, externally defined values and concerns; leaving emic, locally defined concerns out of the picture. Risk assessments which are based on emic criteria focus on risk as it is perceived and evaluated by the lay public. The tendency to ignore perceived risk as a valid component in the assessment of risk is based on the notion that perceived risks are neither objective nor scientifically derived.

The failure here is in not recognizing that *all* notions of risk are culturally constructed based on socially and culturally shaped concepts and statistics. Such a view is not intended to be nihilistic (arguing that there is *no* risk reality) but rather, social constructionist (arguing that concepts such as risk have been constructed in such a way that they appear devoid of ideological content, and therefore are self-evident). Social constructionist theory "assumes that social categories have been constructed through historical and social processes . . . in such a way that the ideological and institutional interests served by a particular construct are erased and the categories appear natural" (Patton 1994, 4).

Social constructionist theory lends itself easily to HIV research because the epidemic is worldwide while the bulk of research and policy comes from the West. The social constructionist questions the categories of epidemiology attempting to demonstrate their culture-bound, political, or moralistic basis or examining their general applicability. In striking contrast to public health risk associations and "prostitution," for example, Patton demonstrates:

> Evaluation of sex worker risk reduction projects suggest that women who sell sex are more likely to adopt prevention measures (especially condom use or avoidance of intercourse) than are women who simply have sex in the context of recreation, love, or other socially condoned sexual arrangements. But the strong separation between sex for hire and sex for "love" also results in a bifurcation of sex workers' risk reduction strategies. Women who sell sex are more likely to engage in prevention behaviors while having sex in the context of "work" than in their domestic relationships. (1994, 53)

The social constructionist argument is that risk categories are only made meaningful in social context and that the categorization systems must be analyzed, not simply adopted.

The Medical (Mis)Use of Ethnography

Taking this approach, I intend in the remainder of this paper to examine the uses of ethnography in the medical construction of African AIDS risk categories, represented in articles and letters found in a variety of medical research journals such as the *Lancet*, the *British Medical Journal, Science*, and the *New England Journal of Medicine*. Focusing on African "high risk activities" these articles use ethnographic information to foreground aspects of traditional culture, emphasizing the failure of Africans to adjust to the conditions of Western civilization. Heavily stereotyped and abstracted from social, historical, or cultural context, these studies condemn traditional culture through an emphasis on the risks intrinsic to such practices as blood brotherhood, ritual scarification, and traditional healing techniques. By highlighting the dialogue on African risk, this chapter will attempt to outline and illustrate the specific cultural misunderstandings found in medical researchers' uses of ethnographic data, misunderstandings which allow research on risk to become a dialogue on neocolonialism.

Although the medical use of ethnographic materials would seem to suggest a sensitivity toward locally constructed perceptions of risk, this is not the case. Ethnographic data—the folklorist's guide to vernacular perception—at the hands of medical researchers appears to become grist for the "real risk" mill. Rather than being constructed as information to be used in weighing gains and losses or being measured statistically in terms of actual incidence of infection, the data is piled into the unexamined "danger category" suggested by Douglas. The inclusion of ethnographic material in these danger areas, while problematic in that it is unweighed, unexamined, and not part of a dialogue with the lay public, might still be an improvement over total ignorance of cultural data, were it based on sound ethnography. The selection of ethnographic material, however, is a significant part of the problem.

Due in part to the demographic profile of the AIDS crisis, the greater awareness of medical consumerism, and the strengthening of voices in the medical humanities and social sciences, medical researchers are becoming increasingly aware of the need to take account of cultural issues in health care and public health education. While this newfound awareness is commendable, it points out problems intrinsic to unskilled collection and interpretation of ethnographic data. Having received no training in the discursive aspects of cultural representation, medical researchers generally are unable to weed out ethnographic accounts which are unsystematic, patchy, inaccurate, or incomplete, and do not recognize the problems inherent in materials which have been collected and interpreted in a context of condemnation. Unfortunately, using such data, they construct images of the diseased or "at risk" cultural "other," and in turn, produce their own seemingly authoritative ethnographic texts.

African AIDS[1]

The literature on African risk for AIDS generated over the last fifteen years is enormous. Most of this literature focuses on what are seen as two very different epidemiological patterns. "Pattern One AIDS," found in the United States and Europe, affects largely the male population at a male to female ratio of 8 to 1. "Pattern Two AIDS," found on the African continent, has a reported sex ratio of 1 to 1 (Hunt 1996, 1345). The contrast between Pattern One and Pattern Two epidemiologies has caused considerable comment on African paths of transmission and risk factors. Further, while 10 percent of the world's population lives in sub-Saharan Africa, it is estimated that about 55 percent of persons with the HIV virus live there, including over 80 percent of the world's seropositive women (Goldin 1994, 1360). While estimates of prevalence of the virus in Africa differ and while the worldwide AIDS statistics are constantly changing, it is clear that the magnitude of AIDS in Africa is significant.

Though the epidemiological statistics suggest heterosexual transmission in Africa, AIDS researchers and writers continually push for more exotic explanations of African AIDS.[2] Simon Watney notes:

> African AIDS must . . . always be presented as sui generis, a completely different disease from AIDS in the First World. Indeed, most commentators have preferred almost any explanation of the 1:1 AIDS ratio of men to women in most African countries other than that of heterosexual transmission. (Watney 1990, 96)

Even when heterosexual transmission is granted as the major route of infection, the construction of risk takes a shape of "otherness." In an article entitled "Reassuring News about AIDS: A Doctor Tells Why You May Not Be at Risk" published in *Cosmopolitan,* Robert E. Gould writes:

> The data I gathered concerning heterosexual intercourse in Africa show marked differences from the way it is usually practiced in the United States . . . Many men in Africa take their women in a brutal way, so that some heterosexual activity regarded as normal by them would be closer to rape by our standards and therefore be likely to cause vaginal lacerations through which the AIDS virus could gain entry into the bloodstream. (1998, 147)

Although the Gould excerpt may appear easy to dismiss by virtue of its publication in a popular magazine, it is indicative of the wider medical picture. A search through computerized medical indexes for articles on AIDS in Africa betrays a widespread evolutionary paradigm. While AIDS researchers clearly recognize that African cultural beliefs and practices have to be accounted for in any discussion of the disease and its African ramifications, the belief and practices which are discussed are stereotyped heavily and are abstracted from any kind of real context. Medical researchers of African birth are continually writing in to the journals to head off overzealous Western researchers making uncontextualized pronouncements about African traditional life and culture. The following controversy, which took place in the letters and commentaries section of the *Lancet* in 1987, is representative of these debates. The first letter, entitled "AIDS and the Witch Doctor," was printed as follows:

> Sir,—The reassurance given by the Medical Acupuncture Society (May 30) about the risk of contracting AIDS is welcome. In Africa, however, the use of non-sterile instruments is widespread among witch doctors, who are often consulted initially by patients.

Many patients presenting to hospital with pain or swelling are seen with small lacerations over the affected area, indicating that the witch doctor has been at work. One patient recently seen with chest pain . . . had 150 of these markings.

Witch doctor induced gastrointestinal disorders are commonly seen in this hospital, but many psychiatric patients benefit from seeing the witch doctor. The methods of traditional healers are thought to be similar throughout Africa, and in view of the huge population consulting such healers I suggest their name be added to the possible risk factors for the transmission of HIV infection. (O'Farrell 1987, 166)

A response was published one month later, entitled "AIDS and the African Healer":

Sir—In rural Africa most people who feel ill first consult traditional healers, herbalists or as Dr. O'Farrell calls them witch doctors, who often apply concoctions of herbs, roots, and leaves to skin that has been scarified around the suspected lesion. O'Farrell fears that through use of non-sterile instruments these traditional healers might contribute to the spread of AIDS in Africa.

O'Farrell seems unfamiliar with the methods of traditional healers and the limited capability of HIV to survive outside the human organism. For scarifications only razor blades or similar cutting devises are used, never needles or other hollow instruments where blood might stay inactive for longer. It is very unusual for scarifications to be done on several people one after another, the only way that might permit transmission of HIV. In Tanzania a complete treatment by an herbalist takes 20–60 minutes and by the time the razor blade is used again the retrovirus should be destroyed. (Schmutzhard 1987, 459)

As the second letter points out, the problem with much of the disinformation about Africa and AIDS is a lack of proper contextualization. A piece of social data is simply matched with a risk category.

Issues of sexuality were the focus of many of these articles and controversies, portraying African sexual practices based on questionable ethnographic information or taking a practice recorded at one place and time and generalizing it to the whole of African culture. Again from the *Lancet*, a medical researcher warned:

In his book on the sexual life of people in the great Lakes area of Africa, Kashamura writes: "to stimulate a man or a woman and induce them to intense sexual activity, monkey blood for a man or she-monkey blood for a woman was directly inoculated in the pubic area and also in the thighs and the back. These magic practices would therefore constitute an efficient experimental transmission model and could be responsible for the emergence of AIDS in man. (Noireau 1987, 1499)

While the author of this article is to be commended for considering actual ethnographic studies of African life and culture in his commentary, the study he has chosen is based on observations reported in 1927 with no more recent data. The data is not given its proper historical context, but rather presented as current practice.

Geographical generalizations provide the same difficulty. Africa is taken as one culture without variation over time and space. Little attention is paid to urban and rural differences, differences by district, or differences within populations. Debates over female circumcision have focused on exactly this issue. The journal *Science* published the following debate:

> The high incidence of AIDS among men and women in Africa has led to the suggestion that a different mode of transmission may be at work there. Colin Norman echoes this view in his summary of the international Symposium on African AIDS. In fact the spread of the disease among heterosexuals in Africa and homosexuals in the West may point to a common factor in their sexual practices. Contact with blood during intercourse is thought to be largely responsible for the transmission of the virus among homosexuals in the United States. The same principle may apply to heterosexuals in central Africa, where female circumcision is still a widespread practice. In its most extreme form referred to as infibulation, the operation consists of the removal of some or all of the vulval tissue, after which the two sides of the wound are sewn together, leaving only a small opening for the passage of urine and menstrual blood. Subsequent vaginal intercourse is therefore difficult if not impossible and is chronically associated with tissue damage, tears and bleeding. Anal intercourse is a common recourse for heterosexual partners. . . . Understanding the pattern of AIDS in Africa will probably first require understanding the cross cultural differences in sexual practices. (Linke 1986, 203)

It would appear that the author of this letter, anthropologist Uli Linke, has generalized the geographical context of the practice of infibulation. One of his colleagues responded:

> Uli Linke's letter about AIDS in Africa suggests that contact with blood during intercourse may be an indirect consequence of the African practice of female circumcision. It then describes an extreme and rare form of female circumcision—infibulation. Infibulation is found only in a part of Northeastern Africa outside the region where AIDS has been reported and is very different in its social and biological effects from the kind of female circumcision that is practiced more widely in Africa. A secondary

problem with the logic of hypothesizing that AIDS is transmitted by traditional custom is that in Africa it appears to be primarily an urban disease, as it is in the United States. Traditional customs, such as female
circumcision have their origins in the rural sector. I think it would be
most productive to look at data pertaining to life in African cities and to
examine such phenomena as male labor migration, often described as
being disruptive to marriage and family life. (Burton 1986, 1236)

In relation to the geographical generalization of African AIDS issues,
Simon Watney argues:

> ... the notion of "African AIDS" already obscures the specific character-
> istics of the different AIDS epidemics in these countries, constructing
> them in the spurious unity of an "Africa" which is immediately denied
> any of the cultural, social, economic, and ethnic diversity which is taken
> for granted in Europe and North and South America." (Watney 1990, 94)

What is clear from the literature on Africa and AIDS is that much of the
data which is used to describe cultural practices takes a part of the story and
confuses it with the whole. AIDS researchers in Africa, knowing that they are
dealing with a very different lifestyle, have gone looking through the ethnographic data for cases of "risky behavior." In this sense the literature searches
out the deviant and uses it to understand the health needs of the entire culture.
Reports are taken at face value, with little thought given to how the data was
collected, by whom, and under what circumstances. The researchers do not
recognize that ethnographic data, like scientific data, is not all methodologi-
cally sound. One must understand the methodological orientation before
adopting it as a source of factual information. Much of the data used in these
discussions were originally collected and interpreted in a context of condemnation, emphasizing the failure of Africans to adjust to the conditions of
Western society. The data tend to be patchy and unsystematic in nature, and yet
the health and lives of an entire country are being tied to its implications. The
data exclude the less exotic, more mundane sexual behaviors and by so doing
target the unusual for health education efforts and health development policy.

But another problem with the portrayal of African sexual culture in this
literature has to do with the issue of how normalcy, deviance, and risk are
defined. Prostitution, said to be widespread in African culture, is frequently
defined in the medical literature as sexual exchange with a monetary component (Packard and Epstein 1991), but clearly the risks of such an exchange are
based on the numbers of partners and on the practice of unsafe sex. A
woman, paid by one man who is only sexually active with her, would according to such definitions still be classified as a prostitute. While such a case may

seem unlikely, it points to the more widespread limitations of risk involved with prostitutes who service a small regular cliental versus those who engage in such services with an unknown larger public. Clearly the risks are different, perhaps indicating one of the reasons why urban populations must be dealt with differently than rural populations. Cross-cultural researchers need to consider the issue of what counts as equivalent phenomena. The well-known association of African sexuality with polygamy is a good example. While polygamous relationships do increase the number of partners one has, the assumption, seen regularly in the medical literature, that polygamy constitutes promiscuity, is unjustifiable. While numbers of partners exceed those considered the norm in Western society, individuals are not necessarily active outside of those relationships, and such activities do not in themselves constitute a risk.

Folk Culture as Risk

I am not suggesting here that such risk behaviors do not occur or that they are not potential avenues for HIV infection, but I am suggesting that medical evidence concerning AIDS in Africa has been constructed to fit preexisting notions about African sexuality and disease, and to fit preexisting notions of the exoticism of traditional cultures. Western research on AIDS had already defined AIDS as a behavioral problem associated with "aberrant" lifestyles; perhaps this provided a predisposition to looking for deviance in an African setting. The result, however, is a discourse which privileges those patterns of social intercourse suggesting that Africans have multiple sexual partners or inject monkey blood, and excludes from discussion the broader patterns of sexuality found on a day-to-day basis.

This search for the exotic invariably leads medical researchers to folklore and particularly customary practice. In Africa, risk becomes associated with traditional healing, children's games, and initiations such as those associated with blood brotherhood. Daniel B. Hrdy writes in *Review of Infectious Diseases*:

> Factors thought to influence sexual transmission in Africa include
> 1) promiscuity, with a high prevalence of sexually transmitted diseases;
> 2) sexual practices that have been associated with increased risk of transmission of HIV (homosexuality and anal intercourse); and 3) cultural practices that are possibly connected with increased virus transmission (female circumcision and infibulation). Other nonsexual cultural practices that do not fit the age distribution pattern of AIDS but may expose individuals to HIV include 1) practices resulting in exposure to blood (medicinal bloodletting, rituals establishing blood brotherhood and possibly ritual

and medicinal enemas; 2) practices involving the use of shared instruments (injection of medicines, ritual scarification, group circumcision, genital tattooing and shaving of body hair; and 3) contact with nonhuman primates. (1987, 1109–10)

The discussion of African AIDS and risk is part of an authoritative and sophisticated medical discourse of control and exclusion, which uses folklore as an index to socialization and traditional culture as a flag of physical danger. The new wrapping paper on this old evolutionary argument, though, is outwardly biomedical and scientific and, as such, passes for nonideological and neutral.

Central to the perception of African health issues is the evolutionary image of the "primitive native" making a difficult adjustment to conditions of a "civilized" industrial world. The development discourse of which this is a part is much older than the battle with AIDS. In 1963 the director of Kenyan medical services stated:

> The African in his rural setting is strictly bound by tribal patterns of behavior, beliefs and customs. He is an integral part of his community and his thinking tends to be communal. . . . With the transposition to the town he forsakes the communal life for an individualistic life, unsupported by tribal rules and regulations. While forsaking these supports, he is not yet ready to adopt the codes and rules which have brought social stability to western civilizations. Furthermore, he is abandoning ingrained centuries of agricultural and pastoral tradition and learning the technical skills of an industrial world quite strange to him. (Fendell 1963, 574)

What is perhaps most interesting about the concentration on exotic tribal customs of the natives is that while tribal life is seen as uncivilized and risky, it is simultaneously discussed as protective and constrained. The dilemma is fascinating. One researcher indicated:

> As people leave rural villages and migrate to urban areas, the general level of promiscuity increases. This increase may be attributable in part to the relaxation of traditional village values. . . . (Hrdy 1987, 1112)

RISK REDUCTION

What I have presented here is meant neither to oppose the efforts of those researchers attempting to slow the rate of HIV infection in Africa, nor to attack the attempts made to allow for the consideration of cultural issues in AIDS education and policy making. Quite the reverse is true. It *is* meant, however, to argue that shoving health care workers in the direction of ethnographic material is not enough. We must raise awareness of the need to understand the methodologies of cultural study and their radical impact on health issues. Understanding sexual and cultural issues cannot be a process of deviance seeking or risk seeking. It must be a process of investigating a range of cultural issues which bear on sexual behavior, a range which may include marriage, divorce, kinship, fertility beliefs, initiation rites, gender roles, child rearing, and so on. But it must also be a process of trying to understand not just the exotic, but also the mundane.

We must, as health researchers and as social scientists, place more value on the subtleties of ethnographic research. Is the data contextualized historically, geographically, or in terms of groups and subgroups? What are the political, social, and economic ideologies which motivated ethnographic collection? Is a part of a behavioral complex being taken for the whole? Is cultural difference being taken to constitute danger or commanding a focus which obscures more pervasive mundane threats? Are very different types of health behavior with different degrees of risk being assumed to constitute equivalent phenomena?

More to the point, we must involve the lay public in the identification of risk, if for no other reason than to have them articulate community *perceptions*. At worst, such information could provide public health needs analysis. At best, it could indicate a whole new set of unknown risks or put to rest those based on exoticism.

We should not lose track of the special skills which are required in the treatment of cultural information. Without those skills, epidemiology may become neocolonialist ideology and risk might become what we take when we steer physicians in the direction of ethnography. Dressed up as biomedicine and couched in a discourse of risk, even colonialist ethnography passes for neutral and nonideological.

Notes

1. The phrase "African AIDS" is intended here to refer to the discursive construction of AIDS in Africa. Simon Watney (1990) cites Cindy Patton as initially coining the phrase in "Inventing African AIDS" (1988).

2. Simon Watney notes:

   As a cultural and psychic construction, "African AIDS" exhibits at least five consistent aspects. First, it speaks of a peculiar and special affinity between a virus and a continent. Second, it reads the modes of transmission of HIV as signs of a generalized and homogenous African "primitiveness" whether sexual or medical. Third, it singles out the alleged "misreporting" of African HIV and AIDS statistics as further evidence of "backwardness" and "unreliability." Fourth, it equates black Africans and Western gay men as willful "perverts" who are equally threatening to "family values." Fifth, it regards "Africa" as the source of the HIV infection in the sense of origin and of *cause*. (1990, 94)

References

Burton, M. 1986. AIDS and female circumcision. *Science* 231 (4743): 1236.

Douglas, Mary. 1992. *Risk and blame: Essays in cultural theory.* London: Routledge.

Fendell, N. 1963. Public health and urbanization in Africa. *Public Health Reports* 78: 574.

Goldin, Carol S. 1994. Stigmatization and AIDS: Critical issues in public health. *Social Science and Medicine* 39 (9): 1359–66.

Gould, Robert E. 1998. Reassuring news about AIDS: A doctor tells why you may not be at risk. *Cosmopolitan,* January, 147.

Hrdy, Daniel B. 1987. Cultural practices contributing to the transmission of human immunodeficiency virus in Africa. *Review of Infectious Diseases* 9 (6): 1109–19.

Hunt, Charles. 1996. Social vs biological: Theories on the transmission of AIDS in Africa. *Social Science and Medicine* 42 (10): 1345–1456.

Linke, Uli. 1986. AIDS in Africa. *Science* 231 (4735): 203.

Noireau, F. 1987. HIV transmission from monkey to man. *Lancet,* 27 June, 1498–99.

O'Farrell, N. 1987. "AIDS and the witch doctor." *Lancet,* 18 July, 166.

Packard, Randall, and Paul Epstein. 1991. Epidemiologists, social scientists, and the structure of medical research on AIDS in Africa. *Social Science and Medicine* 33 (7): 771–94.

Patton, Cindy. 1988. Inventing African AIDS. *City Limits* 363: 85.

———. 1994. *Last served? Gendering the HIV pandemic.* London: Taylor and Francis.

Schmutzhard, Erich. 1987. AIDS and the African traditional healer. *Lancet,* 22 August, 459.

Seidel, Gill. 1993. The competing discourses of HIV/AIDS in sub Saharan Africa: Discourses of rights and empowerment vs discourses of control and exclusion. *Social Science and Medicine* 36 (3): 175–94.

Stoffle, Richard, Michael Traugott, John Stone, Paula McIntyre, Florence Jensen, and Carla Davidson. 1991. Risk perception mapping. *American Anthropology* 93 (3): 611–35.

Watney, Simon. 1990. Missionary positions: AIDS, "Africa" and race. In *Out there: Marginalization and contemporary cultures,* ed. Russell Ferguson and Martha Gever, 89–103. New York: New Museum of Contemporary Art and MIT Press.

the new age dilemma

7

THE NEW AGE SWEAT LODGE

WILLIAM M. CLEMENTS

The 10 August 1997 issue of the *Westchester Weekly*, a section of the Sunday *New York Times*, includes an article entitled "Prayer Group in Patterson Follows Rituals of Indian Purifying" (Fullam 1997). The piece recounts the use of the Lakota Indian sweat lodge ritual accompanied by a "drum ceremony" adapted from the Micmacs by a group of suburbanites who call themselves the "Red Road." Though some of the participants state that they have been adopted by Native American families, "the closest thing to an actual American Indian in the group" is a person of Italian and Shoshone descent (the latter four generations removed) who studied with Ed McGaa, a Lakota spiritual leader who works with participants in contemporary alternative spirituality. The group, who share such common problems as "divorce, addictions, [and] grandchildren thrust on us in our later years" which the Christianity into which they were enculturated does not effectively address, sweats once a week and operates out of White Buffalo, a craft shop run by a woman of Greek-Portuguese descent. The *Times* reporter notes the effects of their participation in the sweat lodge experience: "While all members claimed to have had changes in their personal lives as a result of their American Indian spiritual practices, some also claimed more awareness in their political lives," especially in regard to issues affecting Native Americans. The location of the Red Road sweat lodge, though, is kept secret out of fear of reprisals from Native Americans who object to non-Indians "co-opting" their ceremonies. The use of American Indian ceremonies for healing and other spiritual ends in Westchester County represents a practice whose roots go back to the beginning of contact between Europeans and their predecessors in the Western Hemisphere. But it has grown exponentially during the last decade or so, often associated with protocols of alternative spirituality which are usually placed under the general rubric "new age."[1] Accounts of sweat lodge use, for example, abound in literature by and about adherents of alternative spirituality. One person has written of her experience at a sweat ceremony at a Unitarian Universalist retreat and camp in western Massachusetts (Fairclough 1992); paying guests at the Open Spoke Ranch near Stillwater, Oklahoma, can enjoy the experience of sweat lodge hot tubs (Lee 1995, 254); the sweat lodge experience is among the amenities offered to guests who stay at some vegetarian-oriented bed and breakfast hostelries (Ryan 1996); students at Worcester Polytechnic Institute can participate in the sweat lodge as part of a program called "Passages" (Gose 1996); and the "exciting week" offered by the Sunrise Retreat Center of Rimrock, Arizona, begins with a sweat lodge.[2] Examples could be multiplied on end, but the Westchester County example can be considered somewhat paradigmatic of the current popularity of sweat lodge ceremonialism: its association with a commercially oriented arts and crafts venture, the apparent lack of involvement of people with primary cultural roots in Native American societies, its eclectic borrowing of procedures from different Indian ethnic groups, the experience's impact for participants on both personal and social levels, and the recognition that Indians may be uncomfortable—to the point of vaguely conceived "reprisals"—with the adoption and adaptation of traditional spiritual customs by cultural outsiders.

Or consider the testimonial of Colin Pringle regarding his first sweat lodge, which took place at a 1979 Rainbow Gathering. Led by a "Native American medicine man" named Medicine Story, the ritual involved about half a dozen participants. After they had entered the dome-shaped structure and heated rocks had been placed in a pit in the middle of the lodge, Medicine Story said a few words "to help center the energy" while the other people chanted. Pringle reports that the couple of hours spent in the lodge produced sensations "like being in an isolation tank." While the sweat lodge is communal in contrast to the solitary isolation tank, "both experiences tend to give you the we are all one feeling that LSD is known to produce." The lodge has its risks. The intense heat requires the same kind of consciousness alteration needed for coal-walking, Pringle avers. But the result is "a spiritual boost." He testifies to the immediately positive effects that his first experience produced:

> Like other forms of meditation, it clears your mind of all the worries, fears and other distractions of everyday life, and it works without drugs or expensive equipment like isolation tanks or bio-feedback equipment. It's such a simple ritual, yet it's so powerful. I think it gave me the energy to get through a mishap that happened the next day, when I accidently consumed more LSD than I would have liked.[3]

What are students of alternative healing methodologies to make of the Westchester County use of the sweat lodge and of this account, which (except for its references to LSD) represents the experiences of a number of non-Indians who have participated in the sweat lodge? On one hand, glowingly positive testimonials by sweat lodge leaders as well as by satisfied participants appear in a variety of books and articles, on the internet, and in oral tradition. These accounts suggest that for people seeking alternatives to mainline religion and medicine, the sweat lodge seems to be filling some real needs. But at the same time, many traditional Native Americans and individuals who perceive themselves as their spokespersons see new age uses of the sweat lodge and other manifestations of Native American spirituality as another instance of the five-hundred-year-old appropriation of things Indian by Europeans and Euro-Americans. The purpose here is not to assume sides in what is an often passionate, sometimes acrimonious debate. Instead, I am concerned with the "logics" that inform the use of the sweat lodge outside its original cultural contexts as a method for healing in the broadest sense of that term for people who have turned to spiritual and medical alternatives to making themselves and their environment whole.

Ceremonial sweating may be the most widely known ritual healing practice in native North America. The earliest contact documents report the use of sweat baths for hygienic and therapeutic purposes, sometimes for specific ailments but often as a general cure-all. Not confined to any ethnic group or culture area, sweating occurred among native communities in virtually every part of the continent (Vogel 1970, 254–57). Methods of administering sweat baths varied, of course, as did the degree to which the practice had spiritual significance. The approach to sweating that has exerted the most influence in contemporary alternative spirituality is that of the Lakota of the northern Plains, probably because of the influence of Joseph Epes Brown's book *The Sacred Pipe* (1953; Bucko 1998, 51–53), which presents a detailed description of the Lakota sweat lodge ritual, or *inipi*, recorded from the Oglala Lakota spiritual leader Nicholas Black Elk. The reputation that Black Elk developed as a result of John G. Neihardt's poetic presentation of his life history in *Black Elk Speaks*, which has enjoyed considerable popularity since the 1960s especially in the new age movement, undoubtedly contributed to the foregrounding of Lakota ceremonialism in alternative spirituality. Moreover, the high visibility of two Lakota spiritual practitioners, Wallace Black Elk (a spiritual, though not genealogical descendant of Nicholas Black Elk) and Ed McGaa (Eagle Man), has contributed to the prominence of the Lakota version of the sweat lodge. The popular reception of Richard Erdoes's treatment of the life history of John Fire Lame Deer is another relevant factor. Undoubtedly, the Lakota prominence in popular culture images of the generic "Indian" must be taken into account as well.

Considerable variation characterizes even Lakota sweating; in fact, the more punctilious a sweat lodge leader is about the exactness of procedures, the more likely he or she has derived knowledge of those procedures from new age publications rather than traditional Lakota sources. In general terms, though, the ceremony does follow a standardized pattern. The venue for the ceremony is a dome-shaped structure, whose frame usually consists of pliable saplings secured into the earth and bent together. A single door may be directionally oriented toward either east or west. The sweat lodge (sometimes simply referred to as a "sweat," also a term for the ceremony itself) is covered with hides, blankets, tarpaulins, or plastic. The object is to capture and retain as much heat and to exclude as much light as possible. The sweat lodge may be a relatively permanent structure; leaders, both traditional Lakota and new age, may have lodges erected in their backyards. Often, though, participants will be expected to assist in constructing a lodge for a particular sweat, the result being a structure that is disassembled as soon as the ceremony concludes.

The ceremonial leader or an assistant heats rocks on a fire built outside the lodge (hence the alternate term "stone-people lodge"). Some ceremonialists insist that a certain number of rocks be heated, while others make no specific recommendations. Igneous rocks of some sort ("lava rocks") are thought to be best for ceremonial purposes. Meanwhile, participants enter the lodge by crawling through the door perhaps after an introductory ritual involving an offering of tobacco smoke. Traditionally, sweat lodge ceremonies seem to have been segregated by gender, in which cases the participants entered the lodge naked. In the mixed sweats that occur among participants in contemporary alternative spirituality, men and women are likely to wear bathing suits or other light garb.

Participants position themselves around a central indentation in the earth into which the fire tender introduces some of the heated rocks. Water poured over the rocks produces steam which begins to heat the darkened enclosure. As the temperature builds, the leader may intone a prayer to Wakan tanka, Tunkashila, Mother Earth, or another animatistic deity. Each participant will have his or her turn at prayer, which both traditionally and in new age contexts often begins with the Lakota phrase *Mitákuye oyás'* (all my relatives). Prayers may be for personal needs, though the community (defined as ranging from the immediate reference group to the cosmos in general) usually receives some attention. After a period of time, the door of the lodge will be opened and participants given the chance to drink some water. The process may be repeated for several rounds (or "endurances"), four being a frequent number. Often sage is sprinkled over the heated stones, and a pipe filled with tobacco is passed among the participants.[4]

Europeans apparently adopted Native American practices of sweating for medicinal purposes very soon after contact. Several early accounts by missionaries and explorers report the authors' participation in or observation of the ceremony. An example appears in the work of Moravian missionary John Heckewelder, whose 1819 account of the Lenni Lenape (Delawares) continues to receive high marks for its ethnographic value. In a chapter entitled "Remedies," Heckewelder notes, "The sweat oven is the first thing that an Indian has recourse to when he feels the least indisposed; it is the place to which the wearied traveller, hunter, or warrior looks for relief from the fatigues he has endured, the cold he has caught, or the restoration of his lost appetite" (1819, 225). The missionary provides a fairly good description of procedures in the "oven" and more to the present purpose offers the following account of its use by a Euro-American:

> In the year 1784, a gentleman whom I had been acquainted with at Detroit, and who had been for a long time in an infirm state of health, came from thence to the village of the Christian Indians on the Huron river, in order to have the benefit of the sweat oven. It being the middle of winter, when there was a deep snow on the ground, and the weather was excessively cold, I advised him to postpone his sweating to a warmer season; but he persisting in his resolution, I advised him by no means to remain in the oven longer that fifteen or at most twenty minutes. But when he once was in it, feeling himself comfortable, he remained a full hour, at the end of which he fainted, and was brought by two strong Indians to my house, in very great pain and not able to walk. He remained with me until the next day, when we took him down in his sleigh to his family at Detroit. His situation was truly deplorable; his physicians at that place gave up all hopes of his recovery, and he frequently expressed his regret that he had not followed my advice. Suddenly, however, a change took place for the better, and he not only recovered his perfect health, but became a stout corpulent man, so that he would often say, that his going into the sweat oven was the best thing he had ever done in his life for the benefit of his health. (1819, 226–27)

Heckewelder encountered the man fifteen years later, when he claimed to have suffered no illness at all in the interim. He died "at an advanced age," some thirty years after his sweating experience (1819, 227). Similar accounts can be gleaned from such sources as Heckewelder: occasional instances of Europeans or Euro-Americans who enjoy relief from some ailment as a result of ceremonial sweating. These seem, though, to be isolated cases and exemplify individuals who were willing to take advantage of any available curative procedures. To my knowledge, in early accounts one does not encounter attempts to spread the use of the sweat lodge beyond the immediate community.

That is just what began to happen in the 1970s with the emergence of new age consciousness. Some alternative religious communities during the 1960s may have adopted the sweat lodge into their ceremonial agendas, but one does not hear of widespread new age use until the next decade when examples such as those reported at the beginning of this essay become more and more commonplace. The period also marks the emerging visibility of Native American (often Lakota) promoters of their indigenous spirituality (or modified versions thereof) to non-Indian populations.

Commentators on new age spirituality have noted the eclecticism and volatility of the "movement." During the quarter-century or so that has passed since alternative spirituality emerged into the mainline, various points of stress have become foregrounded and then receded to a less visible position as new emphases replace them. While the 1970s were marked by an emphasis on Eastern religions, especially those from India, and on the methodology of channeling spiritual entities from the past, more recently environmental concerns have come to the fore and spiritual agendas adapted from native America and the Celtic cultures of northern Europe have received increased attention (Lewis 1992, 10). This does not mean that these emphases have not always been a part of contemporary alternative spirituality, just that fluctuations in prominence have occurred. For example, *The Teachings of Don Juan* (Castaneda 1968) has been an influence on alternative spirituality virtually since its publication, but Native Americana did not become one of the *prominent* new age themes until about a decade later. While sweat lodge ceremonialism adopted from Lakota and other American Indian groups may have been conducted in new age contexts thirty years ago, now they have become rather standard features of new age spiritual experiences. The emergence of figures such as Vincent La Duke, Ed McGaa, Jamie Sams, and Wallace Black Elk as ostensible guides for non-Indians into Native American spirituality had brought the sweat lodge (and other adapted Native American ceremonies) into prominence by the 1980s. La Duke, a Chippewa who used the name "Sun Bear" in his role as spiritual leader, focused much of his attention on orienting followers (members of what he called the "Bear Tribe") with the cosmic forces of earth using the medicine wheel. In the Bear Tribe, the sweat lodge offers individuals an opportunity to undergo ritual purification before the medicine wheel ceremonies.[5] McGaa (a Lakota who is also called "Eagle Man") works with a "Rainbow Tribe," whose membership extends to non-Indians. His earth-oriented spirituality adapts the seven rites which Nicholas

Black Elk had described to Brown in *The Sacred Pipe* so that the focus will be upon environmental consciousness and so that their accessibility will extend to non-Indians. Less coherent in polity than the others, Wallace Black Elk nevertheless sees the sweat lodge as part of what "Earth People" should be doing in order to reestablish their harmony with the earth.

The work of these ceremonial leaders has engendered some vociferous responses, and the new age sweat lodge because of its prominence has received special attention from critics, most of whom are either Indians or persons sympathetic to traditional Indian cultures. Though the reaction of some Native Americans to the use of the sweat lodge by non-Indians in the new age movement has been indifferent or even sometimes favorable, a vocal group of spokespersons has been adamantly opposed to what they consider appropriation of Indian spirituality by non-Indians—hence, the perceived need to conceal the location of their sweats by the Red Road group in Westchester County, New York. Many have extended their criticism especially to other Indians such as Wallace Black Elk and Ed McGaa who have been responsible for introducing new agers to the sweat lodge and other manifestations of Native American spirituality.

The principal charges involve the "selling" of Indian ceremonies—that is, the fact that some practitioners, Indian and non-Indian, charge fees for conducting the sweat lodge (Shaw 1995, 86). The website for the Earth Circle Association's sweat lodge (www.sfin.com/org/earthcircle/sweatlodge.html) suggests that participants make "a donation comparable to a doctors [*sic*] visit" to defray ceremonial expenses and "to the support of the ceremonial leader." Frequently, though, according to critics, those leaders have little in the way of traditional credentials or claims to expertise. While Euro-Americans who lead sweats almost invariably claim to have received instruction and authorization from a tribal teacher, many traditionalists hold that assuming a leadership role requires that one have previously participated in other Lakota ceremonies such as the Sun Dance or at least have the ability to speak Lakota (Bucko 1998, 64, 102). Those who fail these tests lack the "confirmation of the [traditional Indian] community" for their role as spiritual leader (Hobson 1979, 106). They are, in the frequently cited words of Ward Churchill, one of the leading critics of the new age movement's use of things Indian, "plastic medicine men" (1996, 355–65) whose principal motivation is financial.

But criticisms extend to issues more fundamental than commercialism and credentialing. For one thing, critics argue that the sweat lodge has meaning only within a larger religious context—that of Lakota or other specifically tribal spirituality (St. Pierre and Long Soldier 1995, 35, 207). There is indeed a tendency to "mix and match" elements of various Native American religious systems as if they together comprised a coherent whole (Bell 1997), a process exemplified by the use of Lakota and Micmac ceremonialism by the Westchester County Red Road group. For another instance, the "Seven Day Native American Spiritual Journey" offered by the Sunrise Retreat Center of Arizona offers not only the sweat lodge (using the Lakota term *inipi* to refer to the experience), but also the "Cherokee and Navajo Prayer Way."[6] Extracting the sweat lodge from its traditional context, argue critics, renders it meaningless and perhaps even dangerous. New agers who enter the sweat lodge without perceiving it as part of a larger ceremonial continuum trivialize the experience, and that has ramifications for the very real role that the sweat lodge is playing in the revival of traditional spirituality. Sweats have come to figure into situations of crisis which contemporary Native Americans face. They play a role in treatments for dependency, for example, and prisons with significant Native American populations have sometimes provided sweat lodges as part of their rehabilitation programs (Farnsworth 1996; Johnson 1997). New agers "playing Indian" by entering the sweat lodge undercut the power of the sweat lodge experience for Native Americans who are trying to come to terms with their own cultural identity, a nebulous view of which may contribute to drug abuse and criminal behavior. For Lakota and some other Indians, the sweat lodge has a role in cultural identity similar to that of the sauna among Finnish Americans (Lockwood 1977). Consequently, its use by people from other ethnicities seems inappropriate. According to Cynthia R. Kasee,

> While the "franchising" of Indian religions would deal a death blow to cultures practiced collectively by Native people, the loss of group identity conveyed by these faiths would devastate those who also rely on them as the Red Road to recovery. If Indian religions can be bought by any dilettante with a credit card, they lose their ability to require commitment, reform, and dimunition of ego. In other words, the practicing Indian Traditionalist is the antithesis of the Ramada Inn Sweatlodge Yuppie. (1995, 86)

According to this view, the new age sweat lodge is but another instance of Euro-American theft from Native Americans, part of a continuing pattern that began with land and continues through spirituality. Religious historian Martin E. Marty has characterized the behavior of what he calls "Boulder types" (from the Colorado city that is a locus for much new age activity) who "believe that they can and should jump out of their cultural skin and can simply take over the elements of the 'other.' They will do thus at whatever cost to the integrity of the borrowed-from, or stolen-from" (1994, 564). A suggestion frequently made by critics of the new age use of Native American spirituality is that Euro-Americans in search of spiritual fulfillment should instead explore the mystical tradition of Western Christianity (Shaw 1995, 89).

Critics also note the physical distress—on a few occasions to the point of fatality—that has sometimes affected non-Indians who are unprepared for the intense heat and potentially claustrophobic atmosphere of a sweat (D'Antonio 1992, 55). The spiritual powers which the sweat invokes may also be too much for the uninitiated to handle.

Finally, new age use of the sweat lodge is perceived by Native American critics as being too oriented to individual interest in self-actualization. When such ceremonialism occurs within the context of contemporary alternative spirituality, participants tend to downplay the community orientation that figures into traditional enactments. Christopher Jocks has noted, "Typically, practices that seem to involve 'mystical' individual experiences are promoted, while other elements considered equally or more important by Native partic-ipants are ignored: elements such as kinship obligations, hard work, suffering, and the sometimes crazy realities of everyday reservation life" (1996, 418). The tendency has been to use Indianness as represented in borrowed ceremonies as a way of finding "personal solutions to the question of living the good life" (Deloria 1998, 174).

My failure to evaluate and then either to endorse or refute these criti-cisms does not necessarily mean that I agree or disagree with them.[7] My pur-pose here is to note their existence before exploring the context of the use of the Lakota sweat lodge in contemporary alternative spirituality. That context lies in a healing logic that involves historical precedent both in terms of the role of sweating in Western medicine and the contact relationships between Native Americans and Europeans and in the general new age search for per-sonal fulfillment and for a sense of holistic community.

Indeed, the new age use of the Lakota sweat lodge constitutes an instance in a recurrent phenomenon in the contact history of Indians and Europeans, the incorporation of cultural material from the former into the belief and behavioral systems of the latter—what is dismissively referred to as "playing Indian" for purposes of revelry and rebellion, of assertion of a dis-tinctly Euro-*American* identity and artistic inspiration, of ecological sensitiv-ity and spiritual renewal (Deloria 1998). One impetus for that incorporation came from the economics of survival: the Indians had already adopted suc-cessful lifestyle strategies to the environments into which Europeans were intruding. Incorporating at least some native hunting, gathering, and horti-cultural techniques made practical sense. On the medical front, the inclusion of Indian pharmacopeia into European-based healing systems also made sense, as the plants and other natural substances from which palliatives might be derived were often unfamiliar to new arrivals. This inclusion contributed to the use of Native American imagery in the promotion of patent medicines during the nineteenth century. The "Indian medicine show," in fact, endured as late as into the 1970s. The technique was to advertise a product, largely consisting of alcohol, by connecting it by name with a Native American origin and by association with the show's performers, who donned Indian costume and sang and danced in what were perceived as Indian rhythms (Green 1988, 40).

The contemporary image of the Indian as healer in new age contexts has ample historical precedent, but the persistent presence of Indian influences in Euro-American life, long after adjustments to European lifeways had made them adaptive to the "New World," suggests something that transcends the prosaically practical. Much has been written about the attraction of the "primitive" to people jaded by the artificialities of Western civilization (for example, Torgovnick 1990). The discovery of Indians in the Americas by Columbus and his successors revealed real people to whom the idealized concept of the primitive could be attached. Though an anti-image which equated savagery with bestiality was often concurrent, one prevailing image of the American natives characterized them as representing what all of mankind had once been: natural philosophers, living in harmony and at ease with their environment. This concept of the "noble savage," which may have first been connected with American Indians by Montaigne, had a particular appeal for the Enlightenment and romantic philosophies which contributed to the formative moments in the American republican experience. In broad outline, the ethical aspects of the noble savage concept for overcivilized humanity held that a person who had become enervated by the unnecessary complexities of the institutions of European-derived society could experience physical, intellectual, and spiritual regeneration by learning from the Indian (Slotkin 1973). Based on generations of living close to a specific tract of earth, the Indian as noble savage intuitively sensed the higher truths of existence. While one should avoid the excesses of unbridled license that could emerge in the savage state (especially among people for whom that state was something adopted after already being corrupted by civilized artificiality), a person could become healthily harmonious with the cosmos by learning from an Indian. A common figure in American literature and popular culture is the Indian "sidekick" who provides a Euro-American protagonist with the spiritual (and often other) support needed to become fully human. Chingachgook plays this role in classic American literature for Natty Bumppo, for example, as does Tonto for the Lone Ranger in more recent expressive culture. Particularly relevant to new age spirituality is a reading of Castaneda's *The Teachings of Don Juan* that places it within this tradition: the Yaqui shaman as guide for the spiritual maturation of the young Western anthropologist (Clements 1985). That new agers, disgruntled with the mainline Judeo-Christian heritage and already opened to alternatives by their contacts with Eastern religious influences, would find native Americana attractive seems inevitable. Not only do Indian cultures offer a primitivistic answer to the over-civilization that may be responsible for new age anomie, but they do so from an American perspective. One need not turn to the exotic East—for spirituality coming from those who have spoken for the "spirit of the continent," in D. H. Lawrence's words (quoted in Deloria 1998, 3), has roots in *this* portion of Mother Earth. Those who are dissatisfied with what the mainstream offers can turn to a source of autochthonous spirituality and cite many precursors in Euro-American–Native American contact history for doing so.

That new agers are concerned about establishing a spiritual identity with American roots is evident in the claims made by some Euro-American partic-ipants in contemporary alternative spirituality that they had, in fact, been Native Americans in previous lives (Bucko 1998, 230–31; Smith 1991). They consequently justify their use of spiritual and healing procedures such as the sweat lodge by asserting that they are reclaiming what was once their proper cultural inheritance. Of course, other Indian ceremonials besides the sweat lodge can and are being reinterpreted by new agers, but none to the extent of the Lakota sweat lodge. This spiritually based healing ritual has several advan-tages: unlike a Navajo sing, it is relatively easy to conduct and it requires little in the way of specialized ritual paraphernalia; unlike the vision quest, it can be extracted from its distinctive spiritual context and introduced into a variety of new age and even mainstream Judeo-Christian environments (as well as into secular contexts); unlike the Sun Dance, it does not call for intense and painful sacrificial commitment; and it does have some forerunners as a healing pro-cedure in Western medicine.

Though mainstream medicine now regards sweating primarily in terms of its role in regulating body temperature, this physiological process has a long history as a purificatory and healing procedure in the Western tradition. Humoralism, for instance, which advocated a holistic approach to preventing and responding to disease, made use of sweating as one way of regulating the balance between such physiological states as moist and dry, hot and cold. Hildegard of Bingen, a twelfth-century religious whose writings on a medicine grounded in humoralism have been enjoying a revival of interest in the 1990s, recommended steam baths for corpulent individuals, "since the humors that are superfluous in them are controlled and lessened" (Flanagan 1996, 117–18; see Malpezzi, this volume). She also advised those suffering from arthritis and lameness as well as from various psychological imbalances to take baths in which the steam had been sweetened with extracts from chestnuts or oats

(Strehlow and Hertzka 1988, 110–11). But while it may have fallen from favor as a purifying mechanism in mainstream Euro-American medicine, folk medicine continues to endorse the beneficial effects of sweating. In addition to the general folk idea that sweating is good for a person and that one who sweats profusely in response to exertion or intense heat is demonstrating a normal, healthy reaction (Hand, Casetta, and Thiederman 1981, 258)—an idea supported by contemporary exercise physiologists (for example, Bailey 1994, 218–19)— sweating receives specific recommendation as a way of breaking a fever. Plant-based folk medicine suggests a variety of teas (such as corn pone or willow bark) as a way of inducing sweating for that purpose (Hand 1961, 188, 191). Tying red onions to the feet and rubbing the body with warm vinegar will also produce a fever-breaking sweat (Hand 1961, 189). Other ailments for which folk medical practitioners have endorsed sweating include cramps and neuralgia (Hand 1961, 163, 239).

Regardless of the role that sweating has played in the therapeutic heritage of the West and of the history of borrowing from American Indians by Europeans and Euro-Americans, the new age movement would not have been attracted to the sweat lodge if it did not serve the ends of alternative spirituality. The roots of the new age lie principally in Western adaptations of Eastern religions, particularly Buddhism and Hinduism. As other sources of spirituality that are compatible with the ways in which new agers have used those religious traditions have become known, they have become part of the movement. One important focus of new age spirituality has been on the transformative nature of religious experience. For the individual, this means growth, continual learning, and a movement toward holistic perfectionism (Lewis 1992). Testimonials about the sweat lodge experience indicate that it has a role in accomplishing these goals. To begin with, some participants stress that the sweat may be part of a regimen of physical healing: "Any illness that needs to be sweated out is so done in the sweat lodge" (Lee 1995, 54). Adolph Hungry Wolf, who was popularizing Native American traditions several years before the dawn of the new age, noted about "sweat bathing": "The expulsion of dirt and germs through profuse sweating literally causes the removal of evil from the body" (1973, 24). The role of sweating in physical healing coincides with the Western notions that the process cleanses the body of toxic substances. Lewis Mehl-Madrona, a physician of Cherokee heritage with an M.D. from Stanford University, includes the sweat lodge in what he calls a "healing intensive" for the chronically ill. Patients usually participate in a seven-day program that combines Native American medicinal practices from various ethnic traditions with Morita therapy from Japan. Mehl-Madrona uses the sweat lodge for purification on the third or fourth night of the program (1997,

254–60). Sweats conducted under the auspices of the Woptura Medicine Society "will prevent common illnesses and begin to heal even chronic illnesses such as all forms of cancer, lupus, Parkinson's disease and even AIDS. The ceremony will purify the organs of the body, the blood, the heart, lungs, liver, kidneys, pancreas, gall bladder and all others."[8]

But new age testimonials about the sweat lodge experience suggest that it contributes to personal growth and healing in ways other than just the physical. Ceremonial sweating can be a *rite de passage* during which one is personally transformed while sharing the fraternal and sororal ritual ambience that Victor Turner has called *communitas* (1969). A common analogy is drawn between sweating and the Christian rites of baptism and being born again (which, of course, in some Christian groups occur concurrently; Lee 1995, 55–56).[9] Beth Moscov, a new age practitioner who has adapted American Indian ceremonials primarily for Euro-American women participants, has stressed this feature of the sweat lodge experience in a poem she wrote in 1993 "after a women-only sweatlodge ceremony on the spring equinox":

> I was born again today.
> I went in on my hands and knees,
> bowing reverence to the many things.
> I came out on my hands and knees,
> This time as a newly born infant seeing the world for the first time.[10]

Common imagery about the lodge itself stresses its womb-like nature: the circular shape, the narrow passage through which one enters and exits, the darkness, and the moistness. It is perceived as "the moist womb of Mother Earth" (McGaa 1992, 83). And, of course, it is more than just the physical sensations, which may require considerable fortitude and endurance from participants, that contribute to the passage aspects of the experience. The prayers, which often involve frank revelations of their sense of self, afford participants a kind of group therapy (Garrett and Osborne 1995). As Wallace Black Elk has described the experience of healing and rebirth in the sweat lodge,

> This little guy [the spiritual force encountered in the sweat] goes inside and investigates everything. He sees everything. So the enemy does damage to the brain or heart or liver or kidney or whatever. He goes there. He sees, like X-ray. He sees it, and he goes there and repairs whatever is damaged. He recreates all the molecules, genes, organics, fibers, or whatever the enemy damages. He recreates and reforms it. That is why he has his name. That is why we call him Creator. So he reconstructs the human mind and physical body. He recreates the human spirit, so that the spirit could wear its robe [physical body] and walk with a clear mind. (Black Elk and Lyon 1990, 41)

Moreover (and in support of this new age emphasis), imagery of rebirth permeates traditional Lakota accounts of sweat lodge participation, and Raymond A. Bucko has published several narratives of "conversion" by Lakota participants which foreground the rite de passage aspects of sweating (1998, 171–96).

The communitas element of the sweat lodge is perhaps most clearly evident in the adoption of the Lakota phrase meaning "all my relatives." Theoretically, the distinctions that categorize people in ordinary existence disappear in a sense of community that includes not only the other human participants, but the nonhuman natural and spiritual realms. Defenders of new age uses of ceremonial sweating and other manifestations of Native American spirituality stress the universal inclusiveness of the phrase: that "relatives" is meant to incorporate not only traditional Lakota religionists but anyone with the proper attitude of humility and sense of community. In fact, one of McGaa's disciples has suggested that the Lakota phrase means "we are related to all things" (1992, 85). Other ways in which communitas becomes apparent in the sweat lodge include the fact that one crawls in an act of personal debasement on hands and knees into the structure, the seating of participants in a nonhierarchical circle around the heated stones, and the leveling nakedness or scanty clothing worn while in the lodge. The darkness contributes to the loss of ordinary identity and the sense of kinship with the other participants. As one is being purged of the toxins that have generated physical illness, one is also emptied of the trappings of structured self. A person emerges from the lodge physically cleansed and receptive to new influences, those from the spiritual powers that the experience has invoked.

The sweat lodge fulfills the new age program for the individual. The person who participates supposedly leaves the lodge as more nearly perfected in body and spirit. The individual fulfillment afforded by the sweat lodge becomes particularly apparent from a couple of sets of divinatory cards that new age practitioners have developed. Jamie Sams has created a set of tarot-like cards called Sacred Path Cards (1990). The second in the series of forty-one is the sweat lodge. If one draws this card, Sams writes in a book explicating the cards, the person "may be asking for a cleansing," subconsciously taking note of the need for purification of the body, mind, or spirit (1991, 11). A similar card set focuses exclusively on the sweat lodge. An internet advertisement for the Lakota Sweat Lodge Cards, designed by Chief Archie Fire Lame Deer and Helene Sarkis (1994), informs the surfer, "Sitting in the sweat lodge, an improvised womb of Mother Earth, you may experiencean [sic] expanded vision of your being and purpose as well as an intimate sense of walking in balance between the conscious world and the world of spirit." The cards use "the timeless medium of divinatory symbols" to direct the user's consciousness toward "the source of personal power, insight, release, and self-awakening."[11]

While critics have suggested that using the sweat solely for personal fulfillment violates traditional values for the ceremony, the appeal of the sweat lodge to new agers does transcend the personal. Especially for those who have come to the sweat through the influence of Native American leaders such as Wallace Black Elk and Ed McGaa, the sweat lodge is part of a program that has cosmic ramifications. As "a medicine man from the Chippewa tribe of the North Plains" told journalist Michael D'Antonio, "'We have a philosophy that says everything has a spirit: trees, rocks, animals. Our way of life has let us develop along the theological lines that give us a responsible role in the world, not ownership. . . . You go in [the sweat lodge], you listen, and we help you participate. . . . When it's over we are spiritually and physically purified. A cleansing takes place, and if it helps people develop a consciousness for the sacred nature of the Earth, that's good too'" (D'Antonio 1992, 48). "Earth spirituality" (or "Earth people philosophy" or "Mother Earth spirituality") holds that "the land on which we live shapes our experience of the sacred and that, in fact, certain religious movements, ceremonies, and artifacts are present in the land itself" (Buhner 1997, 217). The sweat lodge, which "allows a special closeness to Mother Earth" (McGaa 1990, 7), is one of these autochthonous ceremonies. Participants in sweats emulate "red brother and sister caretakers" of the Americas, individuals who developed methods over millennia for achieving oneness with Wakan tanka that are hemisphere-specific (McGaa 1990, 45). McGaa refers to the seven ceremonies, including the sweat lodge, which he has adapted from the rituals described by Nicholas Black Elk to Brown, as "Mother Earth ceremonies" that arise from the "realization that Mother Earth is a truly holy being" (1990, 204). The sweat is particularly effective for attaining oneness with this being because in what McGaa has called a "spiritual sauna," participants are reborn through "the commingling of [their] own lifeblood (sweat) with the lifeblood of the planet" (1990, 7). In a statement published a couple of years later, McGaa reiterated the way in which the sweat lodge is especially important for adherents of Mother Earth spirituality: "Mother Earth is present. You are sitting upon her. Father Sky is present. The sun's heat is within the glowing stones and brings forth your lifeblood, your sweat, to mix with the lifeblood of the world, the water within the bucket beside the lodge leader" (1992, 83). Theoretically, the interior "harmony and balance" that individuals experience in a sweat "will automatically translate outward to encompass the other worlds in which [they] live simultaneously" (McGaa 1992, 84).

Wallace Black Elk's "Earth people philosophy" essentially emphasizes the same point of view: that while sweating heals the individual, it also heals the cosmos. He notes, "The center is the Earth, and on this Earth we build the stone-people-lodge." The experience of the lodge involves all four of the basic constituents that comprise the cosmos: fire, rock, water, and "green"—in other words, the sage, cedar, and sweetgrass that are sprinkled onto the heated rocks (Black Elk and Lyon 1990, 59–60).

Not all sweat lodge leaders stress the community-oriented aspects of the experience, nor do all participants who recount their experience emphasize this aspect of it. But part of the healing logic of the sweat lodge (and at least part of its appeal in new age contexts which might have foregrounded other, non-Indian sweating protocols such as the sauna) lies in its connection with what proponents of contemporary alternative spirituality perceive as ecological awareness.

The logic of the new age sweat lodge, despite its being the target of considerable criticism, stems from at least two historical settings: the role of sweating in Western medicine, particularly that which has posed an alternative to the mainstream, and the fascination with matters Indian that has been a constant feature of Euro-American culture. Meanwhile, proponents of the lodge testify to its role in physical healing—a role that finds enhancement from its evocation of ceremonial patterns such as rite de passage and communitas. Moreover, the sweat lodge has a role in modern manifestations of the nature religion that Catherine L. Albanese has found pervasive in American spiritual life "from the Algonkian Indians to the New Age" (1990). The merging of these forces in one experience creates a powerful healing procedure that works for its adherents on several diachronic and synchronic levels. The Red Road in Westchester County with their tenuous claims to Native American ethnicity and the offense that they give to many American Indians nevertheless are operating from a coherent logic, a set of assumptions and precedents that makes them actors in a continuing subplot in the narrative of the American experience, a subplot that has at times influenced the main currents of the society's life as it seems to be doing more and more among new agers and others at millennium's end and beginning who have turned to the pre-European indigenes of the Western Hemisphere for a way to enhance their own experience in that land.

NOTES

1. The term "new age" is, of course, problematic. Many participants in what outsiders call "the new age movement" reject the term altogether. And it certainly has been used to cover such a vast array of beliefs and practices as almost

to have lost utility. "Alternative spirituality" as a term has the advantage of not being as offensive to those involved, but it also lacks precision. Generally, what I mean are contemporary (in other words, 1990s) beliefs and practices that lie outside the traditions of "great religions," that represent an often eclectic attempt at blending traditions, that are oriented toward personal transformation and fulfillment, and that have some millenarian overtones often couched in ecological diction.

2. On the internet at www.photon.net/sunrise/seven.html, which I accessed 14 May 1998.

3. Pringle's account, "Centering the Energy in a Sweat Lodge," appears on the internet at www.halycon.com/colimp/sweat.htm, which I accessed on 15 April 1998.

4. The most comprehensive treatment of the procedures of the Lakota sweat lodge is Bucko's (1998). My account draws also upon a variety of descriptions by participants in and observers of the use of ceremonial sweating in contemporary alternative spirituality.

5. La Duke published a number of books until his death in 1992. A generally positive account by an outsider to his movement was done by Catherine Albanese (1990, 155–63).

6. On the internet at www.photon.net/sunrise/seven.html (accessed 14 May 1998).

7. For a response to most of these charges, see Buhner (1997, 79–188). Stephen Harrod Buhner, who led a new age religious gathering in Boulder, Colorado, called the Church of Gaia has been one of the most outspoken defenders of non-Indian use of Indian ceremonials. He has had able opponents in the debate in Ward Churchill, for example, and in the editorial staff of the weekly newspaper *Indian Country Today* (formerly the *Lakota Times*). The issues raised by critics and defenders of non-Indian use of Native American ceremonialism find parallels in a variety of cross-cultural borrowings of what are perceived as "traditions": for example, the blues revival of the 1990s, in which white performers have figured prominently and white audiences have dominated (Lornell 1998). A classic example from Indian–Euro-American relations is the dispute over the ethnicity of artists who can sell their products at the Portal of the Palace of the Governors in Santa Fe, New Mexico (Evans-Pritchard 1987). These cases—and many like them—reflect the disparity that may arise from differing views of what constitutes "tradition," a construct more symbolic than substantive, as Richard Handler and Jocelyn Linnekin have suggested (1984).

8. On the internet at www.redroad.com/cc/inipi.html (accessed 20 May 1998).

9. Bucko (1998, 33) gives Charles Alexander Eastman, a Santee Dakota who received a medical degree and wrote a number of books on American Indian subjects during the early twentieth century, credit for first equating the sweat lodge and baptism.

10. Moscov's poem, entitled "Sweat Lodge," appears on the internet at www.west.net/%7Ekesslari/sweat.html (accessed 20 May 1998).
11. On the internet at www.antelicinsights.com/lakota.html (accessed 3 July 1998).

REFERENCES

Albanese, Catherine L. 1990. *Nature religion in America from the Algonkian Indians to the new age.* Chicago: University of Chicago Press.

Bailey, Covert. 1994. *Smart exercise: Burning fat, getting fit.* Boston: Houghton Mifflin.

Bell, Diane. 1997. Desperately seeking redemption. *Natural History* March: 52–53.

Black Elk, Wallace H., and William S. Lyon. 1990. *Black Elk: The sacred ways of a Lakota.* San Francisco: Harper and Row.

Brown, Joseph Epes. 1953. *The sacred pipe: Black Elk's account of the seven rites of the Oglala Sioux.* Norman: University of Oklahoma Press.

Bucko, Raymond A. 1998. *The Lakota ritual of the sweat lodge: History and contemporary practice.* Lincoln: University of Nebraska Press.

Buhner, Stephen Harrod. 1997. *One spirit many peoples: A manifesto for earth spirituality.* Niwot, Colorado: Roberts Rinehart.

Castaneda, Carlos. 1968. *The teachings of Don Juan: A Yaqui way of knowledge.* Berkeley: University of California Press.

Churchill, Ward. 1996. *From a native son: Selected essays on indigenism, 1985–1995.* Boston: South End Press.

Clements, William M. 1985. Carlos Castaneda's *The teachings of Don Juan:* A novel of initiation. *Critique* 26: 122–30.

D'Antonio, Michael. 1992. *Heaven on earth.* New York: Crown.

Deloria, Philip Joseph. 1998. *Playing Indian.* New Haven, Connecticut: Yale University Press.

Evans-Pritchard, Deirdre. 1987. The Portal case: Authenticity, tourism, traditions, and the law. *Journal of American Folklore* 100: 287–96.

Fairclough, Susanne. 1992. All my relations: A spiritual retreat. *EastWest* 1 March: 62–67.

Farnsworth, Clyde H. 1996. A prison where the Great Spirit of healing dwells. *New York Times* 17 July: A4.

Flanagan, Sabina, ed. and trans. 1996. *Secrets of God: Writings of Hildegard of Bingen.* Boston: Shambhala.

Fullam, Anne C. 1997. Prayer group in Patterson follows rituals of Indian purifying. *New York Times* (*Westchester Weekly*) 10 August: 1, 7.

Garrett, Michael Walkingstick, and W. Larry Osborne. 1995. The Native American sweat lodge as a metaphor for group work. *Journal for Specialists in Group Work* 20, 1: 33–39.

Gose, Ben. 1996. Indian rituals, Jung and nature help students face adulthood. *Chronicle of Higher Education* 6 December: A55–A56.

Green, Rayna. 1988. A tribe called Wannabee: Playing Indian in America and Europe. *Folklore* 99: 30–55.

Hand, Wayland D., ed. 1961. *Popular beliefs and superstitions from North Carolina. The Frank C. Brown collection of North Carolina folklore*, vol. 6. Durham, North Carolina: Duke University Press.

———, Anna Casetta, and Sondra B. Thiederman, eds. 1981. *Popular beliefs and superstitions: A compendium of American folklore from the Ohio Collection of Newbell Niles Puckett.* Boston: G. K. Hall.

Handler, Richard, and Jocelyn Linnekin. 1984. Tradition, genuine or spurious. *Journal of American Folklore* 97: 273–90.

Heckewelder, John. 1819. *An account of the history, manners, and customs of the Indian nations, who once inhabited Pennsylvania and the neighbouring states.* Philadelphia: Abraham Small.

Hobson, Geary. 1979. The rise of the white shaman as a new version of cultural imperialism. In *The remembered earth: An anthology of contemporary Native American literature,* ed. Geary Hobson, 100–108. Albuquerque: University of New Mexico Press.

Hungry Wolf, Adolph. 1973. *The good medicine book.* New York: Warner.

Jocks, Christopher Ronwaniän:te. 1996. Spirituality for sale: Sacred knowledge in the consumer age. *American Indian Quarterly* 20: 415–31.

Johnson, Dirk. 1997. Reversing reservation's pattern of hard drink and early death. *New York Times* 23 December: A16.

Kasee, Cynthia R. 1995. Identity, recovery, and religious imperialism: Native American women and the new age. *Women and Therapy* 16: 83–93.

Lame Deer, Chief Archie Fire, and Helene Sarkis. 1994. *The Lakota sweat lodge cards: Spiritual teachings of the Sioux.* Rutland, Vermont: Destiny Books.

Lee, Scout Cloud. 1995. *The circle is sacred: A medicine book for women.* Tulsa, Oklahoma: Council Oaks.

Lewis, James R. 1992. Approaches to the study of the new age movement. In *Perspectives on the new age,* eds. James R. Lewis and J. Gordon Melton, 1–12. Albany: State University of New York Press.

Lockwood, Yvonne R. 1977. The sauna: An expression of Finnish-American identity. *Western Folklore* 36: 71–84.

Lornell, Kip. 1998. The cultural and musical implications of the Dixieland jazz and blues revivals. *Arkansas Review* 29: 11–21.

Marty, Martin E. 1994. Impure faith. *Christian Century* 1–8 June: 562–64.

McGaa, Ed. 1990. *Mother Earth spirituality: Native American paths to healing ourselves and our world.* San Francisco: HarperCollins.

———. 1992. *Rainbow tribe: Ordinary people journeying on the Red Road.* San Francisco: HarperCollins.

Mehl-Madrona, Lewis. 1997. *Coyote medicine.* New York: Scribners.

Ryan, Ellen. 1996. Arise and eat. *Vegetarian Times* March: 106–11.

St. Pierre, Mark, and Tilda Long Soldier. 1995. *Walking in the sacred manner: Healers, dreamers, and pipe carriers, medicine women of the Plains Indians.* New York: Simon and Schuster.

Sams, Jamie. 1990. *Sacred path cards: The discovery of self through native teachings.* San Francisco: HarperCollins.

———. 1991. *The sacred path workbook: New teachings and tools to illuminate your personal journey.* San Francisco: HarperCollins.

Shaw, Christopher. 1995. A theft of spirit? *New Age Journal* July/August: 84–92.

Slotkin, Richard. 1973. *Regeneration through violence: The mythology of the American frontier, 1600–1860.* Middletown, Connecticut: Wesleyan University Press.

Smith, Andy. 1991. For all those who were Indian in a former life. *Ms* November/December: 44–45.

Strehlow, Wighard, and Gottfried Hertzka. 1988. *Hildegard of Bingen's medicine.* Santa Fe, New Mexico: Bear.

Torgovnick, Marianna. 1990. *Gone primitive: Savage intellects, modern lives.* Chicago: University of Chicago Press.

Turner, Victor. 1969. *The ritual process: Structure and anti-structure.* Chicago: Aldine.

Vogel, Virgil J. 1970. *American Indian medicine.* Norman: University of Oklahoma Press.

8

EVERGREEN: THE ENDURING VOICE OF A NINE-HUNDRED-YEAR-OLD HEALER

FRANCES M. MALPEZZI

A blurb on the cover of the June 1998 *Lapidary Journal*, "The Comeback Mystic: Hildegard von Bingen," announces an accompanying article by Si and Ann Frazier entitled "Woman of the Millennium." The website for Wellspring, a company offering products that promote wellness of mind, body, and spirit, touts this same visionary as "A 12th Century Mystic, A 90's Woman" (wellmedia.com/news/week54/mystic.html), and an electronic advertisement for Heinrich Schipperges's *Healing and the Nature of the Cosmos* explains Hildegard "is once again a cult figure with CDs and T-shirts celebrating her popularity" (raw.rutgers.edu/raw/publisher/hist/vonbingen.htm). The plethora of attention devoted to Hildegard of Bingen (1098–1179), a "saint" canonized only through the vox populi, suggests these designations are more than mere hyperbole. A guest at Judy Chicago's *The Dinner Party*, Hildegard is now the subject of two recent novels, an opera, several videos, and a soon-to-be-released film.[1] Nine hundred years after her birth numerous books both by and about Hildegard are readily available. The 1997–98 *Books in Print* lists over two dozen works, ranging from scholarly monographs to new age publications. These include editions of her letters, visions, songs, and drama as well as biographies, critical studies, and works focusing on her regimen for physical and spiritual well-being. Her music is internationally known, and a variety of CDs can be found at most music stores. A publishing company in Bryn Mawr, Pennsylvania, designed to "promote and preserve the music of women composers of the past and present" has been named after her as has an Australian electronic mailing list that serves as a communication channel for teachers involved in science and technology because Hildegard was "probably one of the first women to write about the method of scientific investigations" (edx1.edu.monash.edu.au/projects/hildegard/). And even the most cursory internet search yields an astounding number of items. Hildegard appears on websites devoted to early women writers, female composers, Catholic saints, as well as on sites for alternative and new age medicine.[2] Biographical and bibliographic information about Hildegard and selections from her works can be gleaned from academic websites such as Bonnie Duncan's "Women Writers of the Middle Ages" (www.millersv.edu/~resound/women.html) and "Medieval Women" (www.georgetown.edu.labyrinth/subjects/women/women.html) or at a site devoted to the Benedictine order (www.osb.org/osb/index.html); her illuminations adorn each page of "The Cosmic Egg" web page (www.cltr.uq. oz.au8000/~pandora/welcome.html); "Motherheart: Health and Wholeness" (gnv.fdt.net/~mother/health_index.html), a website for those who believe health involves "nurturing our unified being" includes the illumination *The Tree of Life* "painted by Hildegard of Bingen" and a link to Bonnie Duncan's material; "One Degree Beyond" (www.whidbey.com/onedegreebeyond/perslink.htm) contains links to web pages on new cosmology, on Reiki, and to the Memorial University of Newfoundland Hildegard of Bingen page. One can purchase her books and CDs on a variety of websites. References to her appear on a listserver devoted to the history of brewing because she may have been the first person to describe hopped beer (http://www.pbm.com/~lindahl/hist-brewing/archive/0162.html). The recipe for "St. Hildegard's Cookies of Joy" can be found on a Boston public radio site (www.wgbh.org/wgbh/pages/pri/spirit/specials/recipes/311recipes.html), and her herbal remedies are recommended on a variety of sites. There is even a website for a Generation X young man who believes he is the reincarnation of Hildegard (www.ordovirtutum.com). Wired as well as feted on several continents with concerts, lectures, conferences, and tours in honor of her nine-hundredth birthday, Hildegard indeed seems to be the woman of the millennium in her widespread appeal to a very disparate audience.

Clearly the interest of academicians in the work of this multitalented and complex woman is understandable, especially on the part of those concerned with expanding a heretofore patriarchal canon. However, the profusion of material about her is obviously not limited to dry tomes by medievalists exploring early music and literature nor to mainstream religious studying the history of Benedictine spirituality or Christian mysticism. Hildegard's appeal is neither strictly academic nor elite; it is a mass appeal. Her followers include scholars as well as new age adherents. One academic website bemoans the current popular appropriation of Hildegard: "Less fortunately, Hildegard's visions and music have been hijacked by the New Age movement, whose music bears some resemblance to Hildegard's ethereal airs" (tweedledee.ucsb.edu/~kris/music/Hildegard.html). Although some academics are discomfited by Hildegardian enthusiasts who do not always understand the complexities of her religio-historical context (some, in fact, even assigning her to an incorrect century), one cannot help but be astounded by the international recognition of this woman who until quite recently would not even have been taught in specialized upper-level university classes. For those inspired by her beliefs, admiring of all she accomplished, finding her medical concepts relevant, the voice of this nine-hundred-year-old woman who considered herself a feather on the breath of God resonates in our time.

Details of Hildegard's life can be culled from the numerous letters she left behind; from the biography composed by two monks, Gottfried and Dieter, incorporating memoirs dictated by Hildegard; and from the fragmentary biography produced by Guibert of Gembloux. Condensed biographical information about Hildegard is available on many internet sources and is included in many scholarly studies, such as Peter Dronke's *Women Writers of the Middle Ages* (1984) and Barbara Newman's *Sister of Wisdom: St. Hildegard's Theology of the Feminine* (1989). A fuller study of her life is Sabina Flanagan's *Hildegard of Bingen, 1098–1179: A Visionary Life* (1989). Hildegard's popularity can be attested to by Routledge's 1998 release of a second and revised edition of that work.

The tenth of her parents' children and, thus, their tithe to God as they dedicated her to the religious life when she was only eight years old, Hildegard of Bingen might, at first glance, seem an unlikely figure to capture the imagination and admiration of a twenty-first century popular audience. Even those who would romanticize the medieval past might have difficulty identifying with a child immured to the world when she was placed in the charge of Jutta of Sponheim, an anchoress whose enclosure was attached to the Benedictine monastery at Disibodenberg, Germany. When Jutta's spirituality attracted more disciples, their cell was eventually transformed into a Benedictine convent. Hildegard professed her vows as a young woman of fifteen or sixteen, committing herself to obedience, stability, and conversion of life under the Rule of St. Benedict. With Jutta's death in 1136, Hildegard was the choice of the other nuns to assume the leadership role. In 1141, after first seeking counsel from Bernard of Clairvaux, she responded to a divine imperative to write about the visions of the living Light that she had experienced since childhood. Ultimately, the increase in nuns and divine instigation prompted Hildegard to move the convent to Rupertsbert, in spite of opposition from church hierarchy. Hildegard proved herself a capable administrator and a prolific writer. Her fame and her convent grew until she founded a second convent at

Eibingen. Hildegard recorded her visions in the *Scivias (Know the Ways of the Lord), Liber vitae meritorum (Book of Life's Merits),* and *Liber divinorum operum (Book of Divine Works).* She also supervised illuminations illustrating her visions; these were probably produced by the nuns in the convent's scriptorium. She is responsible for the first extant morality play, the liturgical drama *Ordo virtutum (Play of the Virtues).* She composed a cycle of seventy-seven songs, *Symphonia harmoniae caelestium revelationum (The Symphony of the Harmony of Heavenly Revelations).* She is often designated Germany's first woman doctor and scientist because of her encyclopedic *Subtilitates naturarum diversarum creaturum (The Subtleties of the Diverse Natures of Created Things),* which includes both her *Causae et curae (Causes and Cures)* and *Physica (Natural History)* or *Liber simplicis medicinae (Books of Simple Medicine).* In addition she carried on such an extensive correspondence with religious and secular figures from all walks of life who sought and received her frank advice that she has been likened to a medieval "Dear Abby" (Petroff 1986, 142). She embarked on four preaching tours, wrote a life of Saints Rupert and Disibod, a treatise on the Benedictine Rule and the Athanasian Creed, and is responsible for an invented language.

Far from silent in her own time, Hildegard continues to speak to our age, most notably in her role as healer, a role that in many ways unifies her other roles as prophet, visionary, abbess, composer, scientist, herbalist, and dramatist. Ruth M. Walker-Moskop has argued for the centrality of healing to all Hildegard's works; she asserts that health "is a unifying theme in each of her books" (1985, 19). In her visionary *Scivias* she "outlines the way to health through faith" as she "describes the way to harmony with God, a necessary prerequisite for a person's internal spiritual and physical health" (1985, 20); in the *Physica* and *Causae et curae* she focuses on "how to promote physical health" by providing a "practical handbook on medicine" in the former and a "holistic philosophy of healing" in the latter (1985, 21); in *Liber vitae meritorum* she writes "a prescription to cure a sick soul" (1985, 22); and in *Liber divinorum operum* she "describes the ultimate cosmic bonds on which human health depends" and provides a "guide for healing the body and soul" (1985, 22). Many are specifically interested in the natural remedies she provides in her scientific works. Her *Natural History,* divided into nine sections, contains descriptions of plants (including about three hundred herbs), animals, metals, stones, and minerals, focusing on their medicinal properties; and the *Causes and Cures,* divided into five sections, discusses the origin and treatment of disease with precise "recipes" for natural treatment. Yet, the philosophy of holistic healing that integrates the health of body and soul articulated in these and her other works is a major reason for her current following. As her own illnesses were pivotal factors in her life, healing the body, the spirit, and the mind was Hildegard's life and work. Her hands-on practice of medicine, her writing, her music, her art all focus on this multifaceted concept of health. To understand Hildegard as healer is to recognize that health is more than the absence of disease or a palliating of the symptoms of disease. According to Walker-Moskup, "Hildegard understands health in a broad, holistic sense. For twelfth-century thinkers, health was clearly a multidimensional concept that involved striving for harmony with God, for inner spiritual harmony, for balance among the physical humors, for concord between soul and body, and for harmony between human beings and the cosmos" (1985, 19). Hence, a 1994 edition of *Causae et curae*, an English translation of the German translation of the Latin text, is entitled *Holistic Healing*— taking liberties with the letter but not the spirit of Hildegard's title.

Although there is some disagreement whether her *Natural History* and her *Causes and Cures* are based on visions, on Hildegard's experience as a practicing physician in the tradition of Benedictine medicine, or on some combination of the two, the material in these scientific works as well as her music, the illuminations accompanying her visions, and her philosophy of holistic health lend themselves to the adaptation of those concerned with alternative medicine with its stress on the importance of balance and harmony in life and components such as proper diet, herbalism, aromatherapy, and sound therapy. Moreover, there are those like Matthew Fox who see Hildegard as affecting more than the health of the individual. Fox argues she is a force for healing society and the church:

> Hildegard gifts us today because she *heals*. She awakens and she heals. She awakens Christianity to some of the wisdom of the ancient women's religions and thereby offers healing to the male/female split in religion. She awakens the psyche to the cosmos and thereby offers healing to both. She awakens to the holiness of the earth and thereby heals the awful split between matter and spirit in the West. She awakens art to science and science to music and religion to science. And thereby heals the dangerous rift between science and religion that has dominated the culture the past three hundred years in the West. (1988, 20)

For Fox, disseminating an understanding of Hildegard's philosophy as it is expressed in her writing, her music, and her art has a therapeutic value that is truly transformative.

Although Hildegard often appeals to those dissatisfied with conventional or orthodox medicine and religion, the philosophy Hildegard espouses is one which in its emphasis on the interrelationship of the physical, mental, emotional, and spiritual is wholeheartedly the product of medieval and Renaissance Christianity. Barbara Newman cautions, "The stunning original-ity of her formulations must not be allowed to obscure her fundamental orthodoxy or her classic Benedictine approach to the spiritual life" (1989, xvii). Likewise, Sabina Flanagan notes, Hildegard is far from unconventional in her time: "Contrary to some modern perceptions of Hildegard, her thought was in many ways more conservative than revolutionary, depending on the time-honored methodology and learning of the monastic milieu in which she spent her life" (1996, 2). From the perspective of this worldview, humankind at creation was in harmony with the divine. Sin injected the discordant note, a cacophony that had a range of physical, emotional, mental, spiritual, and social ramifications. The equation between sin and sickness (both physical and spiritual) is consistent throughout the medieval and Renaissance period. Sin debilitates in a variety of ways. One need only consider Dante's graphic tenth *bolgia*, the Valley of Disease, in circle 8 of *The Inferno*; Edmund Spenser's parade of the seven deadly sins—each afflicted with an appropriately corre-sponding physical malady—in the House of Pride in book 1 of *The Faerie Queene*; John Donne's extended treatment of the analogy between physical and spiritual health in his *Devotions upon Emergent Occasions*; or John Milton's catalog of human suffering in Adam's vision of the Lazar-house in book 11 of *Paradise Lost* as the archangel Michael instructs him about the con-sequences for humankind of the intemperance and disobedience of the first parents. Hildegard is part of an extensive Christian tradition that sees illness as a result of the Fall and recognizes health as more than a physical matter. At the same time Hildegard is also part of a Christian tradition that sees creation as a reflection of the Creator and recognizes both the symbolic and practical use of all aspects of creation. As Katharina M. Wilson notes in her introduc-tion to selections from Hildegard in an anthology of medieval women writers, "For a person of the twelfth century, the world was a storehouse of meaning, all its objects and activities referring ultimately to a realm both transcendent and divine" (1984, 118). Hence, herbs, precious stones, and animals have spe-cial application in the healing process of humankind. Heinrich Schipperges maintains Hildegard's "religious teachings contained nothing new; they sim-ply sought to explain and proclaim traditional doctrine" (1997, 4):

> Hildegard's writings show us the structure of the universe as a unified whole—a universe, though, that is out of joint—and how the parts will be conjoined again for the salvation of humankind. The interrelatedness of everything—humankind and the cosmos, body and spirit, nature and grace—and the interdependence of everything were not just so many

empty words to Hildegard. They went to make up a functional holistic picture of the world, down to the minutest detail. Her entire work is characterized by a clear-headed realism that focuses on the history of salvation: the vision of a world created out of nothing; the creation and fall of humanity; the Incarnation of the son of God; and the resurrection of the body at the end of time. (3–4)

Hildegard's worldview of the interconnectedness of Creator and all of creation is wholly consistent with the Christian tradition she is embedded in and underlies her medical practice.

That medical practice itself was based on conventional science. Elisabeth Brooke in her study of the tradition of women healers notes that Hildegard "was familiar with classical authors such as Pliny and Galen, as well as with contemporary medical texts from Salerno and other medical schools" (1997, 23). Timothy P. Daaleman has examined the way Hildegard was influenced by classical medicine and by the tradition of "monastic medicine" which "assimilated the local traditions which existed outside the cloister walls" (1993, 282). The foreword to *Holistic Healing* acknowledges: "*Holistic Healing*, as a handbook providing information and suggestions in matters of sickness and healing, stands foursquare in the tradition of monastic and popular medicine which itself was based on the medical knowledge of antiquity. Added to this are oral traditions and Hildegard's own experience in medicine and care of the sick. The entire book bears the stamp of the author's faith and Christian culture" (Hildegard 1994, xiii). Hildegard's understanding that disease is the result of an imbalance of the humors (though she makes some significant adaptations) comes from the classics, but she also blends into her practice folk and magical traditions—the latter most notably demonstrated through her use of charms and incantations. The power of these is recognized by her followers today and one can find Hildegardian charms on the internet (webs.linkport.com/~grimnir/magichealing/charms.htm) against mental illness, against bewitchment, to heal jaundice, against melancholy, against migraines, against obsessions, and to ease delivery; others are occasionally included in texts such as Elisabeth Brooke's *Medicine Women* (1997, 35–36).

A key Hildegardian concept, *viriditas,* while uniquely expressed, illustrates Hildegard's orthodoxy. Barbara Newman comments: "*Viriditas* for Hildegard was more than a color; the fresh green that recurs so often in her visions represents the principle of all life, growth, and fertility flowing from the life-creating power of God" (1989, 102). Flanagan notes that even some of Hildegard's cures involving trees "derive their effectiveness by association from other qualities of the tree, such as its vigour or *viriditas,* freshness, or tenderness" (1989, 85).

According to Strehlow and Hertzka, "Hildegard uses the word *viriditas* to refer to all living things, the energy of life which comes from God, the power of youth and of sexuality, the power in seeds, the reproduction of cells, the power of regeneration, freshness, and creativity" (1988, xxvii). In contrast, illness is the drying out of this life-force. Because this life-force comes from God, healing must be more than a physical process. Matthew Fox discusses this core component of Hildegard's belief and imagery and finds three sources for her use of viriditas: Scripture, her environment (the lush Rhine Valley), and her own surge of creativity (1985, 32–33). The Judeo-Christian associations of fructification and dessication are long-standing. The withered garden and the burgeoning Eden have long emblematized the physical, spiritual, and creative status of humanity. The psalmist thirsting for God as the hart for flowing streams (Psalms 42), thirsting for God as his flesh fainted for him "as in a dry and weary land where no water is" (Psalms 63) decried the aridity of the soul cut off from the fountain of life. Edmund Spenser's Colin Clout, the shepherd-poet wasting away physically and spiritually in the "December Eclogue" of *The Shepheardes Calender* laments that the flowers which once bloomed in his garden had withered, their roots dried up for lack of dew. He and his poesy are blighted gardens. Having sinned against Nature and God, Coleridge's ancient mariner is surrounded by undrinkable water. His burning thirst on the sea externalizes the spiritual thirst of the man who has cut himself off from God. In our own time, poets such as T. S. Eliot have led readers through heaps of broken images, dead trees, and dry stones, the wasteland of hollow men. Aridity is sickness, sin, sterility. For the heart is the biblical *hortus conclusus*, the enclosed garden. When its center is God, the fountain of life, grace transforms that garden to the restored Eden raised in the waste wilderness of postlapsarian humanity, the paradise within. The seventeenth century British poet-priest George Herbert compared the sterility of the soul to a withered garden in his poem "Grace" (Hutchinson 1941, 60–61), and in "The Flower" (165–167) he describes the spiritual renewal through grace as he rejoices that his "shrivel'd heart" has "recover'd greenesse" (2.8–9). This influx of grace brings with it the creative spirit: "After so many deaths I live and write" (1.37). Like Hildegard, he associates sin not only with dessication but also with disease as his speaker complains in "The Sinner": "I am all ague" (1.1; see Hutchinson 1941, 38). The pattern is a conventional one: the Christian spirit knows both paradise lost and paradise regained in the cyclic fall and spring of the soul. Adamant in sin, the hardened heart is a cursed ground bearing little fruit; or a *hortus* green with energized life. This is the great Christian narrative that spans the arid deserts of the individual's separation from God (bringing with it physical illness and the drought of creativity) as well as the oases of spiritual renewal when the presence of grace brings harmony with the divine and consequent physical, mental, and emotional well-being. The heart of Hildegard's imagery is very traditionally Christian. Both in spite of and because of her own religious and medical orthodoxy, Hildegard's appeal today is to those looking for alternatives to conventional medicine. Some of her followers are devoted Christians who regard Hildegard as a spokesperson for the divine; others are seeking religious as well as medical alternatives and see Hildegard as the wisdom of the past that legitimates the choices they make. In her doctoral dissertation, Sue Spencer Cannon documented the relevance of Hildegard's medicine for a modern audience: "Hildegard's medicine, in many of its facets, is seriously practiced today in Western society as an alternative to Western bio-medicine by a growing number of people" (1993, 124). In Europe this has been formalized in the practice of Hildegard-medicine, primarily as a result of the work of Dr. Gottfried Hertzka and his successor, Wighard Strehlow. Hertzka, a graduate of the University of Vienna medical school, opened the Hildegard Practice in Konstanz and published several books on Hildegard's medicine. Currently there are in Europe a number of societies, journals, and symposia offered for adherents of Hildegard-medicine. For Hertzka, Hildegard-medicine is of value for reasons "based on the considerations, stemming from his Catholic faith, that Hildegard was not an innovative twelfth-century thinker, but rather a mere conduit through which God revealed his medicine to humankind" (Cannon 1993, 147). Hertzka is one of those who interprets Hildegard's medical material to be a direct result of her visions and sees her functioning as the Holy Ghost's secretary (Cannon 1993, 162). For Hertzka and many others, Hildegard-medicine "is desirable to its adherents because it is medicine from the most knowledgeable source possible: humankind's creator. For the faithful, Hildegard-Medicine becomes a comfort whether an ailment is relieved or not because it allows them the conviction that whatever the outcome, it is the will of God and therefore the best for them" (Cannon 1993, 173).

While the impetus for the formalization of Hildegard-medicine stemmed from Hertzka's Catholic faith, the adaptability and applicability of this practice extends beyond such mainline religious beliefs. Hildegard has gained a significant following among those searching for medical and religious alternatives, including new age adherents. This has occurred for several reasons:

(1) Gender.   As a woman who lived in what is perceived to be an extremely restrictive and chauvinistic age, Hildegard accomplished a great deal and was outspoken in her dealings with a number of male authority figures from abbots and bishops to emperors. Further, her visions of the feminine divine in the form of Sapientia and Caritas, while deriving from the ancient Wisdom

tradition, strike a very modern note. Moreover, she not only discusses matters of human sexuality openly in her writings but specifically treats medical matters of concern to women: "conception and birth, complications in childbirth and gynecological diseases, menstruation and menopause are all extensively described" (Hildegard 1994, xix).[3]

(2) Holistic health.   Her approach to health care is a holistic one that encompasses body, mind, spirit, and cosmos. She believes that the individual is a microcosm of the greater world, that the harmony of both was disrupted as a result of the Fall, and that for true health both must be re-tuned to the divine symphony. Health is more than the absence of symptoms of disease but calls for balance and moderation in all aspects of life and cannot be effected without the operation of grace.

(3) Variety.   Her health care methodology incorporates many aspects from which a modern audience can pick and choose: herbalism, aromatherapy, diet and fasting, laying on of hands, therapeutic stones, prayer and incantation, light energy, sound therapy, art therapy, and hydrotherapy. One need only skim through the table of contents for a reference work such as *Alternative Medicine: The Definitive Guide* (1994) to recognize how relevant the many facets of Hildegard's medicine are today.

(4) Ecological consciousness.   As Matthew Fox argues, "Hildegard is deeply *ecological* in her spirituality" (1985, 8). Because she believes in both the sacrality and the interconnectedness of all creation, she respects Nature and recognizes its power. Those interested in Green Power cannot help but find the Hildegardian image of viriditas intriguing.

When Bear and Company, a new age publisher, provided an English translation of Strehlow and Hertzka's work (1988), basic concepts of Hildegard-medicine were made accessible to a larger and specifically new age audience. As Michael D'Antonio has shown in *Heaven on Earth*, healing is "one of the primary concerns of the New Age": "The New Age has also fostered a proliferation of alternative therapies: herbal medicine, acupressure, Reiki massage, enema therapy, even flower essence treatments. In virtually every case, advocates claim these remedies are based on ancient wisdom and that they bring relief without pain" (1992, 67). The introduction to *Alternative Medicine: The Definitive Guide* reinforces this concept that alternative medicine has a significant tradition:

> The underlying concepts of alternative medicine are not new. They represent a return to the principles that have been part of human understanding

of health and disease for thousands of years. Over the centuries, medical wisdom evolved within a framework which linked health to a state of harmony or balance, and disease to a state of disharmony or imbalance, and took into account the factors that contributed to both. (1994, 5)

References to Hildegard often legitimate alternative treatments. As a twelfth-century visionary and "saint" (albeit uncanonized), she is the "ancient wisdom" that lends a stamp of authority to modern practitioners. She is often referred to in advice provided by modern herbalists. For example, Michael Castleman in *The Healing Herbs: The Ultimate Guide to the Curative Power of Nature's Medicines* cites numerous Hildegardian remedies throughout his book and finds her unique as "the only medieval woman who left any account of 'wise woman' healing practices" (1995, 17). He finds her recommendations for a balanced diet and tooth brushing with aloe and myrrh especially sensible (1995, 7). Rosemary Gladstar in *Herbal Healing for Women* cites Hildegard's recommendation of comfrey for wounds (1993, 237), the inclusion of licorice in her materia medica (1993, 247), and the use of valerian as a sedative (1993, 256). On the internet a page on healing herbs recommends vervain to aid digestion, relieve depression, and ease headaches and aches and pains and points out, "The twelfth-century German abbess and herbalist Hildegard of Bingen prescribed a medicinal tea of vervain and vermouth for 'toxic blood' (infections), toothache and 'discharges from the brain to the teeth'" (www.healthyideas.com/healing/herb/her). The same website also cites Hildegard in its recommendation of cinnamon and notes that she used it "as 'the universal spice for sinuses,' and to treat colds, flu, cancer and 'inner decay and slime,' whatever that means." Yet another website from Snow Mountain Botanicals argues for the importance of valerian as a safe and effective medicine by noting, "Hildegard of Bingin [*sic*], famous abbess/herbalist of Germany, used it as a sedative in the twelfth century" (www.pacific.net/~smb/valerian_notes.html). Another website points to Hildegard's recommendation of tansy to treat a cold and includes a passage from Hildegard on the humors (homepage.rconnect.com/Karyn/colds.htm). The resume for the nutritionist Ward W. Bond of Carol Bond Health Foods not only lists his membership in such organizations as the Herb Research Foundation and the Herbalist Guild but also in the International Society of Hildegard von Bingen (www.carolbond.com/ward.htm). The mention of this twelfth century visionary's name confers authority on the advice and advisors of herbal lore. Moreover, she confers not only authority but the authority of a Western rather than Eastern tradition, an important distinction David Frawley makes in his foreword to the English translation of the Strehlow and Hertzka book as he asserts that Hildegard's "knowledge can help Western herbal medicine return itself to an equal level of sophistication with the Eastern systems that are becoming popular today. Hildegard's medicine, therefore, has a special import today for this regeneration of our own older natural-healing tradition" (1988, ix).

Authentication through association with Hildegard occurs not only with herbalists but also with those concerned with the therapeutic use of stones. As Si and Ann Frazier remark, "A small portion of her commentaries describes the medicinal uses of gemstones, a fact that makes Hildegard von Bingen very big among those with a 'metaphysical' interest in minerals, the phenomenon that has put the word 'crystal' into the everyday vocabularies of many people who previously never gave minerals a thought" (1998, 34). The Fraziers note Hildegard's popularity in German and Swiss metaphysical circles and her increasing popularity in the United States. Cannon writes of attending a symposiu:n on Hildegard in Engelberg, Switzerland, in 1991: "I met several people who, following Hildegard's advice, wore pelts or jewelry which they believed had healing and protective qualities. My symposium session neighbor, Frau Grun, who told me that she specialized in Hildegard's lapidary medicine, sincerely believed in the healing powers of semi-precious stones as described by Hildegard" (1993, 170). Hildegard included material on twenty-six precious stones in her *Natural History*. On her use of gems, Frawley comments,

> Like the medieval alchemists with whom she has much in common, Hildegard integrates the use of gems and minerals into her usage of herbs. She recommends such remedies as gold for arthritis, emerald for heart pain, jasper for hay fever or for cardiac arrhythmia, gold topaz for loss of vision, and blue sapphire for eye inflammation. She uses gem wines, similar to the gem tinctures now being used more widely today. (Strehlow and Hertzka 1988, xii)

As with her comments on herblore, her lapidary prescriptions are part of an important Western tradition for those who believe in the medicinal use of crystals and stones today.

For Hildegard, music served an important liturgical function. As a reflection of divine harmony, music could both praise the deity and bring the individual into harmony with God. Fox regards Hildegard's music as "cosmic" and says of *The Symphony of the Harmony of Heavenly Revelations* that Hildegard "expressed musically and poetically her deep mystical experiences of the Cosmic Christ. She believed that singing of words reveals their true meaning directly to the soul through bodily vibrations. Even today these songs evoke mystical experiences in those who sing them" (1988, 110). And, indeed, her music is seen to elicit both mystical and healing experiences. One of the forms of alternative medicine practiced by some Hildegardian followers is sound therapy, a belief in the therapeutic power of sound. A web page maintained by Bison Publishers on Sound and Healing notes,

> Each and every person has a core sound, a vibration or set of vibrations that emanate from our being and our body. Sounding this sound restores us to balance, aligns our energies, releases our powers. When we are diseased, our bodies vibrate in dissonance to our being. We can help ourselves return to health and balance by recalling and reinforcing our natural sound vibrations. You can sing yourself back to health. This is the essence of sound healing.

Arguing that this is not a new concept but one that was recognized by "ancient tribes of humankind," this document also cites Hildegard as an ancient practitioner who "employed these sounds to effect change in the real world of here and now." The site designed "to provide a bibliography of recorded, printed and Web-published resources on the use of sound for healing" includes information about Hildegard's music (www.bison.com/healing.html). The web page of Norma Gentile also testifies to the importance of Hildegard's music as part of a healing methodology. Gentile is a professional singer, vocal coach, and auric healer. She has recorded two CDs of Hildegard's music, *Meditation Chants* and *Unfurling Love's Creation.* In an article from *Continuo* magazine (www.continuo.com/oct97/gentile3.htm), she discusses her discovery of Hildegard's music and her own role as healer and musician. Through Hildegardian chants she experienced "healing currents in sound" and now performs concerts, offers workshops, and leads seminars in the use of sound for healing and meditation. Like Matthew Fox, who sees Hildegard offering a "radical opportunity for global religious ecumenism" (1985, 16), she is impressed by the diversity of those interested in Hildegard, the ecumenical outreach Hildegard encompasses. Gentile writes,

> In the past year I've shared Hildegard's music with a Motherhouse of nuns, a Wiccan conference, a gathering of feminists, members of the Creation Spirituality movement, scholars attending an International Medieval Studies Institute, and religious groups from mainstream Catholics to liberal Protestants and the metaphysical Unity Church. I am amazed by the entry that Hildegard's music allows me into different worlds.

In addition, a website for Healing Yoga classes provides a catalog of music used in these classes. One of the offerings includes Richard Souther's *The Music of Hildegard von Bingen* with the notation that this CD is appropriate for use with the Sun Salutations series (www.io.com/helingyoga/cd.html). Just as Hildegard maintains an active role as healer through her literary work, she also continues to function as healer through her music. Nancy Fierro explains, "The word 'symphonia,' or symphony, had a special meaning for Hildegard. Living in symphony meant living a life of virtue in tune with the harmonious praises of the nine choirs of angels in paradise. Such a life would be inspired, filled with Divine purpose, and so powerful that everything would work together for the person in a harmonious way" (1994, 24). In other words, Hildegard believed music could effect the holistically healthy individual. Many of Hildegard's followers believe that as well and see her music as especially effective in this health process.

The illuminations of Hildegard's visions are also perceived as therapeutic, especially in her use of the mandala, that magic sphere Carl G. Jung—a major influence for many new agers—saw as a "symbolic representation of the 'nuclear atom' of the human psyche" (1964, 213). Jung believed many cultures used the mandala as a healing tool to restore psychic balance, to bring the sick individual "back into harmony with himself and with the cosmos" (1964, 213). Fox perceives Hildegard's mandalas as fulfilling such a healing function for her and for others:

> Readers and pray-ers of Hildegard's illuminations will see many examples of mandalas, those "Maps of the cosmos" developed in East as well as in the medieval West to "liberate the consciousness" and return us to a primeval consciousness which is fundamentally one of unity. Clearly, Hildegard's illuminations played that role with herself, a role of reintegration and holistic relating, which is her intention in sharing them with others that they too may be healed. For Hildegard, her mandalas become a primary means by which the microcosm/macrocosm, the human and the universe, are brought together again. (1985, 16)

Fox points to the way Hildegard through these illuminations enables us to "connect" with an "'essential pattern'" and thus "to find God again, to find salvation or healing for self and others" (1985, 25). Like Fox, others see Hildegardian mandalas as both salubrious and salvific. A website on healing and dreams maintained by Harry Bosma stresses the importance of mandalas (www.xs4all.nl/~hbosma/healing_dreams/mandala.html) and includes a depiction of *Tree of Life* "painted by Hildegard of Bingen" with information on how to access others of her mandalas on the Bonnie Duncan website. "Veriditas: The World Wide Labyrinth Project," developed by Rev. Dr. Lauren Artress of Grace Cathedral in San Francisco, has been much influenced by the illuminations of Hildegard. The project itself is "committed to reintroduce the labyrinth in its many forms as a spiritual tool. Its deeply healing qualities have been lying dormant for centuries so labyrinths need to be established in cathedrals, churches, retreat centers, hospitals, prisons, parks, airports and community spaces around the world" (www.gracecom.org/veriditas/press/sfpresskit.shtml). Dr. Artress presents workshops and lectures worldwide on labyrinths and on Hildegard and planned to conduct a tour in 1998, "Labyrinths of Europe: Walking a Sacred Path," that included a stay at Bingen to participate in the festivities connected with the celebration of Hildegard's nine-hundredth anniversary (www.noetic.org/Travel/labyrinths.html). A licensed psychotherapist, Dr. Artress sees the labyrinth as a mandala that can bring healing change to the individual and society. "Earth Echo," a website maintained by artist Fred Casselman, contains a section on healing images and features "images empowered to assist in our personal and planetary healing" (www.earthecho.com/heal/_healing.html). One of the galleries includes a painting titled *Fires of Saint Hildegard*, dedicated to her with the comment "We love you Saint Hildegard." The Word Gallery has an artistic rendering of the following phrase from Hildegard. The first five lines radiate from a circle formed by the words of the last two lines:

The earth should not be injured
The earth should not be destroyed
As often as the elements, the elements of the world
Are violated by ill-treatment. So God will cleanse them
God will cleanse them thru the suffering, thru the hardships of
    humankind.
God desires that all the world
Be pure in his sight.

At the center of the circle we find the words "Hildegard of Bingen." The image visually illustrates the importance of healing Mother Earth which Matthew Fox sees as one of Hildegard's roles. Information is also included on other websites where one might gain information about Hildegard (www.earth echo.com/words/hild.html). "Earth Echo" affirms the power of art to heal and celebrates the individual, ecological, and cosmic power of Hildegard's healing art.

One of the more remarked upon aspects of Hildegard's life has been her longevity in an age of typically abbreviated life-spans. Even more remarkable is the longevity of her healing practice. Today, through technology, her medical practice may be more extensive than it was in her lifetime as she continues to apply her healing touch through the dissemination of her writing, music, and art. While some may scoff at the popular appropriation of her work by an audience largely incapable of reading her material in the Latin original and not fully aware of the religious, historical, literary, and musical traditions that contextualize her, the same might well be said of her contemporary patients. Hildegard speaks to the learned and the unlearned, to those in the mainstream of religious tradition and those on the periphery. The proliferation of books, CDs, and internet resources clearly indicates the number of people turning to her for healing of the body, of the spirit, and of the earth. Representative of their need is one web page that contains an illumination of Hildegard at work, a depiction of the current Abbey of St. Hildegard in Ibingen, Germany, and an eloquent prayer lamenting the pain of individual souls and of the earth itself. The prayer calls upon Hildegard for help:

> Guide us to participate in the healing of suffering souls. Let us restore the earth and her children to the joy of singing to You. Find the musical tones that once played the Fall. Teach us to sing with the Angels, Saints, and our Ancestors, in the praise and worship of the Trinity. (ourworld.compuserve.com/homepages/PTBrown/)

Viriditas: through the wisdom preserved in her writings, through herbal remedies, charms and lapidary prescriptions, through music and art, the evergreen voice of Hildegard of Bingen endures today as her writings, music, and art provide answers to the prayers of the sick who come to her for holistic healing.

NOTES

1. The novels are Barbara Lachman's *The Journal of Hildegard of Bingen* (1996) and Joan Ohanneson's *Scarlet Music* (1997). The British composer Brian Inglis completed the opera *Hildegard of Bingen* in June 1997 (www.composer.co/uk/composers/inglis.html). An informative video is *Radiant Life: Meditations on the Life of Hildegard of Bingen* from Wellspring Media (1996). The film in progress is the work of Jeanne Spicuzza and her Seasons and a Muse Productions (www.charmrec.com/jeanne/hilde.htm).
2. Two of the best places to discover web resources for Hildegard are the list maintained by the University of Mainz (www.uni-mainz.de/~horst/hildegard/links/links.html) and the links provided with information about the Greenest Branch Conference as part of the celebration of Hildegard's nine-hundredth birthday (www.trinityvt.edu/hildegard/internet.htm). All websites referred to in this chapter were accessed in the summer of 1998.
3. For a fuller treatment of this subject, see Fiero (1994) and Newman (1989).

REFERENCES

Alternative medicine: The definitive guide. 1994. Fife, Washington: Future Medicine Publishing.

Brooke, Elisabeth. 1997. *Medicine women: A pictorial history of women healers.* Wheaton, Illinois: Quest Books.

Cannon, Sue Spencer. 1993. The medicine of Hildegard of Bingen: Her twelfth-century theories and their twentieth-century appeal as a form of alternative medicine. Ph.D. diss., University of California, Los Angeles.

Castleman, Michael. 1995. *The healing herbs: The ultimate guide to the curative power of nature's medicines.* New York: Bantam.

Daaleman, Timothy P. 1993. The medical world of Hildegard of Bingen. *American Benedictine Review* 44: 280–89.

D'Antonio, Michael. 1992. *Heaven on earth.* New York: Crown.

Dronke, Peter. 1984. *Women writers of the middle ages.* Cambridge: Cambridge University Press.

Fiero, Nancy. 1994. *Hildegard of Bingen and her vision of the feminine.* Kansas City, Missouri: Sheed and Ward.

Flanagan, Sabina. 1989. *Hildegard of Bingen, 1098–1179: A visionary life.* London: Routledge.

———. 1996. *Secrets of God: Writings of Hildegard of Bingen.* Boston: Shambala.

Fox, Matthew. 1985. *Illuminations of Hildegard of Bingen.* Santa Fe, New Mexico: Bear and Co.

———. 1988. *The coming of the cosmic Christ: The healing of mother earth and the birth of a global renaissance.* San Francisco: Harper.

Frazier, Si, and Ann Frazier. 1998. Woman of the millennium. *Lapidary Journal,* June, 32–36, 86.

Gladstar, Rosemary. 1993. *Herbal healing for women.* New York: Simon and Schuster.

Hildegard von Bingen. 1994. *Holistic healing.* Ed. Mary Palmquist and John Kulas. Trans. from Latin by Manfred Pawlik; trans. from German by Patrick Madigan. Collegeville, Minnesota: Liturgical Press.

Hutchinson, F. E., ed. [1941] 1945. *The works of George Herbert.* Oxford: Clarendon.

Jung, Carl G., et al. 1964. *Man and his symbols.* New York: Doubleday.

Lachman, Barbara. 1996. *The journal of Hildegard of Bingen.* New York: Crown.

Newman, Barbara. 1989. *Sister of wisdom: St. Hildegard's theology of the feminine.* Berkeley: University of California Press.

Ohanneson, Joan. 1997. *Scarlet music.* New York: Crossroads.

Petroff, Elizabeth Alvilda, ed. 1986. *Medieval women's visionary literature.* Oxford: Oxford University Press.

Schipperges, Henirich. 1997. *Hildegard of Bingen: Healing and the nature of the cosmos.* Trans. John A. Broadwin. Princeton: Markus Wiener Publishers.

Strehlow, Wighard, and Gottfried Hertzka. 1988. *Hildegard of Bingen's medicine.* Trans. Karin Anderson Strehlow. Santa Fe, New Mexico: Bear and Co.

———. 1996. *Radiant life: Meditations on the life of Hildegard of Bingen.* New York: Wellspring Media.

Walker-Moskop, Ruth M. 1985. Health and cosmic continuity: Hildegard of Bingen's unique concerns. *Mystics Quarterly* 11: 19–25.

Wilson, Katharina M., ed. 1984. *Medieval women writers.* Athens, Georgia: University of Georgia Press.

taking it in: the observer healed

9

REFLECTIONS ON THE EXPERIENCE OF HEALING: WHOSE LOGIC? WHOSE EXPERIENCE?

BONNIE GLASS-COFFIN

Once again, the ninth week of a ten-week quarter in introductory anthropology had arrived. For eight weeks I had stressed how comparison and objectivity in anthropological research has helped us make sense of subjects as varied as human evolution and human activity patterns, the logic of kinship, and economic systems. Now it was time to turn from a discussion of anthropology as science to a discussion of anthropology as an interpretive discipline. It was time to focus class attentions on the variety of meanings with which social groups inscribe human experience and on the role of "culture" in shaping these.

I was at once relieved and anxious. Relieved because I was heading into an area that, for me, is familiar territory. With a research emphasis in shamanism and theoretical interests in interpretive anthropology and the anthropology of religion, I felt comfortable in presenting the hermeneutic side of anthropology to my students. Additionally, this was the time of the quarter when I would present accounts of my own fieldwork to my students—when I could speak about the discipline with "ethnographic authority." But, I was also anxious—as I had been in every previous ninth week of every quarter that I had taught Anthropology 101. I was anxious because of the inevitable questions I knew I would be asked as students responded to the presentation of my fieldwork experience. For mine is a fieldwork experience rich in the discussion of spirit entities, of soul loss and recovery, of hexing and curing, and of the envy between friends and family that underlies a desire to seek out sorcerers and to cause intentional harm.

THE ACCOUNT

I began by telling my students how I became interested in studying anthropology while living in Trujillo, a sprawling city located eight hours north of Lima in the heart of Peru's coastal desert. There, as an exchange student for eleven months in 1975 –76, I lived with a middle-class family and attended a Catholic high school. After conquering the culture shock, estrangement, and ennui so commonly experienced by those who step outside the boundaries of their own cultural traditions, I began to feel very much at home in this far-away place. Over the course of my stay I mastered the language and became quite comfortable with the roles of daughter, sister, and student into which I was being socialized. I came to the (premature) conclusion that underneath the veneer of culture, people are pretty much the same wherever you go.

Then one day, a good friend (whom I'll call Sylvia) told me very matter-of-factly that her grandmother had died because of sorcery. According to the account, the grandmother had taken a pitchfork to her neighbor's guinea pigs when they invaded and destroyed her garden. A few weeks later, the neighbor celebrated a birthday and, as is customary, she prepared a feast to entertain all the guests who would drop by her home to extend their best wishes. Sylvia's grandmother, still smarting from the guinea pig incident, didn't go to the celebration. The neighbor, as a kind of "peace offering," sent over a large portion of roast pork from the feast she had prepared for the well-wishers. But, after accepting and eating the pork, Sylvia's grandmother became very ill, suffering stomach pains, nausea, diarrhea, dehydration, and weight loss.

Sylvia hurriedly took her grandmother to the doctor. She suspected that the grandmother was suffering from a food- or water-borne parasitic infection. But the tests revealed nothing. After more tests and a trip to a private clinic to consult a medical specialist, the infectious cause of her suffering was still a mystery. Finally, desperate to help her grandmother, Sylvia took her to a *curandero*—a kind of healer who specializes in diagnosing and treating sorcery.

During the all-night session (called a *mesa*) the curandero—like shamanic healers in other cultural traditions—"saw" behind the veil of ordinary reality and communed with spirit entities who might know the cause of the old woman's suffering. He told Sylvia's grandmother that, wanting revenge, the neighbor had swept up the impression left by the grandmother's footprint and had taken it to a sorcerer. He saw how the sorcerer had given the neighbor *hueso de muerto* (powdered human bone) to slip into the roast pork. He explained that when Sylvia's grandmother ate the pork, she sealed her doom. Unfortunately, according to the healer, the sorcery was *pasado*—it had been done too long before—and he would be unable to undo the harm. As

Sylvia finished recounting the story she sighed deeply, "If only we had gone to a healer earlier we might have saved her. But she died within the month."

In an aside to my students, I described how the healers I've worked with have explained sorcery to me. I told them how, according to their logic (and while under the influence of a hallucinogenic mixture brewed from the San Pedro or *Trichocereus pachanoi* cactus), the curandero would have seen the ritual in which the sorcerer effected the magic that would eventually kill my friend's grandmother. This magic would have consisted of the sorcerer "calling" the grandmother's shadow-soul away from her body. This ability to lure the shadow-soul into leaving the grandmother's body and appearing before the mesa would be possible through the use of sympathetic magic. Like a photograph, the image of her footprint which had been gathered up would serve as a kind of double or "stand-in" for the grandmother and the shadow-soul would come to the mesa because of it. Once her shadow-soul presented itself, the sorcerer would have persuaded one of his allies—probably an *ánima* or spirit of the dead—to imprison the grandmother's shadow so that it couldn't return to her body. The hueso de muerto given to the neighbor would be from a cadaver whose spirit had been unable to rise to heaven because of sins committed in this life. Ingesting this powder would seal the bond between the grandmother's shadow-soul and that of the ánima, so that her shadow-soul would not be able to return to her body. If her soul were not released within a set amount of time by the magical interventions of a healer, the result of this forced separation would be sickness and death. Accordingly, her symptoms would reflect the kind of sorcery she had ingested. Because her shadow-soul was tied to that of a cadaver, she would become more and more emaciated and cadaver-like as her conditions worsened.

THE REACTION

As I had done in previous terms, after finishing the story I looked around the room and tried to read my students' reactions. I asked for "comments, questions, concerns . . . ?" and let the silence that followed do its work. One student—an anthropology major—suggested that we should not be ethnocentric in our assessment of my friend's belief in sorcery. "Even if sorcery doesn't make sense to us, it is part of their culture and we can't judge it by any other standards," the student insisted. Then, several others students who were obviously less indoctrinated in this anthropological paradigm of cultural relativism asked what most students in the room want to know whenever I tell this story. "Does sorcery *really* exist or is a patient's suffering just 'in their heads'? Is it the patient's belief in sorcery that *actually* causes their

affliction or are there *really* spirit powers that sorcerers and healers manip-
ulate? Do *you* believe in it, Dr. Glass-Coffin?"

The First Response: The Logic of Sorcery

These are the questions which underscore my anxiety when I present this
material to my students. In part, the anxiety arises from the fact that I have no
ready answers. The scientific method does not easily lend itself to measuring
the activity of spirit entities and whether observable consequences result from
"good" or "evil" intentions. Translating belief into seemingly culture-free
physiological consequences attributed to placebo and nocebo effects may satisfy the interrogator as to the mechanisms by which sorcery and healing are
translated into body function, but it doesn't negate the fact that underlying
causes for cultural belief may, in fact, exist in the "real" world. Neither does it
explain how sorcery can affect the unbeliever.[1] Also, such reductionistic
responses undermine the very anthropological contributions to human
understanding that makes our discipline important.

Specifically, anthropological theory and practice has shown the power of
cultural belief and tradition in shaping perceptions, not only of our "informants" but also of the researcher and the audience.[2] As Richard Robbins (1997,
80–87) has shown, magic is invoked to explain physical events because of
selective perception, rationalization, secondary elaboration, and appeals to
faith, mystery, or authority. Tanya Luhrmann (1989) has used the term "interpretive drift" to label the process by which people come to view magic as an
efficacious and rational explanation of events (even in the face of contradictory evidence). According to her analysis, interpretive drift includes three elements, which might be summarized as perceptual or cognitive, affective, and
intellectual or analytical. In her model, a ritual participant experiences some
kind of catharsis, revelation, insight, or direct numinous experience that provides emotional rather than cognitive certainty of veracity. Whether preceding, concurrent, or as a consequence of this experience, the participant also
experiences basic shifts in perception and analysis of observable events, and
concludes that human will or spirit power has, indeed, influenced these.
Finally, the participant seeks intellectual strategies to explain the phenomenon
experienced that minimizes dissonance or disjunction between magical and
scientific explanations of observable consequences.

In the account described above (as well as the scores of stories I have been
told by victims in the twenty-plus years since my first encounter with Peruvian
sorcery), interpretive drift can be used to make sense of sorcery as follows:[3] an
individual experiences some kind of suffering and attempts to relieve the

symptoms. If symptoms are somatic, and if the victim has had no previous experience with sorcery, he or she will first rely on home remedies or pharmaceutical products and will seek information about how to alleviate the symptoms from family, friends, or health care professionals. If symptoms do not subside after exhausting all biomedical resources, the victim will pragmatically seek other alternatives. In the search for explanation, the victim will likely be urged by someone who has had a similar experience with symptoms that did not respond to medical treatment to consider sorcery as a possibility.[4]

When they visit a curandero, these suspicions are likely to be confirmed. During the ritual curing session, the healer will often describe how another's envy or unexpressed hostilities towards the victim led them to seek out the services of a sorcerer to cause the suffering. If the narrative fits the victim's already conscious suspicions, or brings to consciousness previously unacknowledged anxieties, the victim will likely experience both catharsis and insight. If the victim did not previously believe in the power of spirits and the evil intentions of family and friends, he or she will probably experience a temporary shift in worldview to accommodate these possibilities. Then, depending on the victim's faith in the healer's ability to undo the sorcery and effect a cure, expectations may be raised, and a wholehearted embrace of the healer's instructions may take place, replacing resignation to suffering with hope and a determination to overcome.[5]

Of course, this process of interpretive drift is not limited to a discussion of the efficacy of shamanic healing for explaining otherwise unexplainable suffering (sorcery) and healing (via participation in a healer's mesa). Similar "shifts" seem to occur in all kinds of "symbolic" healing including psychotherapy (Lévi-Strauss 1963; Scheff 1979; Achterberg 1985; Dow 1986; Torrey 1986). Regardless of healing tradition, these cognitive, affective, and analytical shifts generally include the following elements: first, there is acceptance of both the illness label and the etiology that an expert assigns to the experience of suffering. Second, the victim experiences emotional engagement or catharsis. This leads to an experiential change in consciousness associated with "insight" or "revelation" about the cause of affliction as well as to confidence in the chosen healer and expectation of cure. Finally, the victim's new sense of insight and confidence in the healer who facilitated this shift in awareness leads the victim to have a sense of mastery over the illness.

Thus, interpretive drift provides a very rational explanation for seemingly irrational belief and practice (Luhrmann 1989, 7). However, when researchers invoke this process as a means of dismissing the veracity of magic or the potential harm of sorcery, they sometimes underplay the fact that *all* paradigms—including the kind of observational positivism commonly, glossed as "science"—limit perception. Just as Evans-Pritchard suggested for the magically oriented Nuer (1956), our paradigms work to keep us from having to face contradiction.

The following example will suffice to illustrate this point. In a recent article, C. Roderick Wilson (1994) recounts how one informant, when asked to describe a strongly bluish color card with an indigenous color term, described the card as "leaf-colored." Wilson and a fellow researcher had seen many leaves in the months they had spent with these people but they had never seen blue ones. So, they asked the man to demonstrate just where he had seen a leaf of that color. Without rising, the informant pointed to some trees on a faraway hillside and the two social scientists had to admit that the color matched perfectly. Wilson describes his point as follows:

> As members of scientifically oriented North American culture, [we] "knew" that forested hillsides that appear to be bluish or purplish are in fact "normal" green. Moreover, we both knew that the apparent color change has to do with such phenomena as the diffraction of light, the existence of particulate matter in the air, and so on. To put it another way, we carried around with us scientific explanations of natural phenomena that allowed us to "normalize" observations, to bring observations that ran counter to the usual into conformity with the expected. I have no serious doubt that these particular "scientific" explanations are essentially correct. But still, I am concerned about the fact that my vision is so "normalized" that I could not see what was literally in front of my face. (1994, 199)

THE SECOND RESPONSE: THE LOGISTICS OF SORCERY

While the above paragraphs make sense of magic by problematizing reason, an alternative view has been to assert that the practice of magic has more to do with logistics than with logic. Advanced by social scientists, this response sidesteps altogether a discussion of the relationship between belief and practice. (It can also provide the anxious professor a way to avoid the question about what he or she *personally* thinks). Instead, this response looks at the *utility* of cultural beliefs for solving real-world problems. The "functionalists" assert that magic provides explanations for the otherwise unexplainable or manages the tension between individual desire and social imperative. The "structuralists" assert that magic is invoked to explain and to give shape to an otherwise incoherent reality. The "symbolists" contend that magic is metaphor—a way of expressing meaning poetically.[6]

In the Peruvian case, functional views of sorcery draw attention to the conflict between fierce competition for limited resources and the structured relations of social dependence. In this light, sorcery is seen as a projective mechanism for inexpressible hostilities. Alternatively, because the fear of sorcery can help diffuse expressions of conflict between the individually desirable and the socially necessary, it has been considered a means of social control.

Structural views of sorcery (with their predilection for illuminating the dichotomous categories of deep structure and how these are glossed with meaning) focus on the way Peruvians have accommodated tensions between pre-Columbian and post-conquest worldviews. Before the arrival of Catholicism in the mid 1500s and before the ensuing campaigns to "extirpate idolatries," pre-Columbian cosmologies explained dualism in natural, social, and spiritual relations in terms of a moral code that was both complementary and ambiguous. Both order and chaos, good and evil, culture and nature, man and woman (or any other paired opposite that can be named) were necessary for the proper functioning of the universe. But after the Spanish conquest, an imposed Christian paradigm viewed these universal forces as absolute and contradictory. Both "good" and "evil" were reified, and Peruvian sorcery—at least as we know it today—was born.

Symbolic views of sorcery provide outsiders with a means of "teasing apart" the absolute and the relative in human existence. Suffering and, ultimately, death are universal phenomena, but they are expressed (and experienced) in widely different ways cross-culturally. Symbolic studies of sorcery focus on the meaning that is given to these experiences in specific contexts (physical, social, economic, and political). Thus, they give outsiders insight into the key role played by culture for shaping, contesting, and resisting responses to these realities.

But implicit in all these strategies—whether functional, structural, or symbolic—is an assertion of cultural relativism that smacks of ethnocentrism. Beneath the apparent epistemological generosity of the relativist argument lies a dangerous disclaimer—what may be true for *others* is not at all true for *ourselves*. To draw again from Wilson's article on the subject, he reports the following curious phenomenon: when he brought a Cree medicine man to his classroom to discuss illness etiologies and healing cosmologies, he notes that his students listened with rapt attention and respect. But when he later suggested that shamanic practices are dynamic—that they have a pragmatic basis for their continued practice and should therefore be considered scientifically, his students patently denied this possibility. As he concludes, "Beliefs or practices which can be accorded respect by reasonably enlightened people when encountering aboriginal populations are dismissed from serious consideration within our own intellectual tradition . . . the moment an attempt is made to bring alien beliefs and practices into the arena of scientific investigation, one is dismissed as a crank" (Wilson 1994, 201).

THE THIRD RESPONSE: INTERSUBJECTIVITY IN LOGIC AND EXPERIENCE

What alternatives exist to "explaining away" that which is beyond our vision as delusion, as metaphor, or as simply functionally proscribed? The authors of a recent collection on the anthropology of extraordinary experience recommend taking sacred worldviews seriously. They also ask researchers to entertain the possibility that an informant's explanation of an extraordinary experience might be true instead of dismissing their accounts a priori as fantasy or superstition. This is not the same as wholeheartedly accepting these accounts without skepticism—which is tantamount to "going native" and which negates our ability to translate responses to other audiences. Neither is it the same thing as stepping outside our paradigms when interpreting the world around us, for this is a difficult, if not impossible, task (Pandian 1985). But this response demands awareness that *all* explanations, including our own, are limited by paradigmatic persuasions.

One way to challenge our own perceptions and to come to a closer realization of the intersections of paradigm and practice is through extended fieldwork and firsthand experience of the kinds of phenomena which our informants explain in magical terms. This approach to ethnographic research has been termed "experiential" (Goulet and Young 1994, 304) or "radically empirical" (Jackson 1989). The rationale for this kind of fieldwork stems partly from the assertion that personal experience "becomes a mode of experimentation, of testing and exploring the ways in which our experiences conjoin or connect us with others, rather than the ways they set us apart" (Goulet and Young 1994, 305). In other words, by living and doing as our informants do, we may at least approximate what it is like to see the world through their eyes. By using ourselves as "primary data," we become able to comment on that which is not observable, except through our own experience. In short, experiential fieldwork allows us to explore the possibility (also raised by Luhrmann) that people come to believe in the reality of magic *after* experiencing effective results rather than the other way around.

If an experiential approach to fieldwork allows us to, at least temporarily, step into a new physical (and phenomenological) space, it also moves us to conclude that reality is shaped somewhere in the interstices between external event and the perception or meaning given it. As Goulet and Young put it, interpretation and understanding certainly go hand in hand with that of "experience" (1994, 313). They give the analogy of language acquisition to illustrate their point:

> In the context of repeated and prolonged exposure to members of a linguistic community, a process of assimilation occurs, involving a level of schemata formation of which even the individual who is assimilating the language is unaware. The anthropologist comes to live, as it were, in an acoustic world distinct from that which prevails in his or her own culture. Similarly the anthropologist may come to inhabit other domains of the native speaker's society, be it kinship, economic, or ritual, attending to socially constituted realities that would otherwise remain beyond his or her reach. (1994, 314)

In other words, meaning is "intertwined with intersubjectivity, and communication codes can best be understood in performances where the meaning is created."[7]

In my own fieldwork with northern Peruvian shamans, I came to realize how the intersections of ontological structure, perceived meaning, and intersubjectivity change the lives of both the researcher and the research subject one sunny day in November 1988. On that occasion, an amber-colored bottle that occupied a central space on the healing altar of my primary informant broke. In terms of the event itself, the breakage was a direct result of her taking out the mesa on a day I had asked to photograph the sacred objects on her altar. Had I not intervened in her life, the bottle would not have broken (at least, not at that particular time). At the time of the breakage, she and I both assumed the event to be of little significance. But six months later, while under the influence of the psychoactive San Pedro cactus, she learned that the breakage of that little bottle would shorten her life span by one-third. She exhorted me on that occasion to "make something of your life, so that this event, which has shortened my life and for which you were responsible, will not have been for nothing." Her invocation has stayed with me as a touchstone since that day and has had a profound impact on every aspect of my existence.

Finally, to return to the question of the definition of "rational" scientific inquiry and the way this is often contrasted with "irrational" claims of the veracity of magic, I would remind the reader that, at its root, the scientific method is empirical and that empiricism is based as much in experience as in observation. As Ken Wilber suggests in his latest work, scientific inquiry does not necessarily preclude a serious investigation of the numinous. Instead of dismissing that which is difficult to measure or observe as patently "unscientific," we should seek new ways to measure, replicate, and validate empirical experiences that go beyond those available to a detached, "objective" observer.

Conclusion: Experience Reconsidered

So, what does all this have to do with the question that my students ask and my anxieties about answering it? Does sorcery really exist? And *how* does it work? Is it "just" a question of belief and of neuropsychological processes that result from emotional engagement with a set of symbols? Or is there "really" some essential, yet largely invisible, force that certain individuals have the ability to tap into in order to alter the physical world? And, if this force is nonexistent, why do we have so many recorded instances of so-called supernatural phenomena in folklore and in the anthropological record (Walker 1995)? Called things like god, devil, vital energy, psi, or electromagnetism depending on the worldviews of the one doing the labeling, there are multiple millions of people who share such beliefs. Have they all been duped? In other words, do psychological theories of projective mechanisms, sociological theories of functionalism and social control mechanisms, or cognitive analyses of varying worldviews adequately account for the continued practice of magical rituals among otherwise rational (and highly literate, technologically sophisticated) people?

Based on my own dissertation fieldwork with female curanderas from 1987 to 1989, I know that shifts in perception are personally unconvincing if not accompanied by direct experience. I also know that the reality of magic exists somewhere between the ontology of structure and the inscription of meaning. Did I undergo interpretive drift while in the field? Undoubtedly. Did this interpretive drift influence my perception of external phenomena? Probably. Certainly, I was much more attuned to the night cries of distant animals, the appearance of the night sky, and to meteorological phenomena when I left Peru in 1989 than when I first arrived. I also reconceptualized my own attitudes and values while in the field based on the moral principles of "good" and "evil" which I saw in others (and experienced in myself). I was changed by my fieldwork and I saw sorcery change the lives of many other people.

But during my stay in this enchanted country, I also saw phenomena that I cannot explain, and experienced states that I cannot replicate. I know them to be true as certainly as I know the color of the leaves on the trees outside my office window. Among these events, I have seen a healer produce rain in a cloudless sky and I have also seen the rain cease instantly when commanded. I have witnessed the extinguishing of starlight in the night sky as if at the touch of a light switch.[8] I have seen visions, both under the influence of hallucinogens and in what has been called an "ordinary" state of consciousness.

I also know that I interpret these shared experiences differently than do either the healers or the victims of sorcery that I worked with. This is so because the meaning I give to life experiences comes from my own stock of knowledge which has been gathered in the course of a lifetime of events that predate as well as postdate my immersion into the ethnographic experience. My understanding is as Wagner (1981, 12) has suggested. In his words, "what the fieldworker invents . . . is his own understanding; the analogies he creates are extensions of his own notions and those of his culture, transformed by his experiences in the field situation."[9] Because I have no cultural logic with which to attach these experiences I find sorcery a difficult concept to grasp at a phenomenological level.

Thus, when students ask if sorcery exists, I usually hesitate and then answer in the affirmative, or admit that I do not yet know. For, to suggest that sorcery only exists at the intersection of meaning and experience seems too reminiscent of the culturally relative response that explains away the relevance of sorcery with arguments of functionalism, structuralism, or metaphoric meaning. But to assert that sorcery exists because I experienced phenomena which I can't explain both violates phenomenological principles of my own paradigms and falls short of the standards of validity and reliability which my students mainly share. And so, until I can articulate a model for explaining sorcery that makes sense both to me and to my students without violating the claims of my informants,[10] my "ninth-week anxiety" will not (and should not) abate. My students will have to learn to live with the ambiguities of empiricism. And, as researchers, we should continue to consider the role of experience in anthropology—as both science and interpretive discipline.

NOTES

I extend my heartfelt thanks to Erika Brady, David Hufford, Bonnie O'Connor, Barre Toelken, Barbara Walker, and all the fine faculty fellows of the Fife Folklore Conferences who have inspired my thinking on this topic over the years. To Maruja Barrig, Mario Chiappe, Luis Dragunsky, Iris Gareis, John Gillin, Donald Joralemon, Luis Millones, Carmen Pimentel Sevilla, Mario Polía, Douglas Sharon, Donald Skillman, Rafael Vásquez Guerrero, and all the other investigators who have contributed to our understanding of Peruvian sorcery, I also extend my thanks. I am also immensely grateful to all the Peruvians, healers, patients, friends, and "family," who have shared their lives with me (and, thus, become part of my life) over the last twenty-five years. Finally, my thanks to Joralemon and Sharon for including me in a grant which made my dissertation research possible and to the many colleagues and students and various Utah State University offices which have since supported and encouraged my research.

1. Although the people I interviewed (both patients and healers) assert that belief in the power of sorcerers and healers certainly underlies the petitioner's susceptibility to harm and likelihood of a cure, I also encountered many patients who claimed to experience the effects of sorcery *before* they ever believed in its power. In fact, a common disclaimer among first-time patients to healers was that "I never believed in sorcery until it happened to me."

2. For a good review of the scope of anthropological responses to "magic," see Luhrmann (1989, 8–10) and Goulet and Young (1994), from which the following summary is drawn.

3. The following summary is based on my own research (Glass-Coffin 1984) in urban and peri-urban Trujillo, where multiple health resources are readily available. In rural areas, where access to biomedical resources is more limited, alternative health care options tend to be invoked earlier in the process of health decision making.

4. For reasons I have more fully described elsewhere (Glass-Coffin 1991), sorcery beliefs are common in northern Peru. One element of this belief asserts that there exist two categories of illness—those with natural causes and those caused by sorcery. While the former are best cured by a doctor, the latter never respond to biomedical intervention. If symptoms are not somatic, but rather economic (a thriving business suddenly fails), relational (a family member suddenly becomes abusive or distant), or affective (one experiences an otherwise unaccountable change in behavior or personality), the victim will likely suspect sorcery as the cause of their sudden turn of bad luck early in the diagnostic process.

5. Of course, it is difficult to unravel whether this felt experience of healing precedes or follows these changes in perception and emotional engagement. Most theories of symbolic healing (discussed following) suggest that the emotional engagement precedes the physical consequence, but I am inclined to support Luhrmann's suggestion that belief often follows practice. I say this because of the number of people I have encountered in Peru who assure me that they never would have believed in sorcery as an explanation for their afflictions if they hadn't experienced it directly for themselves. Certainly, belief and practice, experience and analysis are mutually important ingredients when considering the efficacy of symbolic healing.

6. For a good introduction to these orientations in anthropological theory, see Langness (1987). In the following text, I have summarized functional, structural, and symbolic contributions of over fifty years of research into northern Peruvian sorcery in other publications. For discussion, see Glass-Coffin (1991, 1996, 1998, 1999).

7. This quote is a paraphrase of Victor Turner's assertion, as quoted in Bastien (1987) and cited in Goulet and Young (1994, 319).
8. These perceptions were not experienced alone, but in the company of other patients and ritual participants. Additionally, the rain incidents occurred before the start of the ritual, and before the ingestion of any psychoactive substances that might alter perception. The starlight incident occurred after the ritual was in progress, but was simultaneously commented on by at least a dozen other ritual participants at the instant of its occurrence.
9. As quoted in Goulet and Young (1994, 322).
10. See Young (1994) for a discussion of this approach to modeling that which is outside the investigator's "reality."

REFERENCES

Achterberg, Jeanne. 1985. *Imagery in healing: Shamanism and modern medicine.* Boston: Shambhala and New Science Library.
Dow, James. 1986. Universal aspects of symbolic healing. *American Anthropologist* 88 (1): 56–69.
Evans-Pritchard, E. E. 1956. *Nuer religion.* Oxford: Oxford University Press.
Glass-Coffin, Bonnie. 1984. Health-care decision-making among an urban middle-class population. Master's thesis, University of California, Los Angeles.
———. 1991. Discourse, *daño*, and healing in north coastal Peru. *Medical Anthropology* 13 (1–2): 33–55.
———. 1996. Male and female healing in northern Peru: Metaphors, models and manifestations of difference. *Journal of Ritual Studies* 10 (1): 63–91.
———. 1998. *The gift of life: Female spirituality and healing in northern Peru.* Albuquerque: University of New Mexico Press.
———. 1999. Engendering Peruvian shamanism through time: Insights from ethnohistory and ethnography. *Ethnohistory* 46 (2): 205–38.
Goulet, Jean-Guy, and David Young. 1994. Theoretical and methodological issues. In *Being changed by cross-cultural encounters: The anthropology of extraordinary experience,* ed. David E. Young and Jean-Guy Goulet, 298–335. Peterborough, Ontario: Broadview.
Jackson, Michael. 1989. *Paths toward a clearing: Radical empiricism and ethnographic inquiry.* Bloomington: Indiana University Press.
Langness, Lou L. 1987. *The study of culture,* revised ed. Novato, California: Chandler and Sharp.
Lévi-Strauss, Claude. 1963. *Structural anthropology.* New York: Basic Books.
Luhrmann, Tanya M. 1989. *Persuasions of the witch's craft: Ritual magic in contemporary England.* Cambridge, Massachusetts: Harvard University Press.
Pandian, Jacob. 1985. *Anthropology and the western tradition: Toward an authentic anthropology.* Prospect Heights, Illinois: Waveland.

Robbins, Richard H. 1997. *Cultural anthropology: A problem-based approach*. 2nd ed. Itasca, Illinois: F. E. Peacock.

Scheff, T. J. 1979. *Catharsis in healing, ritual, and drama*. Berkeley: University of California Press.

Torrey, E. Fuller. 1986. *Witchdoctors and psychiatrists: The common roots of psychotherapy and its future*. New York: Harper and Row and Perennial Library.

Wagner, Roy. 1981. *The invention of culture*. Chicago: University of Chicago Press.

Walker, Barbara, ed. 1995. *Out of the ordinary: Folklore and the supernatural*. Logan: Utah State University Press.

Wilber, Ken. 1998. *The marriage of sense and soul: Integrating science and religion*. New York: Random House.

Wilson, C. Roderick. 1994. Seeing they see not. In *Being changed by cross-cultural encounters: The anthropology of extraordinary experience*, ed. David E. Young and Jean-Guy Goulet, 197–208. Peterborough, Ontario: Broadview.

Young, David E. 1994. Visitors in the night: A creative energy model of spontaneous visions. In *Being changed by cross-cultural encounters: The anthropology of extraordinary experience*, ed. David E. Young and Jean-Guy Goulet, 166–94. Peterborough, Ontario: Broadview.

10

The Hózhó Factor: The Logic of Navajo Healing

Barre Toelken

Before entering into this discussion, I need to make clear that these comments and observations are not made by a Navajo but by a non-Navajo who has spent more than forty years as an adopted member of a Navajo family, the Yellowmans. This does not confer on me any special right to speak for or represent the Navajos in general or the Yellowman family in particular; it does not entitle me to dispense Navajo ritual "secrets," or to claim that I am providing the reader with an inside view of Navajo spiritual healing. Indeed, I regard all books by non-Natives which make such claims to be exploitative and destructive frauds. This essay does not offer anything more complicated than some perspectives formed from years of acquaintance, respect, and love for the people who first became known to me when they saved my life (I had come down with pneumonia while camped near their home in Montezuma Creek Canyon in southeastern Utah). They made the simple (but expensive) decision to hire a *hataałii*, literally, a singer or chanter, to treat my illness.

At that moment, I was transformed from a stranger to a guest, from an odd prospector camping nearby in a flimsy tent to a familiar, coughing, fever-ridden resident in their one-room hoghan; from a hopeful employer of Navajo guides to a panicked consumer of Navajo medicine; from a harmless curiosity to a burden and a health threat; from a benevolent exploiter of Navajos to a desperate participant-observer of Navajo culture—a prime candidate, in other words, for achieving an experience-centered perspective on healing whether I wanted to or not.

Little Wagon, the elderly father-in-law of Hugh Yellowman, had dropped by at my camp a number of times to squint at all the strange equipment and to satisfy himself that indeed there was a white person who was actually being paid to look for *tsé* (stones) in the desert. One day he found me barely able to sit up (my prospecting partner had gone to Salt Lake City some days before), and promptly (and roughly) hauled me to the back end of his wagon, dumped me in, and later—with a witty remark about having bagged a *bilagáana* (white person)—deposited me at the feet of his white-haired wife, who looked away with a stricken "Oh, God, now there's one right here in our own home" expression.

Little Wagon's daughter, Helen, and her husband, Yellowman, and several of their children also lived in the large, circular traditional hoghan (which is made of logs, branches, and rocks, covered with mud). The four adults and six children (sometimes more, when the older ones were home from boarding school) were now joined in their cozy circle by a sick man. Why did they take me in? Why did they go to the considerable expense of bringing in, first, a diagnostician, and then a hataałii? What did he do for me, medically, and how did it all work out? These are not only questions which I posed to myself at the time, but they are also important medical and cultural questions which lead us to some interesting observations about the validity of another form of healing. In trying to account for and understand what happened to me personally, I willy-nilly have to make sense of Navajo healing logic—or else conclude that I was coincidentally healed by a chance group of ignorant and untrained Indians. Naturally, in this case, it would be easier to end this account with the line used by so many storytellers and yarn-spinners when their young audiences demand, "What happened then, Grandpa?" "Well, I died." But it's a bit more difficult to account for an experience which initially makes no sense in one's own mind: in order to achieve an understanding, one must do what all folklorists and anthropologists do, and that is to place the event fairly within the supporting frameworks of its own culture to find out not only what it "means," but how it means. An experience-centered discussion, then, is not simply an exercise in self-indulgent validation of the participant-observer method, but rather must be viewed as an attempt to clarify and account for (1) an occurrence one might otherwise not have witnessed or been conscious of except for having been a participant, (2) utilizing the perspectives and nuances of the experience itself (not invented or imposed by the observer), (3) in a way that is true to the logical constellations of those among whom the event occurred and who understand its principal parts, and (perhaps most difficult of all) (4) articulated in such a way that the participant-observer brings the whole concept across as illustrative of something worth learning. It does us no good for someone to describe a fascinating cultural encounter and then just drop the subject as if it's just too, too impossible to grapple with.

A serious account of this sort entails the responsibility to report not only the event's surface features, but to examine fairly the system of thinking and believing that renders the cultural occurrence normal and valid rather than inexplicable or nonsensical. An experience-centered discussion of Navajo healing requires me to look seriously at their assumptions about health and sickness, and it should provide me with a level of understanding which lies at least as close to their voice as it does to my theory. In my attempt to make sense of the way my adopted family healed me, I began by asking questions of the singer, and I had the luxury of augmenting my perceptions in ongoing conversations with the Little Wagon and Yellowman families. These perspectives have been enlarged through the years by a continual return to issues which were not quite clear to me, and slowly by this means, a traumatic personal experience has yielded a tremendous richness of insight into Navajo worldview. One of several things I have learned in this process is that experience-centered discovery can be profound; another is that it apparently never includes closure on the ramifications of the subject. Another is that such learning is not bounded or controlled by deadlines: the pace is measured in years, not in months. In 1954, I began the process by asking the hataałii what it was he had done; I am still processing the layers of information and cultural nuance as I write this essay.

A hataałii is the cultural equivalent of our doctor, but is often referred to in English by the primitive term "medicine man." Suffice it to say, neither the term nor the practitioner is limited by gender. Most singers are indeed men, but this is mostly due to the years it takes an apprentice to learn a ceremony fully. There is no impediment to a woman becoming a singer, but since women own the children, the home, and most of the livestock, they seldom care to leave their position of power (where a husband can be divorced simply by his wife leaving his personal effects outside the door) to follow some older singer around—with little or no pay—for twenty years or so learning the words, tunes, rituals, sand paintings, and medicines necessary to the mastery of any one of the several hundred healing "ways" employed in Navajo healing. Besides, as several Navajo women have told me, men need something important to do in the world.

Actually, there are several kinds of healers in addition to the singers: diagnosticians (the most common employ hand trembling [*ndishniih*], or crystal gazing [*déest'íí' 'áshlééh*]), who determine not only what ailment the patient has, but what particular ritual would offer the most appropriate response; herbalists, whose own expertise is shared with singers and with others in need of a symptomatic cure (a colleague of mine, a sociologist doing field research on the Navajo reservation, came down with a sudden asthmatic condition and was cured immediately by a Navajo woman who had an herbal remedy on hand); and rare, talented practitioners who act somewhat like faith

healers. Only the last of these would come anywhere near the standard definition of shaman, by strict definition a person who—usually by having died and
come back to life—has the magical or personal power to affect the health of
others (for better or for worse).

Shamans are rare in Navajo culture except for the *yenaaldlooshi* (literally "evil trotting canine-like"), the Navajo embodiment of evil, or "skinwalker"
as such a person is usually called in English. This is a Navajo who studies a
kind of reverse medicine which is used to injure or kill others in the belief that
in so doing the perpetrator gains personal health, power, or property. There is
no doubt that there are such people: I have met a few of them and have seen
the results of their work. While stories about them make up much of the legendary repertoire of young Navajos, the yenaaldlooshi themselves are not typical of Navajo medical thought (except insofar as they validate Navajo beliefs
by contrast, working in opposition to the kinds of healing logic I will discuss
in this paper). That's as much as I want to say or think about the skinwalkers;
I do not care to come any closer to them than reading about them in a Tony
Hillerman novel. Most Navajo healers, from informal herbalists to carefully
practiced singers, learn their profession through years of intense education in
and memorization of medicines, songs, arts, psychology, and ritual practice.
It's medicine, not magic, and it constitutes the core of Navajo religious practice in general, since virtually every Navajo ritual focuses on a patient and a
singer-doctor.

Of course, I did not know any of this in the winter of 1954, as I lay—
dying, I supposed—on the dirt floor of Little Wagon's family's hoghan.
Coughing uncontrollably one night, I was nudged by Yellowman, who was
trying to offer me something out of a small container, shining a small flash-
light's yellow beam on it so I could see what it was. It was a tin of Sucrets
cough lozenges, but how it got into that remote canyon—or how long it had
been there—was a complete mystery to me. Yellowman kept saying, "*Nizee'!
Nizee'!*" which means "your medicine," but—because of the tonal possibilities
in Navajo which allow for puns in almost any circumstance—also means
"your mouth," or, "shut up!"

Leaning on my elbow in the dark hoghan, I unwrapped one of the cough
drops and got it into my mouth. My next memory is of waking—apparently a
day or so later, also at night—and sensing that the hoghan was full of people.
I had been dragged or carried to the west side of the hoghan opposite the
door. I noticed that the door was open, the space filled by a white sheet that
billowed back and forth as the wind blew outside. Next to my head sat a man
I didn't recognize, singing a chant I didn't understand. From somewhere else
in the hoghan I could hear another voice or two joining in. Occasionally, some

bitter liquid was poured in my mouth, and I was at least partly relieved to see that the bowl was then passed around so everyone else could share its contents. But I remember thinking I must be at the end of things; I would die in this roadless desert canyon and my folks in Massachusetts would never know the details.

As I learned later on, the ceremony which had now focused on me was the Red Antway, which had been recommended by the hand trembler diagnostician during a previous ceremony held while I was unconscious or asleep. Red Antway is usually used for lower intestinal complaints and maladies associated in Navajo custom with inadvertently breaking the taboo against urinating on ant hills, so why it was chosen for my upper respiratory problems I cannot say. My Navajo family later suggested that perhaps my camp had disturbed the ants somehow, and that was why the imagery came to the hand trembler. The ceremony made constant (and very effective) use of emetics, accompanied by songs which described evils being expelled from my lips, and so there was also the possibility that the ceremony was aimed at some form of witchery which had affected me. Later, I was told that the purgatives which made me vomit onto sand paintings of Horned Toad were expelling Red Ant People (later rephrased as "antness") from me.

There was a succession of sand paintings depicting variously colored Ant People, Horned Toad, Sunray Girl, Pollen People, and Corn People (all of them icons of sacred living aspects of nature). I was bathed several times with yucca suds, required to crawl through a succession of hoops outside the hoghan door, and on one occasion was frightened out of my wits by the sudden appearance of a "bear," a man blackened with soot and decorated with bear footprints who jumped at me from concealment behind a blanket. Although the Red Antway often lasts for eight or nine nights, mine ended on the morning of the sixth day, and was followed by a short protection rite from the Blessingway. My fever was gone and, although I was too weak to walk around much, I was able to breathe better and was coughing less each day.

Now, in terms of medicines, I have no doubt that what I was given to drink, to chew, to swallow whole, and on one occasion to smoke, must have had actual healing properties. Some of them tasted like pine tar, one concoction had a light mold on it and a moldy taste, and the "mountain tobacco" I smoked caused my nose to run uncontrollably and loosened the mucous in my throat.

The ritual activities were somewhat more difficult for me to understand, and I cannot claim to this day that I have a full intellectual command of their logical principles. But I can come close. Navajo rituals are said to create or to restore the quality of hózhó, a term which means something like a combination of beauty, stability, balance, and harmony. The medicines are believed to have the capacity of addressing the symptoms of illness, but not of curing the illness itself more than superficially, for it is thought to be the direct result of imbalances and disharmonies brought about by accident, by inattention to proper behavior, by reckless or immoderate actions (including excessive competitiveness), or by the ill will of others (including skinwalkers).

The sand paintings used during the ceremonies provide visual icons of the natural forces one must heed in order to be receptive to the restoration of balance and harmony; the songs and prayers (usually characterized by quadruple repetition of phrase, color, and action representing the four cardinal directions) set up a vocal context of redundant, interactive, circular patterns which are thought to reestablish normal reciprocative balances in the mind of the patient. Characters like the Red Ant People (living beings of the very first world in the Navajo Emergence story) represent the basic natural subterranean powers that epitomize the earth's "inner being," for which those who live on the surface constitute the "outer being" (yet another balanced, reciprocative model for natural relationships). When the patient is placed on a sand painting, he or she actually becomes part of, indeed an actor in, this sacred icon; when the colored sands are swept up and thrown away outside before sundown, the focused symbols are atomized, returned to their generalized presence in the universe, and the patient thus envisions the sickness, too, physically being taken out of the hoghan and redistributed in the world instead of concentrated in the individual. Movement within the hoghan is always circular, almost always sunwise. In other words, virtually all actions, words, tunes, movements, colors, and places are phrased in such a way as actually to *articulate* and dramatize the desired condition of balance for the patient (and by extension, all those present) in the setting of the natural world and universe. This reestablishment of hózhó is no more beautifully expressed than in the songs sung at dawn on each morning of the ceremony, with great detail on the last morning: the dawn is first described as a horizontal thin white line (indeed what the very first moment of dawn looks like in the desert); then dawn is depicted as spreading, then moving upwards, then passing overhead, then becoming complete; then the sunrise itself is described as it moves to completion; and then—in the formula so familiar to students of the Navajo—hózhó, or beauty, is described as spreading out around us in all directions, ahead of us, behind us, on all sides of us, above us and below us; finally, beauty has settled everywhere around us.

To understand the impact of such imagery on Navajos (of course it's admittedly powerful for anyone), we need to remember that Navajos do not see language as merely describing reality: rather, language creates the reality in which we live. With these images being sung close behind you, you experience the moment of dawn as the conclusion of a healing ritual and the symbol of restoration (in fact, in some ceremonies, like the *Hózhó-jí*, or Beauty Way, the patient faces the dawn at the moment the thin white line appears and actually "breathes it in"); it is a powerful combination of personal experience and the ritual articulation of restoration.

This intersection of ritual, language, action, and reality is rarely found in Anglo-American medical practice, or at least so the Navajos feel. In fact, traditional Native people often encounter its principles in macabre reversal when they visit a non-Navajo medical doctor. Blood and urine samples, skin scrapings, and other "specimens" are taken away into other rooms (just what skinwalkers might do with them); long objects like needles, tongue depressors, thermometers, and doctors' fingers are pointed at them in gestures exactly like those which indicate an intention to kill; and language is directed at them for its information capacity, not for its restorative powers. To be sure, times have changed, and Navajo people have been abroad in the world enough to have become sophisticated about such things: they may register such outrages today more as impolite behavior than as traumatic miscarriages of healing power. Nonetheless, especially for older patients, the aggregate impact of "Anglo medicine" can be quite frightening. And if it is true that the psychological state of the patient has a substantial effect on the healing process, we can say that much of what passes as healing logic for non-Navajos not only strikes the Navajos as deranged and dangerous, but indeed becomes an actual impediment to healing.

In this regard, I cannot think of a better example of the power of language to inhibit healing than the time I was asked to visit a physician to find out why he was "trying to kill" his elderly Navajo patient. The old man had refused to go back to his doctor, and indeed appeared close to terrified even at the thought of it. The doctor's opinion was that the old man was endangering his own life by stubbornly refusing to take his medicine regularly (he was being treated for diabetes). "I told him right out, if he didn't take his medicine, he was going to die." I pointed out that in the worldviews of many Native peoples, speaking of something created a reality, and that probably the old man had been frightened by the doctor's phrasing. "Well, what am I supposed to do? Hug him and tell him he's a wonderful old man and just let him die? My obligation is to tell him the truth: and the truth is, if he doesn't take his medicine, he's going to die." I said, "Why couldn't you tell him: 'If you do take your medicine, you're going to live and be with your grandchildren'?" "Never thought of that," he said. I mention this episode not only because it illustrates how language may function differently in such situations (in one case, the language is a vehicle of information—sterile, incontrovertible fact; in the other, language is a creative, powerful force which actually had a palpable impact on the patient), but also to show how near we often are to each other without realizing it. Worldview differences can sometimes act like walls, but more often they are veils; realizing this might lead us to see these differences as exciting resources rather than as problems.

A psychiatrist doing research on the psychological dimensions of Navajo healing once remarked to a group of friends that while he was interviewing an elderly medicine man he himself had suddenly received something just short of a visionary experience. The old man was in the midst of recalling how many years he had "followed," studied under, various elderly singers, each of whom in his own lifetime had spent years learning the words, songs, medicines, and ritual movements of several healing ceremonies. The old singer noted how difficult it had been to learn all the phrasing exactly, so that the depth of knowledge and power in the ceremonies would not erode over the years. The psychologist-researcher suddenly realized that he was listening to an oral account of unbroken medicinal and psychological practice and theory which had already been ancient when Freud and Jung were developing the modern field of psychology in which he himself had been trained.

Doctors at the Indian Health Service hospital in Tuba City, Arizona, told me that they had started "allowing" Navajo chanters to visit patients in the hospital, in the hopes that hearing a trusted and familiar voice would make them feel more at home and relaxed. Indeed it did, and the doctors had a sense that healing rates and successful treatments had gone up. They were not prepared to discover one day that the chanters also were able to bring Navajos out of comas almost every time (unless there had been massive brain damage). A chanter would sit at the head of the patient's bed and quietly sing and talk to the comatose Navajo for hours on end, taking a break now and again, until the person came out of the coma. I am not aware of any formal study being made of this process, but one doctor friend of mine said that his impression was that the chanters had about an 80 percent rate of success.

What logic accounts for this? In the absence of data "readable" by Western science, we have the tendency to grasp for ideas like "coincidence," but that would not account for a score of 80 percent—or even 40 percent for that matter. The Navajos do have a logic for this phenomenon, and it is based in part on their concept of the spirit or soul, *nílch'i*, literally wind, air, breeze. This is a living entity residing within us which relates us to the larger wind outside. It is shaped and mediated by our mouths when we speak (which is one of the reasons speaking is thought to have a direct effect on outer reality); but more to the point, it animates us in ways that are not under our conscious control. In other words, it functions not only as a life-force which ties us to the rest of nature, but it also acts very much like what we call the unconscious. Navajo singers have told me that even when the body is incapacitated (as in a coma) or unconscious (as in sleep), the nílch'i is still alive and functional as long as the patient is breathing. The singer contacts the wind-spirit through the patient's ear, and, in effect, encourages it to reanimate the body. I have been told by non-Navajo friends who have experienced comas that they remember much of what was said around them, even though they could not respond, so it seems that the experience is not isolated to Navajos, though the logical assumption that the minds of comatose patients can be reached with therapeutic results is apparently more advanced among the Navajos than it is among us.

Other culturally constructed phenomena are not so easy to account for. One of the doctors at Tuba City hospital told me about the teenage boy they had taken in as a burn victim on one occasion. He had been repairing his motorcycle, and the gasoline he was using to cut the grease had exploded and burned him over much of his body. He was convinced the incident was no accident, and that it had been precipitated by an old lady in his neighborhood who was suspected of being a witch, a skinwalker. He had accidentally backed into her propane tank some months earlier, and she had threatened to get even with him. He begged the doctors and nurses to make sure the old woman did not get to him in the hospital. The doctors assured him they would protect him, assured him the old woman was not a witch, assured him that he was on the mend. His burns, while serious, were responding to treatment, and he was feeling better every day. Nonetheless, the old woman was discovered roaming the hospital corridors, and was noisily ejected by the staff on several occasions. And while everyone was sure she had never reached the boy's room, he died in his bed suddenly of undetermined causes.

The Navajo concept of witchcraft understands it as operating in opposition to healing: it separates and alienates, it kills and injures, it destabilizes and deharmonizes—all usually under the command of someone who thinks to gain power (or revenge) by destroying the health of another. A witch is characterized by aggressive behavior, by serious personal competition, by antisocial actions of any sort. The logic of it—especially in contradistinction to the logic of Navajo healing—is clear enough. But my intellectual appreciation of this neat, bifurcated symmetry does not allow me to penetrate the mystery of the burned boy in Tuba City. I could dismiss it as one of those many puzzles I will never understand were it not for the fact that the young man was the father of my Navajo daughter's first child, a baby boy who also died inexplicably soon after birth.

As we might expect, the Navajo assumptions about balance and harmony also work on a much larger scale than just the human. In fact, it seems clear to me that the concepts of hózhó, "harmony," "beauty," and "balance," that inform the logic of healing are the local manifestations of conditions thought to be ideally present in the whole of the universe. When these balances in nature are threatened or destabilized, the result can be devastating for everyone, as was richly illustrated in the Four Corners area in 1993, when healthy Navajos began dying of a mysterious flu-like illness. The Associated Press quoted local and Indian Health Service doctors who theorized that the "baffling syndrome" was some kind of plague, and in an attempt to capture the Native perspective, AP quoted Navajo elders' explanations that the illness was a signal from nature that Navajos were neglecting their traditional values.

Scientists discovered that the virus was being carried by rodents, and the Center for Disease Control in Atlanta eventually identified the culprit as the hantavirus, named after the Hantaan River, where an outbreak had caused many casualties during the Korean War. Apparently, flooding and the bombing campaigns during the war had driven thousands of rodents from their homes and into the paths of humans, who picked up the virus from dust which carried dried mouse urine and droppings. In 1993 the southwestern United States had experienced unusually heavy and extended rains, one result of which was that the pinyon trees bore a tremendous harvest of nuts—attracting both the rodents and human gatherers into the same area.

Navajo tradition holds that when rodents, especially mice, become so numerous that people become aware of them at night running over their bedding, then all clothes and bedding should be immediately taken outside and burned. Navajo singers recalled that in 1918 and 1933 there had been similar years: heavy rains, large pinyon nut harvests, numerous mice, and—as one might expect—a pulmonary affliction that killed many people. The disease was considered to be the result of the imbalance in nature. By ignoring the older custom of burning clothes and bedding when such an infestation occurred in 1993, modern Navajos had indeed endangered their lives. And even before the scientists had isolated and identified the virus, the Navajo singers had already placed the event in the context of customary anecdote, oral history, and healing practice—to say nothing of understanding the phenomenon in terms of changes in the natural setting. Hantavirus is in fact the result of environmental imbalances, and is not simply a plague spread by human-to-human contact. While the Navajo understanding of this situation cannot be used as a claim that they somehow know something which the rest of us do not, it certainly stands as an example of how another culture's logic of health can generate insights as reliable as our own.

Some years ago, it was common to see Navajos wearing strings of colored glass beads and juniper seeds around their necks and wrists. Called "ghost beads" by white tourists to whom they were also sold in souvenir stands along the highways, these items were called *gad bi náá'* (literally, "juniper's eyes") by the Navajo. It was said that they represented in physical form the network of cooperation and reciprocation which could bring about harmony and balance in one's life: the juniper tree supplied the berries; the small ground animals collected them, taking them to their burrows and worrying the cap off one end so they could get to the tiny nut meat inside; the Navajo children gathered them from the animals' burrows, keeping only those which had already been opened (so they would not deprive the animals of food). The beads, worn around some part of the body, represented a physical surrounding by the interactive components of the natural world—the plants, animals, and people. To wear them was to feel enclosed in a symbol of environmental balance, of hózhó.

One doesn't see the juniper necklaces as much these days (except on tourists), and I cannot help but feel that their absence from the scene may signal a departure—an apostasy, if you will—from the logical assumptions which gave them intense meaning for many previous generations. Sadly enough, during the hantavirus episode in 1993, many Navajo young people went to their doctors instead of to their singers, no doubt because their willingness to accept the validity of their own cultural logic had been undermined or denigrated by the culture around them, the culture which now dominates their education, their economy, their environment, and, alas, their sense of science. It seems to me that one advantage of study in the field of culturally constructed medicine—especially in the mode of what David Hufford has called "experience-centered" scholarship—is that we can help to foster the idea that cultural diversity in thinking is neither a virtuous political exercise nor a threat to science but a rich and underestimated source of insight for humankind in general.

NOTES

A personal essay of the sort attempted here is not dependent on secondary sources which can be footnoted. Nonetheless, a number of works provide further illustration and explanation for basic issues brought up here which have been dealt with more extensively by scholars of the Navajo, noted by anthropologists and other students of Native American cultures, and reported in the news media. Readers may wish to consult Leland C. Wyman, *The Red Antway of the Navaho* (Santa Fe, New Mexico: Museum of Navajo Ceremonial Art, 1965) for a fuller description of several versions of the central healing ritual discussed here. The complexity of

Navajo language, with special reference to worldview and logical assumptions, is explored by Gary Witherspoon in *Language and Art in the Navajo Universe* (Ann Arbor: University of Michigan Press, 1977). A basic and thorough study of Navajo healing thought is Gladys A. Reichard, *Navaho Religion: A Study of Symbolism* (New York: Bollingen Foundation, 1950; republished in one volume by Princeton University in 1974). The principal healing ritual of the Navajos, from which all others are said to branch, is discussed by Leland C. Wyman in *Blessingway* (Tucson: University of Arizona Press, 1970). The idea of cultural apostasy or despiritualization was put forward by Calvin Martin in an essay about the erosive effects of European disease and religion on the Micmacs of northeastern Canada, "The European Impact on the Culture of a Northeastern Algonquian Tribe: An Ecological Interpretation" (*William and Mary Quarterly* 31 (1974): 3–21). The hantavirus epidemic was discussed in Associated Press releases across the country in June 1993, followed by a special editorial in the *Baltimore Sun* on 28 July 1995. "All Things Considered" aired a lengthy interview on the subject on National Public Radio on 11 February 1995 (I am indebted to Bert Jenson of Vernal, Utah, for bringing the latter two instances to my attention). The reader of these notes may be relieved to know that "Navajo" is the Spanish spelling of a word which is still under contentious debate. During the 1930s and 1940s, wishing to downplay the Hispanic look of the word, the tribe and most scholars used the spelling "Navaho," but in recent years the preference has been for "Navajo"; hence, one finds both spellings of the term in the literature. The Navajos call themselves Diné, which means "people" or "humans."

further investigation

Bibliography

FOLKLORE AND MEDICINE

MICHAEL OWEN JONES AND ERIKA BRADY,
WITH JACOB OWEN AND CARA HOGLUND

Any bibliography treating a topic so complex, addressed in the literature of so many disciplines, must finally be a selective one. The criterion used in compiling this list has been the inclusion of representative works of greatest interest and utility to two groups of readers: cultural specialists (especially folklorists), and those in the healing professions. With these readers in mind, we have adapted the structure of the excellent bibliography found in *Herbal and Magical Medicine*, which should also be consulted (Kirkland et al. 1992, 197–233). As with this work, we have not attempted to cross-reference entries; the reader should check all categories pertinent to the topic. Unlike the previous bibliography, however, in those entries involving a practice common within a particular population we have given categorical priority to the community rather than the practice. In searching for information concerning African-American practice relating to childbirth, for example, the first place to look is 3B, then 1G for more general references on the topic, and possibly 4C for information concerning African origins. This choice was made to assist those in medical settings who are often called upon to address clinical issues relating to practice common within a specific population. We also suggest that the reader review the references cited in the articles included in this collection.

The ancillary areas of medical sociology and medical anthropology are merely touched on; the reader is encouraged to consult bibliographies available in the standard works in those fields. Researchers should also investigate the extensive and growing resources available electronically through the internet, which range from the biomedical mainstay MEDLINE to eccentric and highly individual web pages devoted to the most esoteric of healing practices.

The entries in this bibliography are included because they elucidate nonconventional health practice within cultural systems of belief. Readers interested solely in scientifically supported data concerning pharmaceutical efficacy or potential negative interaction with conventional treatment should investigate sources such as Mark Blumenthal's compendium, *The Complete German Commission E Monographs* (Austin Texas: American Botanical Council; Boston: Integrative Medicine Communications, 1998) or *The Physicians Desk Reference for Herbal Medicines* (Montvale, NJ: Medical Economics Company, 2000), or the online database NAPRALERT.

The references found in this bibliography were compiled by Michael Owen Jones. Erika Brady was responsible for their organization into the present format, with the assistance of Jacob Owen and Cara Hoglund.

Bibliography Outline

I. Traditional and alternative beliefs and practices
  A. Ethnobotany and herbalism
  B. Magic, witchcraft, shamanism, and charms
   (a) Practitioners
   (b) Practices
  C. Religious healing in Vodou, Santería, Lucumí, Candomblé, Spiritism, and Spiritualism
  D. General religious and faith healing
  E. Psychosomatic conditions and hypnosis
  F. Ethnopsychiatry, psychotherapy, and symbolic healing
  G. Menstruation, pregnancy, childbirth and children, and midwifery
  H. Home remedies, popular beliefs, and superstitions
  I. Evil eye
  J. Burn healing, blood stopping, wart healing, and thrash cures
  K. Metaphor, narrative, and ritual
  L. Powwow
  M. Veterinary healing practices
  N. Geophagy
  O. Homeopathy and holistic healing
II. North American folk medicine: Regional variations
  A. Southwestern
  B. Northeastern
  C. Southern
  D. Midwestern
  E. Western
  F. Urban
III. Ethnomedical traditions in North America
  A. American Indian
  B. African, African American, Afro-Caribbean
  C. Hispanic or Latino

D. Pennsylvania German
E. Asian American
F. Canadian
IV. World ethnomedical traditions
A. Latin American
B. Caribbean
C. African
D. Asian
E. British
F. European
G. Judaic and biblical
V. History of medicine
VI. General studies
VII. "Quackery"
VIII. Specific pathologies

BIBLIOGRAPHIC LISTINGS

I. *Traditional and alternative beliefs and practices*

I.A. *Ethnobotany and herbalism*

Alpers, William G. 1915. Remarks on digitalis. *Cleveland Medical Journal* 14: 99–112.

Angier, Bradford. 1978. *Field guide to medicinal wild plants*. Harrisburg, Pennsylvania: Stackpole Books.

Balick, M. J. 1990. Ethnobotany and the identification of therapeutic agents from the rainforest. *Ciba Foundation Symposium* 154: 22–31.

Bergen, Fanny D. 1892. Some bits of plant lore. *Journal of American Folklore* 5: 19–22.

———. 1899. *Animal and plant lore collected from the oral tradition of English speaking folk. Memoirs of the American Folk-Lore Society*. Vol. 7. Boston and New York: n.p.

Berman, Alex. 1956. A striving for scientific respectability: Some American botanics and the nineteenth century plant materia medica. *Bulletin of the History of Medicine* 30 (1): 7–31.

Browner, Carole H. 1985. Criteria for selecting herbal remedies. *Ethnology* 24: 13–32.

Campa, Arthur L. 1950. Some herbs and plants of early California. *Western Folklore* 9: 338–47.

Castleman, Michael. 1995. *The healing herbs: The ultimate guide to the curative power of nature's medicines*. New York: Bantam Books.

Chiej, Roberto. 1984. *The Macdonald encyclopedia of medicinal plants*. London: Macdonald.

Crellin, John K., and J. Philpott. 1990. *Herbal medicine past and present*. 2 vols. Durham, North Carolina: Duke University Press.

Croom, Edward M. 1983. Documenting and evaluating herbal remedies. *Economic Botany* 37: 13–27.

de Laszlo, Henry, and Paul S. Henshaw. 1954. Plant materials used by primitive peoples to affect fertility. *Science* 119: 626–30.

Dixon, Royal, and Raymond Comstock. 1914. Wicked or irreligious plants and their superstitions. Part 2 of The folk-lore of plants. *Trend* 8 (1): 124–27.

Duke, James. 1995. Assessment of plants as medicines: A tale of two tales. *Journal of Alternative and Complementary Medicine* 1 (1): 9–13.

Etkin, Nina L. 1988. Ethnopharmacology: Biobehavioral approaches in the anthropological study of indigenous medicines. *Annual Review of Anthropology* 17: 23–42.

———. 1993. Anthropological methods in ethnopharmacology. *Journal of Ethnopharmacology* 38: 93–104.

Farnsworth, Norman R., Akerel Olayiwola, Audry S. Bingel, Djaja D. Soejarto, and Zhengang Guo. 1985. Medicinal plants in therapeutics. *World Health Organization Bulletin* 63 (6): 965–81.

Feil, Harold. 1957. Story of the foxglove. *Bulletin of the Cleveland Medical Library* 4 (4): 59–64.

Fletcher, Robert, M.D. 1896. The witches' pharmacopoeia. *Bulletin, Johns Hopkins Hospital* 7 (65): 147–56.

Foote, John, M.D. 1916. Trees in medicine. *American Forestry* 22: 648–53.

Gibbs, R. D. 1974. *Chemotaxonomy of flowering plants.* Montreal: McGill-Queen's University Press.

Gray, M. A. 1996. Herbs: Multicultural folk medicines. *Orthopaedic Nursing* 15 (2): 49–56.

Grieve, Maud. [1931] 1971. A modern herbal: The medicinal, culinary, cosmetic, and economic properties. In *Cultivation and folk-lore of herbs, grasses, fungi, shrubs, and trees with all their modern scientific uses.* 2 vols. New York: Dover.

Harborne, Jeffrey B., and H. Baxter, eds. 1993. *Phytochemical dictionary: A handbook of bioactive compounds from plants.* London and Washington, D.C.: Taylor and Francis.

Hoffman, F. A., and D. Eskinazi. 1995. NIH Office of Alternative Medicine Conference: Federal agencies explore the potential role of botanicals in U.S. health care. *Journal of Alternative and Complementary Medicine* 1 (3): 303–8.

Houghton, Peter J. 1995. The role of plants in traditional medicine and current therapy. *Journal of Alternative and Complementary Medicine* 1: 131–43.

Hung, O. L., R. D. Shih, W. K. Chiang, L. S. Nelson, R. S. Hoffman, and L. R. Goldfrank. 1997. Herbal preparation use among urban emergency department patients. *Academic Emergency Medicine* 4 (3): 209–13.

Jagendorf, Moritz A. 1962. Apples in life and lore. *New York Folklore Quarterly* 18: 273–83.

James, R. R. 1928. Ophthalmic leechdoms. *British Journal of Ophthalmology* 12: 401–10.

Kirkland, James, Holly F. Mathews, C. W. Sullivan III, and Karen Baldwin, eds. 1992. *Herbal and magical medicine: Traditional healing today.* Durham, North Carolina: Duke University Press.

Kowalchik, Claire, and William H. Hylton, eds. 1987. *Rodale's illustrated encyclopedia of herbs.* Emmaus, Pennsylvania: Rodale.

Kreig, Margaret. 1966. *Green medicine.* New York: Bantam.

Kyerematen, G. A., and E. O. Ogunlana. 1987. An integrated approach to the pharmacological evaluation of traditional materia medica. *Journal of Ethnopharmacology* 20 (3): 191–207.

Lee, Charles O. 1960. The Shakers as pioneers in the American herb and drug industry. *American Journal of Pharmacy* 132 (5): 178–93.

Lewis, Walter L., and M. P. F. Elvin-Lewis. 1977. *Medical botany: Plants affecting man's health.* New York: Wiley and Sons.

Lipp, F. J. 1989. Methods for ethnopharmacological field work. *Journal of Ethnopharmacology* 25: 139–50.

Lucas, E. H. 1959. The role of folklore in discovery and rediscovery of plant drugs. *Centennial Review of Arts and Science* 3: 173–88.

Maxwell, Hu. 1918. Indian medicines: Numerous popular remedies obtained from forest trees. *Scientific American* 86 (suppl. 2224): 100–103.

McCullen, J. T. 1962. The tobacco controversy, 1571–1961. *North Carolina Folklore* 10 (1): 30–35.

Messer, E. 1991. Systematic and medicinal reasoning in Mitla folk botany. *Journal of Ethnopharmacology* 33 (1–2): 107–28.

Miller, Genevieve. 1959. The sassafras tree. *Bulletin of the Cleveland Medical Library* 6 (1): 3–7.

Moerman, Daniel E. 1977. *American medical ethnobotany: A reference dictionary.* New York: Garland.

———. 1991a. Poisoned apples and honeysuckles: The medicinal plants of Native America. In *The anthropology of medicine: From culture to method,* ed. Lola Romanucci-Ross, Daniel E. Moerman, and Laurence R. Tancredi, 147–57. New York: Bergin and Garvey.

———. 1991b. The medicinal flora of native North America: An analysis. *Journal of Ethnopharmacology* 31: 1–42.

Morton, Julia Frances. 1977. *Major medicinal plants: Botany, culture, and uses.* Springfield, Illinois: Thomas.

———. 1981. *Atlas of medicinal plants of Middle America: Bahamas to Yucatan.* Springfield, Illinois: Charles C. Thomas.

Pang, Z., F. Pan, and S. He. 1996. Ginkgo biloba l: History, current status, and future prospects. *Journal of Alternative and Complementary Medicine* 2 (3): 359–63.

Rainey, Frank L. 1929. Animal and plant lore. *Kentucky Folk-Lore and Poetry Magazine* 4 (1): 8–15.

Relihan, Catherine. 1946. Farm lore: Herb remedies. *New York Folklore Quarterly* 2 (2): 156–58.

Resch, K. L., and E. Ernst. 1995. Garlic (Allium sativum)—A potent medicinal plant. Translated from German. *Fortschritte der Medizin* 113 (20–21): 311–15.

Schweisheimer, Waldemar. 1942. Christmas plants and Christmas trees in medicine. *Medical Record* 155: 541–43.

Silvette, H., P. S. Larson, and H. B. Haag. 1958. Medical uses of tobacco, past and present. *Virginia Medical Monthly* 85: 472–84.

Smitherman, J., and P. Harber. 1991. A case of mistaken identity: Herbal medicine as a cause of lead toxicity. *American Journal of Industrial Medicine* 20 (6): 795–98.

Spjut, R. W., and R. E. Perdue, Jr. 1976. Plant folklore: A tool for predicting sources of antihumor activity? *Cancer Treatment Reports* 60: 979–85.

Stern, E. 1997. Two cases of hepatitis C treated with herbs and supplements. *Journal of Alternative and Complementary Medicine* 3 (1): 77–82.

Swain, T. 1963. *Chemical plant taxonomy.* New York: Academic Press.

Tajonar, L. S. N.d. *Plantas y yerbas curativas de Mexico.* Sucursal, Mexico: Gomez Gomez Hnos.

Thiselton Dyer, T. F. 1889. *The folk-lore of plants.* New York: n.p.

Trotter, R. T., and M. H. Logan. 1986. Informant consensus: A new approach for identifying potentially effective medicinal plants. In *Plants in indigenous medicine and diet: Biobehavioral approaches*, ed. N. L. Etkin, 91–112. New York: Gordon and Breach (Redgrave).

Upton, R. 1997. Herbal monographs push natural medicines into the twenty-first century. *Journal of Alternative and Complementary Medicine* 3 (4): 397–99.

Vestal, Paul K., Jr. 1973. Herb workers in Scotland and Robeson Counties. *North Carolina Folklore* 21: 166–70.

Wilson, Eddie W. 1953. The onion in folk belief. *Western Folklore* 12: 94–104.

Wilson, Miki. 1960a. St. John's wort. *Journal of the Indiana State Medical Association* 53 (2): 316–17.

———. 1960b. Vervain. *Journal of the Indiana State Medical Association* 53 (3): 482–83.

———. 1960c. Rosemary. *Journal of the Indiana State Medical Association* 53 (4): 712–13.

———. 1960d. Hawaii—Rich in lore of medicinal herbs. *Journal of the Indiana State Medical Association* 53 (6): 1206–11.

Young, Kathleen L. 1983. Ethnobotany: A methodology for folklorists. Master's thesis, Western Kentucky University, Bowling Green.

I.B(a).   *Magic, witchcraft, shamanism, and charms: Practitioners*

Atkinson, Jane Monnig. 1992. Shamanisms today. *Annual Review of Anthropology* 21: 307–30.

Charles, Lucile Hoerr. 1953. Drama in shaman exorcism. *Journal of American Folklore* 66: 95–122.

Forbes, Thomas R. 1950. Witch's milk and witches' marks. *Yale Journal of Biology and Medicine* 22: 219–25.

Garcia, R. L. 1977. "Witch doctor?" A hexing case of dermatitis. *Cutis* 19 (1): 103–5.

Guimera, L. M. 1978. Witchcraft illness in the Evuzok nosological system. *Culture, Medicine and Psychiatry* 2 (4): 373–96.

Hand, Wayland D. 1980a. The folk healer: Calling and endowment. In *Magical medicine*, 43–56. Berkeley and Los Angeles: University of California Press.

———. 1980b. Physical harm, sickness, and death by conjury: A survey of the sorcerer's evil art in America. In *Magical medicine*, 215–25. Berkeley and Los Angeles: University of California Press.

———. 1985. Magical medicine: An alternative to "alternative medicine." *Western Folklore* 44: 240–51.

McClenon, J. 1993. The experiential foundations of shamanic healing. *Journal of Medicine and Philosophy* 18 (2): 107–27.

McMillan, D. W. 1932. Witch doctors and their practices. *Journal of the Florida Medical Association* 18: 179–84.

Middleton, John, ed. 1967. *Magic, witchcraft, and healing*. Garden City, New York: Natural History Press (published for the American Museum of Natural History).

Myerhoff, Barbara G. 1966. The doctor as culture hero: The shaman of Rincon. *Anthropological Quarterly* 39: 60–72.

Neki, J. S., B. Joinet, N. Ndosi, G. Kilonzo, J. G. Hauli, and G. Duvinage. 1986. Witchcraft and psychotherapy. *British Journal of Psychiatry* 149: 145–55.

Roberts, A. H. 1952. We aren't magicians, but . . . verbal charms survive in the machine age. *Tennessee Folklore Society Bulletin* 18: 82–84.

Rogers, Spencer L. 1942. Shamans and medicine men. *Ciba Symposia* 4 (1): 1202–14.

Sharon, Douglas C. 1978. *Wizard of the four winds: A shaman's story.* New York: Free Press.

Sharp, P. T. 1982. Ghosts, witches, sickness and death: The traditional interpretation of injury and disease in a rural area of Papua New Guinea. *Papua New Guinea Medical Journal* 25 (2): 108–15.

Thorndike, Lynn. 1929. Magic and medicine. *Medical Life* 36: 148–55.

Weimer, S. R., and N. L. Mintz. 1976. Health practice at the technologic/folk interface: Witchcraft as a culture-specific diagnosis. *International Journal of Psychiatry in Medicine* 7 (4): 351–62.

Wintrob, R. M. 1973. The influence of others: Witchcraft and rootwork as explanations of behavior disturbances. *Journal of Nervous and Mental Disorders* 156 (5): 318–26.

I.B(b).   *Magic, witchcraft, shamanism, and charms: Practices*

Bergen, Fanny D. 1890. Some saliva charms. *Journal of American Folklore* 3: 51–59.

Budge, Sir Ernest Alfred Thomas Wallis. 1930. *Amulets and Superstitions.* London and New York: n.p.

Halpern, Barbara Kerewsky, and John Miles Foley. 1978. The power of the word: Healing charms as an oral genre. *Journal of American Folklore* 91: 103–4.

Hand, Wayland D. 1980a. Folk curing: The magical component. In *Magical medicine,* 1–16. Berkeley and Los Angeles: University of California Press.

———. 1980b. The magical transfer of disease. In *Magical medicine,* 17–42. Berkeley and Los Angeles: University of California Press.

Kanner, Leo. 1939. Mistletoe, magic, and medicine. *Bulletin of the History of Medicine* 7: 875–936.

Lewis, B. S. 1941. Double double: Cauldron bubble. *Journal of the Royal Naval Medical Service* 27 (4): 379–82.

Merrifield, Ralph. 1955. Witch bottles and magical jugs. *Folklore* 66: 195–207.

Van der Geest, S., and S. R. Whyte. 1989. The charm of medicines: Metaphors and metonyms. *Medical Anthropology Quarterly* 3: 345–67.

Vlachos, I. O., S. Beratis, and P. Hartocollis. Magico-religious beliefs and psychosis. *Psychopathology* 30 (2): 93–99.

Wilson, Thomas. 1891. The amulet collection of Professor Belucci. *Journal of American Folklore* 4: 144–46.

Winters, S. R. 1937. Magic medicine. *Hygeia* 15: 630–33.

I.C.   *Religious healing in Vodou, Santería, Lucumí, Candomblé, Spiritism, and Spiritualism*

Alonso, L., and W. D. Jeffrey. 1988. Mental illness complicated by the Santería belief in spirit possession. *Hospital and Community Psychiatry* 39 (11): 1188–91.

Bailey, James A. 1991. *The Yoruba of southwestern Nigeria and Santería in the southeastern United States.* New Bern, North Carolina: Godolphin House.

———. 1996. Santería and Palo Mayombe: The presence of Afro-Cuban artifacts at Wrightsville Beach. *North Carolina Folklore Journal* 43: 128–41.

Bascom, William. 1950. The focus of Cuban Santería. *Southwestern Journal of Anthropology* 6: 64–68.

Berthold, S. Megan. 1989. Spiritism as a form of psychotherapy: Implications for social work practice. *Social Casework: Journal of Contemporary Social Work* (October): 502–9.

Bird, Hector R., and Ian Canino. 1981. The sociopsychiatry of espiritismo: Findings of a study in psychiatric populations of Puerto Rican and other Hispanic children. *Journal of the American Academy of Child Psychiatry* 20: 725–40.

Brandon, George. 1990. Sacrificial practices in Santería, an African-Cuban religion in the United States. In *Africanisms in American culture*, ed. Joseph E. Holloway, 119-47. Bloomington: Indiana University Press.

———. 1991. The uses of plants in healing in an Afro-Cuban religion, Santería. *Journal of Black Studies* 22: 55–76.

Brown, David H. 1989. *Garden in the machine: Afro-Cuban sacred art and performance in New York* City. Ph.D. diss., Yale University, New Haven, Connecticut.

———. 1993. Thrones of the Orichas: Afro-Cuban altars in New Jersey, New York, and Havana. *African Arts* 26 (4): 44–59, 85.

Budiansky, S. 1984. Voodoo on the campus. *Nature* 310 (5980): 718.

Byers, James F. 1970. Voodoo: Tropical pharmacology or psychosomatic psychology? *New York Folklore* 26: 305–12.

Canizares, Raul. 1990. The epiphany and the Cuban Santería. *Journal of Dharma* 15: 309–13.

———. 1993. *Walking with the night: The Afro-Cuban world of Santería*. Rochester, Vermont: Destiny Books.

Craan, A. G. 1988. Toxicological aspects of voodoo in Haiti. *Biomedical and Environmental Sciences* 1 (4): 372–81.

Crapanzano, Vincent, and Vivian Garrison, eds. 1977. *Case studies in spirit possession*. New York: John Wiley.

Curtis, James R. 1982. Santería: Persistence and change in an Afro-Cuban cult religion. In *Objects of special devotion: Fetishism in popular culture*, 336–51. Bowling Green, Ohio: Bowling Green Popular Press.

Davis, E. W. 1983. The ethnobiology of the Haitian zombi. *Journal of Ethnopharmacology* 9 (1): 85–104.

Edwards, Gary, and John Mason. 1985. *Black Gods: Orisa studies in the New World*. New York: Yoruba Theological Archministry.

Finkler, Kaja. 1981. Focus on adherents of spiritualism. Part 2 of Non-medical treatments and their outcomes. *Culture, Medicine and Psychiatry* 5 (1): 65–103.

———. 1985. *Spiritualist healers in Mexico: Successes and failures of alternative therapeutics*. New York: Praeger.

Fisch, Stanley. 1968. Botanicas and spiritualism in a metropolis. *Milbank Memorial Fund Quarterly* 46: 377–88.

Fishman, R. G. 1979. Spiritualism in western New York: A study in ritual healing. *Medical Anthropology* 3: 1–22.

George, Victoria. 1980. Santería cult and its healers: Beliefs and traditions preserved in Los Angeles. Master's thesis, University of California, Los Angeles.

Golden, K. M. 1977. Voodoo in Africa and the United States. *American Journal of Psychiatry* 134 (12): 1425–27.

Gonzales-Wippler, Migene. 1973. *Santería: African magic in Latin America*. Garden City, New York: Doubleday and Anchor.

————. 1982. *The Santería experience.* Englewood Cliffs, New Jersey: Prentice-Hall.

————. 1984. *Rituals and spells of Santería.* New York: Original Publications.

————. 1994. *Santería: The religion.* St. Paul, Minnesota: Llewellyn Publications.

Greenfield, S. M. 1987. The return of Dr. Fritz: Spiritist healing and patronage networks in urban, industrial Brazil. *Social Science and Medicine* 24 (12): 1095–1108.

————. 1992. Spirits and spiritist therapy in southern Brazil: A case study of an innovative, syncretic healing group. *Culture, Medicine, and Psychiatry* 16 (1): 23–51.

Gregory, Steven. 1986. *Santería in New York: A study in cultural resistance.* Ph.D. diss., New School for Social Research, New York.

Guevara-Ramos, L. M. 1982. Espiritismo and medical care. *American Journal of Psychiatry* 139 (9): 1216.

Gustafson, M .B. 1989. Western voodoo: Providing mental health care to Haitian refugees. *Journal of Psychosocial Nursing and Mental Health Services* 27 (12): 22–25.

Hanley, E. 1995. Santería, an alternative pulse (images of Cuba as seen by contemporary photographers). *Aperture* 141 (fall): 30–37.

Harwood, Alan. 1977a. Description and analysis of an alternative psychotherapeutic approach. Part 1 of Puerto Rican spiritism. *Culture, Medicine and Psychiatry* 1: 69–95.

————. 1977b. An institution with preventive and therapeutic functions in community psychiatry. Part 2 of Puerto Rican spiritism. *Culture, Medicine and Psychiatry* 1: 135–53.

————. 1977c. *Rx: Spiritist as needed: A study of Puerto Rican community mental health resources.* New York: Wiley.

Hess, David J. 1994. *Samba in the night: Spiritism in Brazil.* New York: Columbia University Press.

Hohmann, A. A., M. Richeport, B. M. Marriott, G. J. Canino, M. Rubio-Stipec, and H. Bird. 1990. Spiritism in Puerto Rico: Results of an island-wide community study. *British Journal of Psychiatry* 156: 328–35.

Koss, Joan D. 1977a. Religion and science divinely related: A case history of spiritism in Puerto Rico. *Caribbean Studies* 16: 22–43.

————. 1977b. Social process, healing and self-defeat among Puerto Rican spiritualists. *American Ethnologist* 4: 453–69.

————. 1980. The therapist spiritist training project in Puerto Rico: An experiment to relate the traditional healing system to the public health system. *Social Science and Medicine* 14B: 255–66.

————. 1987. Expectations and outcomes for patients given mental health care or spiritist healing in Puerto Rico. *American Journal of Psychiatry* 144 (1): 56–61.

Lachatanere, Romolo. 1942. *Manual de Santería.* Havana: Editorial Caribe.

Lefever, Harry G. 1996. When the saints go riding in: Santería in Cuba and the United States. *Journal for the Scientific Study of Religion* 35: 318–30.

Lichstein, Peter R. 1992. Rootwork from the clinician's perspective. In *Herbal and magical medicine: Traditional healing today,* ed. James Kirkland, Holly F. Mathews, C. W. Sullivan III, and Karen Baldwin, 99–117. Durham, North Carolina: Duke University Press.

Lindsay, Arturo, ed. 1996. *Santería aesthetics in contemporary Latin American art.* Washington, D.C.: Smithsonian Institution Press.

Lubchansky, Isaac, Gladys Egri, and Janet Stokes. 1970. Puerto Rican spiritualists view mental illness: The faith healer as paraprofessional. *American Journal of Psychiatry* 127: 312–21.

Macklin, June. 1974. Belief, ritual and healing: New England spiritualism and Mexican-American spiritism compared. In *Religious movements in contemporary America*, ed. I. I. Zaretsky and M. P. Leone, 383–417. Princeton, New Jersey: Princeton University Press.

Mason, Michael Atwood. 1993. The blood-that-runs-through-the-veins: The creation of identity and a client's experience of Cuban-American Santería-dilogun divination. *Drama Review* 37: 119–30.

———. 1994. "I bow my head to the ground": The creation of bodily experience in a Cuban American Santería initiation. *Journal of American Folklore* 107: 23–39.

Mathews, J. L. 1985. Voodoo and foreign bodies of the stomach. *Gastrointestinal Endoscopy* 31 (6): 408–9.

Mena, Aipy. 1998. Cuban Santería, Haitian Vodun, Puerto Rican spiritualism: A multiculturalist inquiry into syncretism. *Journal for the Scientific Study of Religion* 37: 15–27.

Metraux, A. 1972. *Voodoo in Haiti*. New York: Schocken Books.

Morales-Dorta, Jose. 1976. *Puerto Rican espiritismo: Religion and psychotherapy*. New York: Vantage Press.

Murphy, Joseph M. 1988. *Santería: An African religion in America*. Boston: Beacon Press.

———. 1993. *Santería: African spirits in America*. Boston: Beacon Press.

Newell, William Wells. 1888. Voodoo worship and child sacrifice in Hayti. *Journal of American Folklore* 1: 16–30.

———. 1889. Reports of voodoo worship in Hayti and Louisiana. *Journal of American Folklore* 2: 41–47.

Nunez, Luis Manuel. 1992. *Santería: A practical guide to Afro-Caribbean religion*. Dallas, Texas: Spring Publications.

Oba, Ecun. 1989. *Ita: Mythology of the Yoruba religion*. Miami: Obaecun Books.

Pasquali, E. A. 1994. Santería. *Journal of Holistic Nursing* 12 (4): 380–90.

Perez y Mena, Andres Isidoro. 1991. *Speaking with the dead: Development of Afro-Latin religion among Puerto Ricans in the United States: A study into the interpenetration of civilizations in the New World*. New York: AMS Press.

Polk, Patrick A. 1997. *Haitian vodou flags*. Jackson: University Press of Mississippi.

———, ed. 1998. *Botanica: Art and spirit in Los Angeles*. Los Angeles: UCLA Folk Art Group.

Richard, M. P., and A. Adato. 1980. The medium and her message: A study of spiritualism at Lily Dale, New York. *Review of Religious Research* 22: 186–97.

Rigaud, Milo. 1969. *Secrets of voodoo*. New York: Arco.

Rogers, F. B. 1975. Dr. Thomas W. Fossett (1813–94): Yankee spiritualist. *Journal of the History of Medicine and Allied Sciences* 30 (1): 62–65.

Sanchez Cardenas, Julio. 1993. Santería or orisha religion: An old religion in a new world. In *South and Meso-American native spirituality: From the cult of the feathered serpent to the theology of liberation*, 474–95. New York: Crossroad Publishing.

Sandoval, Mercedes Cros. 1977. Afrocuban concepts of disease and its treatment in Miami. *Journal of Operational Psychiatry* 8: 52–63.

———. 1979. Santería as a mental health care system: An historical overview. *Social Science and Medicine* 13B: 137–51.

———. 1983. Santería. *Journal of the Florida Medical Association* 70: 620–28.

Saphir, J. R., A Gold, J. Giambrone, and J. F. Holland. 1967. Voodoo poisoning in Buffalo, New York. *Journal of the American Medical Association* 202 (5): 437–38.

Sargant, W. 1967. Witch doctoring, zar, and voodoo: Their relation to modern psychiatric treatments. *Proceedings of the Royal Society of Medicine* 60 (10): 1055–60.

Simpson, George Eaton. 1946. Four vodun ceremonies. *Journal of American Folklore* 59: 154–67.

Singer, Merrill. 1984. Indigenous treatment for alcoholism: The case of Puerto Rican spiritism. *Medical Anthropology* 8 (4): 246–73.

Singer, Merrill, and R. Garcia. 1989. Becoming a Puerto Rican espiritista: Life history of a female healer. In *Women as healers: Cross-cultural perspectives*, ed. C. S. McClain, 157–85. New Brunswick, New Jersey: Rutgers University Press.

Snow, Loudell F. 1973. "I was born just exactly with the gift": An interview with a voodoo practitioner. *Journal of American Folklore* 86: 272–81.

———. 1979. Voodoo illness in the black population. In *Culture, curers, and contagion*, ed. Norman Klein, 179. Ovato, California: Chandler and Sharp.

Sosa, Juan J. 1981. La Santería: A new way of looking at reality. Master's thesis, Florida Atlantic University, Boca Raton, Florida.

The spiritualist: Healer and co-therapist. A panel discussion. 1976. *Proceedings of Puerto Rican Conferences on Human Services* (20 October): 181–90.

Stevens-Arroyo, Anthony M., and Andres I. Pérez y Mena, eds. 1995. *Enigmatic powers: Syncretism with African and indigenous peoples' religions among Latinos*. New York: Bildner Center for Western Hemisphere Studies.

Vega, Marta Moreno. 1995. The Yoruba orisha tradition comes to New York City. *African American Review* 29: 201–6.

Ward, Colleen. 1980. Spirit possession and mental health: A psycho-anthropological perspective. *Human Relations* 33: 149–63.

———. 1981. Spirit possession and neuroticism in a West Indian Pentecostal community. *British Journal of Clinical Psychology* 20: 295–96.

Weiss, C. I. 1992. Controlling domestic life and mental illness: Spiritual and aftercare resources used by Dominican New Yorkers. *Culture, Medicine and Psychiatry* 16 (2): 237–71.

Yates, Irene. 1946. Conjures and cures in the novels of Julia Peterkin. *Southern Folklore Quarterly* 10: 137–49.

Zayas, L. H., and P. O. Ozuah. 1996. Mercury use in espiritismo: A survey of botanicas. Letter. *American Journal of Public Health* 86 (1): 111–12.

I.D.   General religious and faith healing

Ahronheim, J. H. 1958. Medicine and religion. *Mississippi Valley Medical Journal* 80: 200–202, 209, 216.

Bilu, Y., and E. Witztum. 1994. Culturally sensitive therapy with ultra-orthodox patients: The strategic employment of religious idioms of distress. *Israel Journal of Psychiatry and Related Sciences* 31 (3): 170–82.

Bram, Joseph. 1958. Spirits, mediums, and believers in contemporary Puerto Rico. *Transactions of the New York Academy of Sciences* 20: 340–47.

Camino, Linda A. 1992. The cultural epidemiology of spiritual heart trouble. In *Herbal and magical medicine: Traditional healing today*, ed. James Kirkland, Holly F. Mathews, C. W. Sullivan III, and Karen Baldwin, 118–36. Durham, North Carolina: Duke University Press.

Corrine, L., V. Bailey, M. Valentine, E. Morantus, and L. Shirley. 1992. The unheard voices of women: Spiritual interventions in maternal-child health. *American Journal of Maternal Child Nursing* 17 (3): 141–45.

Csordas, Thomas J. 1983. The rhetoric of transformation in ritual healing. *Culture, Medicine and Psychiatry* 7: 333–75.

———. 1988. Elements of charismatic persuasion and healing. *Medical Anthropology Quarterly* 2: 121–42.

———. 1994. *The sacred self: A cultural phenomenology of charismatic healing.* Berkeley: University of California Press.

Davis, D. T., A. Bustamante, C. P. Brown, G. Wolde-Tsadik, E. W. Savage, X. Cheng, and L. Howland. 1994. The urban church and cancer control: A source of social influence in minority communities. *Public Health Reports* 109 (4): 500–506.

Etherington, Judy. 1968. Faith healing. *Foxfire* 2 (1): 15–24, 61–70.

Fields, Suzanne. 1976. Folk healing for the wounded spirit. *Innovations* 3 (1): 2–18.

Finkler, Kaja. 1981a. A comparative study of health seekers: Or, why do some people go to doctors rather than to spiritist healers? *Medical Anthropology* 5: 383–424.

———. 1981b. Focus on adherents of spiritualism. Part 2 of Non-medical treatments and their outcomes. *Culture, Medicine and Psychiatry* 5: 65–103.

Frank, Jerome D. 1975. The faith that heals. *Johns Hopkins Medical Journal* 137: 127–31.

Hand, Wayland D. 1980. *Magical medicine: The folkloric component of medicine in the folk belief, custom, and ritual of peoples of Europe and America.* Berkeley and Los Angeles: University of California Press.

Harrell, David Edwin, Jr. 1975. *All things are possible: The healing and charismatic revivals in modern America.* Bloomington: Indiana University Press.

Hieger, Roy R. 1957. Divine healing. The history of faith cures and their status today. *Journal of the Kansas Medical Society* 58 (12): 939.

Hufford, David J. 1977. Christian religious healing. *Journal of Operational Psychiatry* 8: 22–27.

———. 1985. Sainte Anne de Beaupré: Roman Catholic pilgrimage and healing. *Western Folklore* 44: 194–207.

———. 1987. The love of God's mysterious will: Suffering and the popular theology of healing. *Listening* 22: 225–39.

Idler, E. L. 1989. Moral medicine: Symbolic content in nineteenth century Shaker therapeutics. *Culture, Medicine and Psychiatry* 13 (1): 1–24.

Jankovic, S. M., D. V. Sokic, Z. M. Levic, V. Susic, N. Stojsavljevic, and J. Drulovic. 1996. Epilepsy, eponyms and patron saints (history of Western civilization). *Rpski Arhiv Za Celokokupino Lekarstvo* 124 (5–6): 162–65.

Jones, Michael Owen. 1967. Folk belief: Knowledge and action. *Southern Folklore Quarterly* 31: 304–9.

———. 1972. *Why faith healing?* Ottawa: National Museum of Man, Canadian Centre for Folk Culture Studies Mercury Series No. 5.

———. 1998. The aesthetic-emotional aspect of orthodoxy: Interview transcripts, proposed video and possible health implications. Unpublished report, Canadian Museum of Civilization, 93.

———. 1999. On chanting, iconography and emotion: What are some implications for health research? In *From* chantre *to* djak: *Cantorial traditions in Canada,* ed. Robert B. Klymasz. Hull, Ontario: Canadian Museum of Civilization. Forthcoming.

Kong, B. W., J. M. Miller, and R. T. Smoot. 1981. Churches as high blood pressure control centers. *American Journal of Public Health* 71: 1173.

Kurt, D. V. 1982. The Virgin of Guadalupe and the politics of becoming human. *Journal of Anthropological Research* 38: 194–210.

Littlewood, R., and S. Dein. 1995. The effectiveness of words: Religion and healing among the Lubavitch of Stamford Hill. *Culture, Medicine and Psychiatry* 19 (3): 339–83.

Loomis, C. Grant. 1940. Hagiological healing. *Bulletin of the History of Medicine* 8: 636–42.

Mandell, A. 1980. Toward a psychobiology of transcendence: God in the brain. In *The psychobiology of consciousness*, ed. D. Davidson and R. Davidson, 374–464. New York: Plenum.

McDonnell, K. 1976. *Charismatic renewal and the churches.* New York: Seabury Press.

Mickley, J., and K. Soeken. 1993. Religiousness and hope in Hispanic- and Anglo-American women with breast cancer. *Oncology Nursing Forum* 20 (8): 1171–77.

Miller, Joseph L. 1933. The healing gods or medical superstition. *West Virginia Medical Journal* 29: 465–78.

Miller, Russell. 1994. A leap of faith. *New York Times,* 30 January, V8: 1, 24.

Novo Pena, Silvia. 1993. Religion. In *The Hispanic-American almanac,* 367–86. Detroit: Gale Research.

Pedersen, D., and V. Baruffati. 1989. Healers, deities, saints and doctors: Elements for the analysis of medical systems. *Social Science and Medicine* 29 (4): 487–96.

Pimple, Kenneth D. 1995. Ghosts, spirits, and scholars: The origins of modern spiritualism. In *Out of the ordinary: Folklore and the supernatural,* ed. Barbara Walker, 75–89. Logan: Utah State University Press.

Stolley, J. M., H. Koenig. 1997. Religion/spirituality and health among elderly African Americans and Hispanics. *Journal of Psychosocial Nursing and Mental Health Services* 35 (11): 32–38.

Zimmerman, Leo M. 1937. Cosmos and Damian: Patron saints of surgery. *Bulletin of the Society of Medical History* 5: 69–87.

I.E.   *Psychosomatic conditions and hypnosis*

Bevilacqua, J. 1980. Voodoo-myth of mental illness? *Journal of Psychiatric Nursing and Mental Health* 18 (2): 17–23.

Binik, Y. M. 1985. Psychosocial predictors of sudden death: A review and critique. *Social Science and Medicine* 20 (7): 667–80.

Byers, James F. 1970. Voodoo: Tropical pharmacology or psychosomatic psychology? *New York Folklore* 26: 305–12.

Campinha-Bacote, J. 1992. Voodoo illness. *Perspectives in Psychiatric Care* 28 (1): 11–17.

Cannon, Walter B. 1942. "Voodoo" death. *American Anthropologist* 46: 169–81.

Cappannari, S. C., B. Rou, H. S. Abram, and D. C. Buchanan. 1975. Voodoo in the general hospital. A case of hexing and regional enteritis. *Journal of the American Medical Association* 232 (9): 938–40.

Chaturvedi, S. K., P. S. Chandra, M. K. Issac, and C. Y. Sudarshan. 1993. Somatization misattributed to non-pathological vaginal discharge. *Journal of Psychosomatic Research* 37 (6): 575–79.

Cohen, S. I. Voodoo death, the stress response, and AIDS. *Advances in Biochemical Psychopharmacology* 44: 95–109.

D'Andrea, V. J. 1978. Cancer pathomimicry: A report of three cases. *Journal of Clinical Psychiatry* 39 (3): 233–40.

Eastwell, H. D. 1987. Voodoo death in Australian aborigines. *Psychiatric Medicine* 5 (1): 71–73.

Ebert, D., and P. Martus. 1994. Somatization as a core symptom of melancholic type depression. Evidence from a cross-cultural study. *Journal of Affective Disorders* 32 (4): 253–56.

Furnham, A. 1989. Overcoming "psychosomatic" illness: Lay attributions of cure for five possible psychosomatic illnesses. *Social Science and Medicine* 29 (1): 61–67.

Kleinman, A. 1982. Neurasthenia and depression: A study of somatization and culture in China. *Culture, Medicine and Psychiatry* 6 (2): 117–90.

Lex, Barbara. 1974. Voodoo death: New thoughts on an old explanation. *American Anthropologist* 76: 818–23.

Medor, C. K. 1992. Hex death: Voodoo magic or persuasion? *Southern Medical Journal* 85 (3): 244–47.

Pang, K. Y., and M. H. Lee. 1994. Prevalence of depression and somatic symptoms among Korean elderly immigrants. *Yonsei Medical Journal* 35 (2): 155–61.

Ravenscroft, K., Jr. 1965. Voodoo possession: A natural experiment in hypnosis. *International Journal of Clinical and Experimental Hypnosis* 13 (3): 157–82.

Snell, J. E. 1967. Hypnosis in the treatment of the "hexed" patient. *American Journal of Psychiatry* 124: 311–16.

Tung, M. P. 1994. Symbolic meanings of the body in Chinese culture and "somatization." *Culture, Medicine and Psychiatry* 18 (4): 483–92.

Veyrat, J. G., and J. Ferrier. 1989. From Haitian voodoo and Brazilian candomble to European hyperapnea. Applications to psychosomatic medicine. In French. *Annales Medico-Psychologiques* 147 (3): 341–47.

Wintrob, R. M. 1973. The influence of others: Witchcraft and rootwork as explanations of behavior disturbances. *Journal of Nervous and Mental Disorders* 156 (5): 318–26.

I.F.   Ethnopsychiatry, psychotherapy, and symbolic healing

Aneshensel, C. S., and C. A. Sucoff. 1996. The neighborhood context of adolescent mental health. *Journal of Health and Social Behavior* 37 (4): 293–310.

Aneshensel, C. S., V. A. Clark, and R. R. Frerichs. 1983. Race, ethnicity, and depression: A confirmatory analysis. *Journal of Personality and Social Psychology* 44 (2): 385–98.

Angermeyer, M. C., and H. Matschinger. 1994. Lay beliefs about schizophrenic disorder: The results of a population survey in Germany. *Acta Psychiatrica Scandinavica*, suppl. 382, 39–45.

Ardon, R. C., A. J. Rubel, C. W. O'Nell, and R. H. Murray. 1983. A folk illness (susto) as an indicator of real illness. Letter. *Lancet* 2 (8363): 1362.

Barnett, E. A. 1989. Notes on nervios: A disorder of menopause. *Journal of Transcultural Nursing* 10 (2–3): 159–69.

Ben-Amos, D. 1994. Bettelheim among the folklorists. *Psychoanalytic Review* 81 (3): 509–35

Brekke, J. S., and C. Barrio. 1997. Cross-ethnic symptom differences in schizophrenia: The influence of culture and minority status. *Schizophrenia Bulletin* 23 (2): 305–16.

Camas-Diaz, L. 1981. Puerto Rican *espiritismo* and psychotherapy. *American Journal of Orthopsychiatry* 138 (11): 1477–81.

Chopra, M. 1995. Folk medicine and psychiatry. Letter. *Lancet* 345 (8963): 1510.

Cowley, S. 1991. A symbolic awareness context identified through a grounded theory study of health visiting. *Journal of Advanced Nursing* 16 (6): 648–56.

Davidson, J. R. 1985. The shadow of life: Psychosocial explanations for placenta rituals. *Culture, Medicine and Psychiatry* 9 (1): 75–92.

Davison, C., S. Frankel, and G. D. Smith. 1992. The limits of lifestyle: Re-assessing "fatalism" in the popular culture of illness prevention. *Social Science and Medicine* 34 (6): 675–85.

Diagnosis and treatment of depression in late life: The NIH Consensus Development Conference Statement. 1993. *Psychopharmacology Bulletin* 29 (1): 87–100.

Dorta-Morales, José. 1976. *Puerto Rican espiritismo: Religion and psychotherapy.* New York: Vantage Press.

Dow, James. 1986. Universal aspects of symbolic healing: A theoretical synthesis. *American Anthropologist* 88: 56–69.

Edgerton, Robert B., Marvin Karno, and Irma Fernandez. 1970. Curanderismo in the metropolis: The diminished role of folk psychiatry among Los Angeles Mexican-Americans. *American Journal of Psychotherapy* 24 (1): 124–34.

Eisenberg, Leon. 1981. The physician as interpreter: Ascribing meaning to the illness experience. *Comprehensive Psychiatry* 22: 239–48.

Finkler, Kaja. 1980. Non-medical treatments and their outcomes. *Culture, Medicine and Psychiatry* 4: 271–310.

———. 1989. The universality of nerves. *Health Care for Women International* 10 (2–3): 171–79.

Fisch, R. Z. 1992. Psychosis precipitated by marriage: A culture-bound syndrome? *British Journal of Medical Psychology* 65 (4): 385–91.

Flaskerud, J. H., and L. T. Hu. 1992. Relationship of ethnicity to psychiatric diagnosis. *Journal of Nervous and Mental Disease* 180 (5): 296–303.

Frank, Jerome D. 1967. *Persuasion and healing: A comparative study of psychotherapy.* New York: Schocken.

Frerichs, R. R., C. S. Aneshensel, and V. A. Clark. 1981. Prevalence of depression in Los Angeles County. *American Journal of Epidemiology* 113 (6): 691–99.

Gillin, John. 1948. Magical fright. *Psychiatry* 11: 387–400.

Gomez, E. A., and G. E. Gomez. 1985. Folk psychiatry and psychoanalysis. *Journal of the American Academy of Psychoanalysis* 13 (3): 379–90.

Harwood, Alan. 1977a. Description and analysis of an alternative psychotherapeutic approach. Part 1 of Puerto Rican spiritism. *Culture, Medicine and Psychiatry* 1: 69–95.

———. 1977b. *Rx: Spiritist as needed: A study of Puerto Rican community mental health resources.* New York: Wiley.

Herrera, Mary Armstrong. 1972. The miseries and folk medicine. *North Carolina Folklore* 20: 42–46.

Huang, J., J. Fox, C. Gordon, and A. Jackson-Smale. 1993. Symbolic decision support in medical care. *Artificial Intelligence in Medicine* 5 (5): 415–30.

Jayawardene, R. 1993. Illness perception: Social cost and coping-strategies of malaria cases. *Social Science and Medicine* 37 (9): 1169–76.

Karno, M. 1974. Some folk beliefs about mental illness: A reconsideration. *International Journal of Social Psychiatry* 20 (3–4): 292–96.

Karno, M., R. L. Hough, M. A. Burnam, J. I. Escobar, D. M. Timbers, F. Santana, and J. H. Boyd. 1987. Lifetime prevalence of specific psychiatric disorders among Mexican

Americans and non-Hispanic whites in Los Angeles. *Archives of General Psychiatry* 44 (8): 695–701.

Kasper, S., T. A. Wehr, J. J. Bartko, P. A. Gaist, and N. E. Rosenthal. 1989. Epidemiological findings of seasonal changes in mood and behavior. A telephone survey of Montgomery County, Maryland. *Archives of General Psychiatry* 46 (9): 823–33.

Katz, R., and E. Rolde. 1981. Community alternatives to psychotherapy. *Psychotherapy: Theory of Research and Practice* 18: 365–74.

Keefe, S. 1979. Mexican-Americans' underutilization of mental health clinics: An evaluation of suggested explanations. *Hispanic Journal of Behavioral Sciences* 1 (2): 93–115.

Kiev, Ari. 1962. The psychotherapeutic aspects of primitive medicine. *Human Organization* 21: 25–29.

Knight, S., A. Perry, and R. Persaud. 1995. Folk medicine and psychiatry. Letter. *Lancet* 345 (8963): 1510.

Koss, Joan D. 1970. Therapy of a system of a sect in Puerto Rico. *Revista de Ciencias Sociales* 14: 259–75.

———. 1980. The therapist spiritist training project in Puerto Rico: An experiment to relate the traditional healing system to the public health system. *Social Science and Medicine* 14B: 255–66.

———. 1987. Expectations and outcomes for patients given mental health care or spiritist healing in Puerto Rico. *American Journal of Psychiatry* 144 (1): 56–61.

Lee, S. 1996. Reconsidering the status of anorexia nervosa as a Western culture-bound syndrome. *Social Science and Medicine* 42 (1): 21–34.

Leininger, Madeleine. 1973. Witchcraft practices and psychocultural therapy with urban U.S. families. *Human Organization* 32: 73–83.

Lubchansky, Isaac, Gladys Egri, and Janet Stokes. 1970. Puerto Rican spiritualists view mental illness: The faith healer as paraprofessional. *American Journal of Psychiatry* 127: 312–21.

Moerman, Daniel E. 1979. Anthropology of symbolic healing. *Current Anthropology* 20: 59–80.

———. 1983. Physiology and symbols: The anthropological implications of the placebo effect. In *The anthropology of medicine: From culture to method,* 156–67. New York: Praeger.

Mumford, D. B. 1996. The "dhat syndrome": A culturally determined symptom of depression? *Acta Psychiatrica Scandinavica* 94 (3): 163–67.

Neki, J. S., B. Joinet, N. Ndosi, G. Kilonzo, J. G. Hauli, and G. Duvinage. 1986. Witchcraft and psychotherapy. *British Journal of Psychiatry* 149: 145–55.

Omark, R. C. 1980. Nervous breakdown as a folk illness. *Psychological Reports* 47 (3): 862.

Pedersen, P. B., R. T. Carter, and J. G. Ponterotto. 1996. The cultural context of psychology: Questions for accurate research and appropriate practice. *Cultural Diversity and Mental Health* 2 (3): 205–16.

Rips, L. J., and F. G. Conrad. 1989. Folk psychology of mental activities. *Psychological Review* 96 (2): 187–207.

Rogler, Lloyd H., and August B. Hollingshead. 1961. The Puerto Rican spiritualist as psychiatrist. *American Journal of Sociology* 67: 17–22.

Ruiz, Pedro. 1972. Santeros, botánicas and mental health: An urban view. *Transcultural Psychiatric Research Review Journal* 9: 176–77.

Ruiz, Pedro, and John Langrod. 1976. The role of folk healers in community mental health services. *Community Mental Health Journal* 12: 392–98.

Sammons, Robert. 1992. Parallels between magico-religious healing and clinical hypnosis therapy. In *Herbal and magical medicine: Traditional healing today*, ed. James Kirkland, Holly F. Mathews, C. W. Sullivan III, and Karen Baldwin, 53–67. Durham, North Carolina: Duke University Press.

Sandoval, M. C. 1979. Santería as a mental health care system: An historical overview. *Social Science and Medicine* 13B (2): 137–51.

Sargant, W. 1967. Witch doctoring, zar, and voodoo: Their relation to modern psychiatric treatments. *Proceedings of the Royal Society of Medicine* 60 (10): 1055–60.

Shimoji, A. 1991. Interface between shamanism and psychiatry in Miyako Islands, Okinawa, Japan: A viewpoint from medical and psychiatric anthropology. *Japanese Journal of Psychiatry and Neurology* 45 (4): 767–74.

Singer, Merrill. 1984a. Indigenous treatment for alcoholism: The case of Puerto Rican spiritism. *Medical Anthropology* 8 (4): 246–73.

———. 1984b. Spiritual healing and family therapy: Common approaches to the treatment of alcoholism. *Family Therapy* 11: 155–62.

Skevington, S. M. 1986. Psychological aspects of pain in rheumatoid arthritis: A review. *Social Science and Medicine* 23 (6): 567–75.

Slavney, P. R. 1992. Belief and behavior: The role of "folk psychology" in psychiatry. *Comprehensive Psychiatry* 33 (3): 166–72.

The spiritualist: Healer and co-therapist. A panel discussion. 1976. *Proceedings of Puerto Rican Conferences on Human Services* (20 October): 181–90.

Stich, S., and I. Ravenscroft. 1994. What is folk psychology? *Cognition* 50 (1–3): 447–68.

Sue, S., D. C. Fujino, L. T. Hu, D. T. Takeuchi, and N. W. Zane. 1991. Community mental health services for ethnic minority groups: A test of the cultural responsiveness hypothesis. *Journal of Consulting and Clinical Psychology* 59 (4): 533–40.

Swerdlow, M. H. 1992. "Chronicity," "nervios" and community care: A case study of Puerto Rican psychiatric patients in New York City. *Culture, Medicine and Psychiatry* 16 (2): 217–35.

Tousignant, M. 1984. Pena in the Ecuadorian Sierra: A psychoanthropological analysis of sadness. *Culture, Medicine and Psychiatry* 8 (4): 381–98.

Waldram, J. B. 1993. Aboriginal spirituality: Symbolic healing in Canadian prisons. *Culture, Medicine and Psychiatry* 17 (3): 345–62.

Ward, Colleen. 1980. Spirit possession and mental health: A psycho-anthropological perspective. *Human Relations* 33: 149–63.

———. 1981. Spirit possession and neuroticism in a West Indian Pentecostal community. *British Journal of Clinical Psychology* 20: 295–96.

Weclew, Robert V. 1975. The nature, prevalence, and level of awareness of "curanderismo" and some of its implications for community mental health. *Community Mental Health Journal* 11: 145–54.

Weiss, Carol I. 1992. Controlling domestic life and mental illness: Spiritual and aftercare resources used by Dominican New Yorkers. *Culture, Medicine and Psychiatry* 16: 237–71.

Wessels, W. H. 1985. The traditional healer and psychiatry. *Australian and New Zealand Journal of Psychiatry* 19 (3): 283–86.

Westermeyer, J. 1985. Psychiatric diagnosis across cultural boundaries. *American Journal of Psychiatry* 142 (7): 798–805.

———. 1988. National differences in psychiatric morbidity: Methodological issues, scientific interpretations and social implications. *Acta Psychiatrica Scandinavia Supplementum* 344: 23–31.

Westermeyer, J., and J. Kroll. 1978. Violence and mental illness in a peasant society: Characteristics of violent behaviours and "folk" use of restraints. *British Journal of Psychiatry* 133: 529–41.

Westermeyer, J., and R. Wintrob. 1979. "Folk" criteria for the diagnosis of mental illness in rural Laos: On being insane in sane places. *American Journal of Psychiatry* 136 (6): 755–61.

I.G.   *Menstruation, pregnancy, childbirth and children, and midwifery*

Adolph, C., D. E. Ramos, K. L. Linton, and D. A. Grimes. 1995. Pregnancy among Hispanic teenagers: Is good parental communication a deterrent? *Contraception* 51 (5): 303–6.

Barnett, E. A. 1989. Notes on nervios: A disorder of menopause. *Journal of Transcultural Nursing* 10 (2–3): 159–69.

Cattermole-Tally, Frances M. 1978. From the mystery of conception to the miracle of birth: An historical survey of beliefs and rituals surrounding the pregnant woman in Germanic folk tradition, including modern American folklore. Ph.D. diss., University of California, Los Angeles.

Corrine, L., V. Bailey, M. Valentin, E. Morauntus, and L. Shirley. 1992. The unheard voices of women: Spiritual interventions in maternal-child health. *American Journal of Maternal Child Nursing* 17 (3): 141–45.

Davidson, J. R. 1985. The shadow of life: Psychosocial explanations for placenta rituals. *Culture, Medicine and Psychiatry* 9 (1): 75–92.

Davis, D. L. 1988. Folk images of health and menstrual patterns among Newfoundland outport women. *Health Care for Women International* 9 (3): 211–23.

Davis-Floyd, Robbie E. 1987. The technological model of birth. *Journal of American Folklore* 100: 479–95.

———. 1992. *Birth as an American rite of passage.* Berkeley and Los Angeles: University of California Press.

de Laszlo, Henry, and Paul S. Henshaw. 1954. Plant materials used by primitive peoples to affect fertility. *Science* 119: 626–30.

DeSantis, Lydia, and Janice T. Thomas. 1990. The immigrant Haitian mother: Transcultural nursing perspective on preventive health care for children. *Journal of Transcultural Nursing* 2 (1): 2–15.

Etherington, Judy. 1952. Old wives on new lives: A study of prenatal superstitions. *Public Health Nursing* 44 (10): 537–41.

Fishman, C., R. Evans, and E. Jenks. 1988. Warm bodies, cool milk: Conflicts in post partum food choice for Indochinese women in California. *Social Science and Medicine* 26 (11): 1125–32.

Forbes, Thomas R. 1957. Early pregnancy and fertility tests. *Yale Journal of Biology and Medicine* 30: 16–29.

———. 1959. The prediction of sex: Folklore and science. *Proceedings of the American Philosophical Society* 103: 537–44.

———. 1962a. Midwifery and witchcraft. *Journal of the History of Medicine and Allied Sciences* 17: 264–83.

———. 1962b. Perette the midwife: A fifteenth century witchcraft case. *Bulletin of the History of Medicine* 36: 124–29.

———. 1963. Chalcedony and childbirth: Precious and semi-precious stones as obstetrical amulets. *Yale Journal of Biology and Medicine* 39: 390–401.

———. 1964. The regulation of English midwives in the sixteenth and seventeenth centuries. *Medical History* 8: 235–44.

Fox, S. A., and R. G. Roetzheim. 1994. Screening mammography and older Hispanic women: Current status and issues. *Cancer* 74 (suppl. 7): 2028–33.

Frankel, Barbara. 1970. Childbirth in the ghetto: Folk beliefs of Negro women in a north Philadelphia hospital ward. Master's thesis, Temple University, Philadelphia.

———. 1977. *Childbirth in the ghetto: Folk beliefs of Negro women in a north Philadelphia hospital ward.* San Francisco: R and E Research.

Gray, S., S. Lawrence, A. Arregui, N. Phillips, R. Bell, T. Richards, T. Fukushima, and H. W. Taeusch. 1995. Attitudes and behaviors of African-American and Mexican-American women delivering newborns in inner-city Los Angeles. *Journal of the National Medical Association* 87 (5): 353–58.

Johnson, T. M. 1987. Premenstrual syndrome as a Western culture-specific disorder. *Culture, Medicine and Psychiatry* 11 (3): 337–56.

Jordan, Brigitte, ed. 1993. *Birth in four cultures: A cross-cultural investigation of childbirth in Yucatan, Holland, Sweden, and the United States.* Prospect Heights, Illinois: Waveland Press.

Kanner, Leo. 1931. Born with a caul. *Medical Life* 38: 528–48.

Keeler, Teresa. 1984. Narrating, attitudes, and health: The effects of recounting pregnancy and childbirth experiences on the well-being of the participants. Ph.D. diss., University of California, Los Angeles.

Kelly, Isabel. 1965. *Folk practices in north Mexico: Birth customs, folk medicine, and Spiritualism in the Laguna Zone.* Institute of Latin American Studies, University of Texas Press, Austin.

Kelly, K. J., J. Neu, B. M. Camitta, and G. R. Honig. 1984. Methemoglobinemia in an infant treated with the folk remedy glycerated asafoetida. *Pediatrics* 73 (5): 717–19.

Kendall, L. 1987. Cold wombs in balmy Honolulu: Ethnogynecology among Korean immigrants. *Social Science and Medicine* 25 (4): 367–76.

Koniak-Griffin, D., S. Lominska, and M. L. Brecht. 1993. Social support during adolescent pregnancy: A comparison of three ethnic groups. *Journal of Adolescence* 16 (1): 43–56.

Krajewski-Jaime, E. R. 1991. Folk-healing among Mexican-American families as a consideration in the delivery of child welfare and child health care services. *Child Welfare* 70 (2): 157–67.

Layne, L. L. 1996. "How's the baby doing?": Struggling with narratives of progress in a neonatal intensive care unit. *Medical Anthropology Quarterly* 10 (4): 624–56.

Lewis, M. A., C. E. Lewis, B. Leake, G. Monahan, and G. Rachelefsky. 1996. Organizing the community to target poor Latino children with asthma. *Journal of Asthma* 33 (5): 289–97.

Lipton, May. 1969. The history and superstitions of birth defects. *Journal of School Health* 39: 579–82.

Lock, M. 1982. Models and practice in medicine: Menopause as syndrome or life transition? *Culture, Medicine and Psychiatry* 6 (3): 261–80.

Long, E. Croft. 1963. The placenta in lore and legend. *Bulletin of the Medical Library Association* 51: 233–41.

Marquez, Mary N., and Consuelo Pacheco. 1964. Midwifery lore in New Mexico. *American Journal of Nursing* 64 (9): 81–84.

McDaniel, Walton Brooks. 1948. The medical and magical significance in ancient medicine of things connected with reproduction and its organs. *Journal of the History of Medicine* 3: 525–46.

Mennella, J. A., and G. K. Beauchamp. 1993. Beer, breast-feeding, and folklore. *Developmental Psychobiology* 26 (8): 459–66.

Mikhail, B. I. 1994. Hispanic mothers' beliefs and practices regarding selected children's health problems. *Western Journal of Nursing Research* 16 (6): 623–38.

Newman, Lucille F. 1969. Folklore of pregnancy: Wives' tales in Contra Costa County, California. *Western Folklore* 28: 112–35.

Noall, Claire. 1944. Superstitions, customs, and prescriptions of Mormon midwives. *California Folklore Quarterly* 3: 102–14.

Oberg, C. N., and A. Deinard. 1984. Marasmus in a seventeen-month-old Laotian: Impact of folk beliefs on health. *Pediatrics* 73 (2): 254–57.

Oyejide, C. O., and G. A. Aderinokun. 1991. Teething myths in Nigerian rural Yoruba communities. *African Dental Journal* 5: 31–34.

Radbill, Samuel X. 1964. The folklore of teething. *Keystone Folklore Quarterly* 9: 123–43.

———. 1965. Teething in fact and fancy. *Bulletin of the History of Medicine* 39: 339–45.

Radecki, S. E. 1991. A racial and ethnic comparison of family formation and contraceptive practices among low-income women. *Public Health Reports* 106 (5): 494–502.

Richardson, J. L., B. Langholz, L. Bernstein, C. Burciaga, K. Danley, and R. K. Ross. 1992. Stage and delay in breast cancer diagnosis by race, socioeconomic status, age, and year. *British Journal of Cancer* 65 (6): 922–26.

Rogers, Martha E. 1953. Responses to talks on menstrual health. *Nursing Outlook* 1: 272–74.

Rosenthal, Ted. L., Ronald W. Henderson, Arline Hobson, and Maure Hurt. 1969. Social strata and perception of magical and folk-medical child-care practices. *Journal of Social Psychology* 77: 3–13.

Rubio, E. L., B. R. Ekins, P. D. Singh, and J. Dowis. 1987. Hmong opiate folk remedy toxicity in three infants. *Veterinary and Human Toxicology* 29 (4): 323–25.

Sandler, A. P., and L. S. Chan. 1978. Mexican-American folk belief in a pediatric emergency room. *Medical Care* 16 (9): 778–84.

Snapper, I. 1963. Midwifery, past and present. *Bulletin of the New York Academy of Medicine* 39: 503–32.

Snow, Loudell F., and Shirley M. Johnson. 1977. Modern day menstrual folklore: Some clinical implications. *Journal of the American Medical Association* 237 (25): 2736–39.

Snow, Loudell F., Shirley M. Johnson, and Harry E. Mayhew. 1978. The behavioral implications of some old wives' tales. *Obstetrics and Gynecology* 51: 727–32.

Stein, J. A., S. A. Fox, and P. J. Murata. 1991. The influence of ethnicity, socioeconomic status, and psychological barriers on use of mammography. *Journal of Health and Social Behavior* 32 (2): 101–13.

Sullivan, C. W., III. 1992. Childbirth education and traditional beliefs about pregnancy and childbirth. In *Herbal and magical medicine: Traditional healing today*, ed. James

Kirkland, Holly F. Mathews, C. W. Sullivan III, and Karen Baldwin, 170–79. Durham, North Carolina: Duke University Press.

Ugarriza, D. N. 1992. Postpartum affective disorders: Incidence and treatment. *Journal of Psychosocial Nursing and Mental Health Services* 30 (5): 29–32.

Wolf, Z. R. 1993. Nursing rituals: Doing ethnography. *NLN Publications* 19 (2535): 269–310.

Wood, P. J., and L. S. Giddings. 1991. The symbolic experience of hysterectomy. *Nursing Praxis in New Zealand* 6 (3): 3–7.

Zambrana, R. E., and S. C. Scrimshaw. 1997. Maternal psychosocial factors associated with substance use in Mexican-origin and African American, low-income, pregnant women. *Pediatric Nursing* 23 (3): 253–59.

Zambrana, R. E., C. Dunkel-Schetter, and S. C. Scrimshaw. 1991. Factors which influence use of prenatal care in low-income racial-ethnic women in Los Angeles County. *Journal of Community Health* 16 (5): 283–95.

I.H.   *Home remedies, popular beliefs, and superstitions*

Alpers, William C. 1907. History and uses of soap in pharmacy and medicine. *Journal of the Society of Chemical Industry* 26: 594–95.

Attebery, Louie W. 1963. Home remedies and superstitions. In *Idaho reader*, ed. Grace Edgington Jordan, 92–100. Boise, Idaho: n.p.

Bassin, A. 1984. Proverbs, slogans and folk sayings in the therapeutic community: A neglected therapeutic tool. *Journal of Psychoactive Drugs* 16 (1): 51–56.

Bergen, Fanny D., W. M. Beauchamp, and W. W. Newell. 1889. Current superstitions. *Journal of American Folklore* 2: 12–22, 105–12, 203–8.

Brown, Allen L., Steve Whaley, and Watson C. Arnold. 1981. Acute bicarbonate intoxication from a folk remedy. *American Journal of Diseases of Children* 135: 965.

Brown, C. M., and R. Segal. 1996. The effects of health and treatment perceptions on the use of prescribed medication and home remedies among African American and white American hypertensives. *Social Science and Medicine* 43 (6): 903–17.

Curtis, E. K. 1990. The string and the doorknob: Profile of a popular approach to dental extraction. *Journal of Oral and Maxillofacial Surgery* 48 (10): 1084–92.

Dehn, M. A. 1990. Vitamin C, chicken soup, and amulets: Students view self-care practices. *Nurse Educator* 15 (4): 12–15.

Edgar, Irving I. 1962. Superstition and therapeutics in medicine. *Journal of the Michigan State Medical Society* 61 (2): 214–16.

Etherington, Judy. 1968. Home remedies. *Foxfire* 2 (1): 10–14.

Forbes, Thomas R. 1972. Lapis Bufonis: The growth and decline of a medical superstition. *Yale Journal of Biology and Medicine* 45: 139–49.

Forsythe, Warren E. 1947. Fallacies about health. *Hygeia* 25: 512–13.

Fulkerson, C. B. 1908. Medical fallacies. *Journal of the Michigan State Medical Society* 7: 170–75.

Funk, William D. 1950. Hiccup cures. *Western Folklore* 9: 66–67.

Gibson, John M. 1950. Superstition and disease. *Health Pilot* 6–7, 11.

Inman, W. S. 1946. Styes, barley, and wedding rings. *British Journal of Medical Psychology* 20 (4): 331–38.

Kahn, Max, M.D. 1913. Vulgar specifics and therapeutic superstitions. *Popular Science Monthly* 83: 81–96.

Kanner, Leo. 1931. Superstitions connected with sneezing. *Medical Life* 38: 549–75.

Labarbera, Michael. 1964. An ounce of prevention, and Grandma tried them all. *New York Folklore Quarterly* 20: 126–29.

Lalayan, E. 1898. Popular medicine. *Ethnographic Review* 4: 96–100.

Long, Eleanor. 1973. Aphrodisiacs, charms, and philtres. *Western Folklore* 32: 153–63.

Loomis, C. Grant. 1944. Lapidary medicine. *Bulletin of the History of Medicine* 16: 319–24.

MacDonald, Flora. 1956. Home remedies. *North Carolina Folklore* 4 (2): 17–18.

Mieder, Wolfgang. 1993. "An apple a day keeps the doctor away": Traditional and modern aspects of medical proverbs. In *Proverbs are never out of season*, 152–72. New York: Oxford University Press.

Murphree, Alice H., and Mark V. Barrow, M.D. 1970. Physician dependence, self-treatment practices, and folk remedies in a rural area. *Southern Medical Journal* 63: 403–8.

Neal, Janice C. 1955. Grandad—Pioneer medicine man. *New York Folklore Quarterly* 11: 277–91.

Page, Mrs. Marion T. 1954. Superstitions at home. *Tennessee Folklore Society Bulletin* 20: 53–56.

Pritchard, Frank H., M.D. 1901. Some odd remedies and superstitions in the treatment of disease. *Hahnemannian Monthly* 36: 558–61.

Radford, E., and M. A. Radford. 1961. *Encyclopaedia of Superstitions*, ed. Christina Hole. London: Hurchinson.

Shalinsky, Audrey C. 1985. Thermal springs as folk curing mechanisms. *Folklore Forum* 18: 32–58.

Snow, Loudell F., Shirley M. Johnson, and Harry E. Mayhew. 1978. The behavioral implications of some old wives' tales. *Obstetrics and Gynecology* 51: 727–32.

Stahl, William Harris. 1937. Moon madness. *Annals of Medical History* 9: 248–63.

Taylor, Walter. 1957. Home remedies for arthritis. *Proceedings of Texas Folklore Society* 27: 192–200.

Townsend, Barbara Ann, and Donald Allport Bird. 1970. The miracle of string measurement. *Indiana Folklore* 3: 147–62.

Trotter, R. T., II. 1985. Greta and Azarcon: A survey of episodic lead poisoning from a folk remedy. *Human Organization* 44 (1): 64–72.

True, Rodney H. 1901. Folk materia medica. *Journal of American Folklore* 14: 105–14.

Walker, W. R., and D. M. Keats. 1976. An investigation of the therapeutic value of the "copper bracelet"—Dermal assimilation of copper in arthritic/rheumatoid conditions. *Agents and Actions* 6: 454–59.

Westermeier, Therese S. 1953. Old-time commercial cure-alls. *Western Folklore* 12: 257–65.

Whitehouse, M. W. 1976. Ambivalent role of copper in inflammatory disorders. *Agents Actions* 6 (1–3): 201–6.

Wright, Sue, Mick Myra Wright, and Nellie Engelke. 1960. Superstitions and remedies. *West Virginia Folklore* 10: 63–68.

I.I.   Evil eye

Gifford, Edward S., Jr., M.D. 1957. The evil eye in medical history. *American Journal of Ophthalmology* 44 (2): 237–43.

———. 1960. The evil eye in Pennsylvania medical history. *Keystone Folklore Quarterly* 5 (3): 3–8.

Gordon, Benjamin L. 1939. Oculists and occultists: Demonology and the eye. *Archives of Ophthalmology* 22: 25–65.

———. 1961. The evil eye. *Hebrew Medical Journal* 34: 291–361.

Hand, Wayland D. 1980. The evil eye in its folk medical aspects: A survey of North America. In *Magical medicine*, 239–49. Berkeley and Los Angeles: University of California Press.

Helman, Cecil G. 1978. "Feed a cold, starve a fever"—Folk models of infection in an English suburban community, and their relationship to medical treatment. *Culture, Medicine and Psychiatry* 2: 107–37.

Jones, Louis C. 1951. The evil eye among European-Americans. *Western Folklore* 10: 11–25.

McDaniel, Walton Brooks. 1918. The *Pupula duplex* and other tokens of an "evil eye" in the light of ophthalmology. *Classical Philology* 13: 335–46.

Naff, Alixa. 1965. Belief in the evil eye among the Christian Syrian-Lebanese in America. *Journal of American Folklore* 78: 46–51.

Potts, Albert M. 1960. The mind's eye. Some concepts of vision in the ancient and primitive world. *Bulletin of the Cleveland Medical Library* 7 (1): 5–14.

I.J.   Burn healing, blood stopping, wart healing, and thrash cures

Anderson, John Q. 1968. Special powers in folk cures and remedies. *Proceedings of the Texas Folklore Society* 34: 163–74.

Bett, W. R. 1951. Wart, I bid thee begone. *Practitioner* 166 (991): 77–80.

Dorson, Richard M. 1947. Blood stoppers. *Southern Folklore Quarterly* 11: 105–18.

———. 1952. *Bloodstoppers and bearwalkers: Folk traditions of the Upper Peninsula.* Cambridge: Harvard University Press.

Halpert, Violetta. 1949. Indiana wart cures. *Hoosier Folklore* 8: 37–43.

Kirkland, James. 1992. Talking fire out of burns: A magico-religious healing tradition. In *Herbal and magical medicine: Traditional healing today*, ed. James Kirkland, Holly F. Mathews, C. W. Sullivan III, and Karen Baldwin, 41–52. Durham, North Carolina: Duke University Press.

Simmons, Frank. 1938. The wart doctor. *Proceedings of the Texas Folklore Society* 14: 192–94.

Unusual ritual burns of the hand. 1996. *Burns* 22 (5): 409–12.

Webb, Wheaton Phillips. 1946. The wart. *New York Folklore Quarterly* 2: 98–106.

I.K.   Metaphor, narrative, and ritual

Borkan, J., W. Miller, and S. Reis. 1992. Medicine as storytelling. *Family Practice* 9: 127–29.

Bornstein, E. 1988. Therapeutic storytelling. In *Relaxation and imagery: Tools for therapeutic communication and intervention*, ed. R. Zahourek, 101–20. Philadelphia: Saunders.

Burnside, I., and B. Haight. 1994. Reminiscence and life review: Therapeutic interventions for older people. *Nurse Practitioner* 19 (4): 55–61.

Csordas, Thomas J. 1997. *Language, charisma, and creativity: The ritual life of a religious movement.* Berkeley: University of California Press.

DeLuca, E. K. 1995. Reconsidering rituals: A vehicle for educational change. *Journal of Continuing Education in Nursing* 26 (3): 139–44.

Fiese, B. H. 1992. Dimensions of family rituals across two generations: Relation to adolescent identity. *Family Process* 31 (2): 151–62.

Hahn, K. 1987. Therapeutic storytelling: Helping children learn and cope. *Pediatric Nursing* 13: 175–78.

Hand, Wayland D. 1980. *Magical medicine: The folkloric component of medicine in the folk belief, custom, and ritual of peoples of Europe and America.* Berkeley and Los Angeles: University of California Press.

Heiney, Sue P. 1988. Assessing and intervening with dysfunctional families. *Oncology Nursing Forum* 15: 585–90.

———. 1995. The healing power of story. *Oncology Nursing Forum* 22: 899–904.

Johnson, D. R, S. C. Feldman, H. Lubin, and S. M. Southwick. 1995. The therapeutic use of ritual and ceremony in the treatment of post-traumatic stress disorder. *Journal of Traumatic Stress* 8 (2): 283–98.

Jones, A. 1995. Reflective process in action: The uncovering of the ritual of washing in clinical nursing practice. *Journal of Clinical Nursing* 4 (5): 283–88.

Joralemon, Donald. 1986. The performing patient in ritual healing. *Social Science and Medicine* 23: 841–45.

Kerfoot, K., and G. Sarosi. 1993. Hero making through storytelling: The nurse manager's challenge. *Nursing Economics* 11: 107–12.

Klein, R. 1990. Pain control interventions of Milton H. Erickson. In *Brief therapy: Myths, methods, and metaphors,* ed. J. Zeig and S. Gilligan, 273–87. New York: Brunner and Mazel.

Krietmeyer, B., and S. Heiney. 1992. Storytelling as a therapeutic technique in a group for school-aged oncology patients. *Children's Health Care* 21 (1): 14–20.

Levine, E. 1980. Indirect suggestions through personalized fairy tales for treatment of childhood insomnia. *American Journal of Clinical Hypnosis* 23 (1): 57–63.

McGuire, M. B. 1988. *Ritual healing in suburban America.* New Brunswick, New Jersey: Rutgers University Press.

McQuellon, R. P., and G. Hurt. 1993. The healing power of cancer stories. *Journal of Psychosocial Oncology* 11 (4): 95–108.

Mills, J., and R. Crowley. 1986. *Therapeutic metaphors for children and the child within.* New York: Brunner and Mazel.

Newman, P. J., Jr., and M. R. Nelson. 1996. Mainstream legitimization of homosexual men through Valentine's Day gift-giving and consumption rituals. *Journal of Homosexuality* 31 (1–2): 57–69.

Robertson, M., and F. Barford. 1970. Story-making in psychotherapy with a chronically ill child. *Psychotherapy: Theory, Research and Practice* 7 (2): 104–7.

Rosen, George. 1962. Psychopathology in the social process: Dance frenzies, demonic possession, revival movements and similar so-called psychic epidemics. An interpretation. *Bulletin of the History of Medicine* 36 (1): 13–44.

Sidenvall, B., C. Fjellstrom, and A. C. Ek. 1996. Ritualized practices among caregivers at meals in geriatric care. *Scandinavian Journal of Caring Sciences* 10 (1): 53–61.

Sontag, Susan. 1978. *Illness as metaphor.* New York: Farrar, Straus and Giroux.

Strange, F. 1996. Handover: An ethnographic study of ritual in nursing practice. *Intensive and Critical Care Nursing* 12 (2): 106–12.

Thompson, K. 1990. Metaphor: A myth with a method. In *Brief therapy: Myths, methods, and metaphors,* ed. J. Zeig and S. Gilligan, 247–57. New York: Brunner and Mazel.

Vezeau, T. 1993. Storytelling: A practitioner's tool. *MCN: The American Journal of MaternalChild Nursing* 18: 193–96.

Wall, L. L. 1996. Ritual meaning in surgery. *Obstetrics and Gynecology* 88 (4): 633–37.

Wenckus, E. M. 1994. Storytelling: Using an ancient art to work with groups. *Journal of Psychosocial Nursing and Mental Health Services* 32 (7): 30–32.

Wrenshall, Letitia Humphreys. 1902. Incantations and popular healing in Maryland and Pennsylvania. *Journal of American Folklore* 15: 268–74.

I.L. *Powwow*

Aurand, A. Monroe, Jr. 1929. *The pow-wow book: A treatise on the art of "healing by prayer" and "laying on of hands," etc., practiced by the Pennsylvania Germans and others, etc.* Harrisburg, Pennsylvania: Aurand Press.

Byington, Robert H. 1964. Powwowing in Pennsylvania. *Keystone Folklore Quarterly* 9: 111–17.

Frazier, Paul. 1952. Some lore of hexing and powwowing. *Midwest Folklore* 2: 101–7.

Hohman, John George. 1930. *Long lost friend, or book of pow-wows; A collection of mysterious and invaluable arts and remedies for man as well as animals . . .*, ed. A. Monroe Aurand, Jr. Harrisburg, Pennsylvannia: n.p.

Reimensnyder, Barbara Lou. 1982. Powwowing in Union County: A study of Pennsylvania German folk medicine in context. Ph.D. diss., University of Pennsylvania, Philadelphia.

Yoder, Don. 1966. Twenty questions on powwowing. *Pennsylvania Folklife* 15, 4 (summer): 38–40.

I.M. *Veterinary healing practices*

Davidson, Thomas. 1956. Elf-shot cattle. *Antiquity* 30: 149–55.

———. 1960a. The amuletic and transfer charm cure of cattle and horses. *British Veterinary Journal* 116 (6): 205–17.

———. 1960b. The cure of elf-disease in animals. *Journal of the History of Medicine and Allied Science* 15: 282–91.

———. 1960c. A survey of some British veterinary folklore. *Bulletin of the History of Medicine* 34: 199–232.

Hunter, Earl D. 1962. Folk remedies on man and beasts. *Kentucky Folklore Record* 8: 97–108.

I.N. *Geophagy*

Cooper, M. 1957. *Pica.* Springfield, Illinois: Charles C. Thomas.

Halsted, J. A. 1968. Geophagia in man: Its nature and nutritional effects. *American Journal of Clinical Nutrition* 21: 1384–93.

Hunter, J. M. 1973. Geophagy in Africa and the United States. *Geographical Review* 63: 170–95.

Laufer, Berthold. 1930. Geophagy. Field Museum of Natural History. *Anthropological Series* 18 (2).

Reid, R. M. 1992. Cultural and medical perspectives on geophagia. *Medical Anthropology* 13: 337–51.

Vermeer, D. E. 1979. Geophagia in rural Mississippi: Environmental and cultural contexts and nutritional implications. *American Journal of Clinical Nutrition* 32(10): 2129–35.

I.O.   Homeopathy and holistic healing

Berlinger, H. S., and J. W. Salmon. 1980. The holistic alternative to scientific medicine: History and analysis. *International Journal of Health Services* 10: 133–47.

Bullock, M. L., A. M. Pheley, T. J. Kiresuk, S. K. Lenz, and P. D. Culliton. 1997. Characteristics and complaints of patients seeking therapy at a hospital-based alternative medicine clinic. *Journal of Alternative and Complementary Medicine* 3 (1): 31–37.

Dale, R. A. 1996. New developments in Cuban holistic medicine: A personal view. *Journal of Alternative and Complementary Medicine* 2 (2): 299–305.

Mattson, Phyllis H. 1982. *Holistic health in perspective.* Palo Alto, California: Mayfield Publishing.

Ross, A. G. Gordon. 1978. *Homeopathic green medicine.* Wellingsborough: Thorsons.

Sommer, S. J. 1996. Mind-body medicine and holistic approaches: The scientific evidence. *Australian Family Physician* 25 (8): 1233–37.

van Galen, E. 1995. Exploring homeopathic resources on the internet: HOMEOWEB. *Journal of Alternative and Complementary Medicine* 1 (4): 387–91.

II. *North American folk medicine: Regional variations*

II.A.   *Southwestern*

Anderson, John Q. 1968a. Magical transference of disease in Texas folk medicine. *Western Folklore* 27: 191–99.

———. 1968b. Popular beliefs in Texas, Louisiana, and Arkansas. *Southern Folklore Quarterly* 32: 304–19.

———. 1970. *Texas folk medicine: 1333 cures, remedies, preventives, and health practices.* Austin, Texas: Encino.

Bourke, John G. 1894. Popular medicine, customs, and superstitions of the Rio Grande. *Journal of American Folklore* 7: 119–46.

Carrasco, S. 1974. Curanderismo in south Texas. *School Health Review* 5 (5): 7.

Curtin, L. S. M. 1930. Pioneer medicine in New Mexico. In *Folk-say: A regional miscellany,* ed. B. A. Botkin, 186–96. N.p.

Graham, Joe S. 1976. The role of the curandero in the Mexican American folk medicine system in west Texas. In *American folk medicine: A symposium,* ed. Wayland D. Hand, 175–89. Berkeley and Los Angeles: University of California Press.

Hatfield, Sadie. 1943. Folklore of Texas plants. *Proceedings of the Texas Folklore Society* 18: 157–62.

Kay, M. A. 1979. Health and illness in a Mexican American barrio. In *Ethnic medicine in the Southwest,* ed. E. H. Spicer. Tucson: University of Arizona Press.

Keegan, L. 1996. Use of alternative therapies among Mexican Americans in the Texas Rio Grande Valley. *Journal of Holistic Nursing* 14 (4): 277–94.

Kraus, A., G. Guerra-Bautista, and D. Alarcon-Segovia. 1991. Salmonella Arizona arthritis and septicemia associated with rattlesnake ingestion by patients with connective tissue diseases. A dangerous complication of folk medicine. *Journal of Rheumatology* 18 (9): 1328–31.

Marquez, Mary N., and Consuelo Pacheco. 1964. Midwifery lore in New Mexico. *American Journal of Nursing* 64 (9): 81–84.

Quesada, G. M., and P. L. Heller. 1977. Sociocultural barriers to medical care among Mexican Americans in Texas: A summary report of research conducted by the Southwest Medical Sociology Ad Hoc Committee. *Medical Care* 15 (suppl. 5): 93–101.

Scheper-Hughes, Nancy. 1983. Curanderismo in Taos County, New Mexico—A possible case of anthropological romanticism? *Western Journal of Medicine* 139 (6): 875–84.

Spicer, Edward, ed. 1977. *Ethnic medicine in the Southwest.* Tucson: University of Arizona Press.

Trotter, R. T., II. 1982. Contrasting models of the healer's role: South Texas case examples. *Hispanic Journal of Behavioral Sciences* 4: 315–27.

———. 1985. Folk medicine in the Southwest. Myths and medical facts. *Postgraduate Medicine* 78 (8): 167–70, 173–76, 179.

Waterman, S. H., G. Juarez, S. J. Carr, and L. Kilman. 1990. Salmonella Arizona infections in Latinos associated with rattlesnake folk medicine. *American Journal of Public Health* 80 (3): 286–89.

II.B. Northeastern

Baker, Ronald L. 1969. Folk medicine in the writings of Rowland E. Robinson. *Vermont History* 37: 184–93.

Barrick, Mac E. 1964. Folk medicine in Cumberland County. *Keystone Folklore Quarterly* 9: 100–110.

Bayard, Samuel P. 1938. Witchcraft, magic and spirits on the border of Pennsylvania and West Virginia. *Journal of American Folklore* 51: 47–59.

II.C. Southern

Anderson, John Q. 1968. Popular beliefs in Texas, Louisiana and Arkansas. *Southern Folklore Quarterly* 32: 304–19.

Anderson, Urban. 1937. A comparative study of some of the older beliefs and usages of east Tennessee. *Tennessee Folklore Society Bulletin* 3: 1–7.

Babb, E. M. 1935. Survivals of medical magic and superstitions in southside Virginia. *Bulletin of the (Richmond, Virginia) Stuart Circle Hospital* 5: 39–47.

Bacon, A. M. 1896. Conjuring and conjure-doctors in the southern United States. *Journal of American Folklore* 9: 224–26.

Brandon, Elizabeth. 1976. Folk medicine in French Louisiana. In *American folk medicine,* ed. Wayland D. Hand, 215–34. Berkeley and Los Angeles: University of California Press.

Browne, Ray B. 1958. *Popular beliefs and practices from Alabama,* 9. Folklore Studies, University of California Publications, Berkeley and Los Angeles.

Campbell, Marie. 1953. Folk remedies from south Georgia. *Tennesse Folklore Society Bulletin* 19: 1–4.

Cavender, A. P. 1992. Theoretic orientations and folk medicine research in the Appalachian South. *Southern Medical Journal* 85 (2): 170–78.

Clements, William M. 1976. Faith healing narratives from northeast Arkansas. *Indiana Folklore* 9: 15–39.

Cook, C., and D. Baisden. 1986. Ancillary use of folk medicine by patients in primary care clinics in southwestern West Virginia. *Southern Medical Journal* 79 (9): 1098–1101.

Evans, David K., Don Stephen Rice, and Joanne Kline Partin. 1968. Parallels in West African, West Indian, and North Carolina Folklore. *North Carolina Folklore* 17: 77–84.

Flaskerud, J. H. 1980. Perceptions of problematic behavior by Appalachians, mental health professionals, and lay non-Appalachians. *Nursing Research* 29 (3): 140–49.

Harder, Kelsie B. 1956. Home remedies in Perry County, Tennessee. *Tennessee Folklore Society Bulletin* 22: 97–98.

Harris, Bernice Kelly, ed. 1968. *Southern home remedies.* Murfreesboro, North Carolina: Johnson Publishing.

Hawkins, John. 1907. Magical medical practice in South Carolina. *Popular Science Monthly* 70: 165–74.

Jones, Michael Owen. 1967. Toward an understanding of folk medical beliefs in North Carolina. *North Carolina Folklore Journal* 15: 23–27.

Levenson, Beverly, and Myron H. Levenson. 1960. Some southern folk remedies and related beliefs. *North Carolina Folklore* 8 (2): 26–31.

Lewis, Gabe. 1938. Old-time remedies from Madison County. *Proceedings of the Texas Folklore Society* 14: 267–68.

Long, Grady M. 1962. Folk medicine in McMinn, Polk, Bradley, and Meigs Counties, Tennessee, 1910–1927. *Tennessee Folklore Society Bulletin* 28: 1–8.

Martin, Roxie. 1947. Old remedies collected in the Blue Ridge Mountains. *Journal of American Folklore* 60: 184–85.

Mason, James. 1957. Home remedies in West Virginia. *West Virginia Folklore* 7: 27–32.

Mathews, Holly F. 1987. Rootwork: Description of an ethnomedical system in the American South. *Southern Medical Journal* 80 (7): 885–91.

McLean, Patricia S. 1972. Conjure doctors in eastern North Carolina. *North Carolina Folklore* 20: 21–29.

Mullins, Gladys. 1973. Herbs of the southern Highlands and their medicinal uses. *Kentucky Folklore Record* 19: 36–41.

Murphree, Alice H. 1965. Folk medicine in Florida: Remedies using plants. *Florida Anthropologist* 18: 175–85.

Norris, Ruby R. 1958. Folk medicine of Cumberland County. *Kentucky Folklore Record* 4: 101–10.

O'Dell, Ruth W. 1951. Before you call your doctor. *Tennessee Folklore Society Bulletin* 17: 29–31.

Parr, Jerry S. 1962. Folk cures of middle Tennessee. *Tennessee Folklore Society Bulletin* 28: 8–12.

Reynolds, Hubert. 1950. Grandma's handbook. *Tennessee Folklore Society Bulletin* 16: 13–14.

Ritter, M. R. 1992. Take two spider webs and call me in the morning: Southern folk medicine. *North Carolina Medical Journal* 53 (5).

Rogers, James C. 1968. Talking out fire. *North Carolina Folklore* 16: 46–52.

Ross, R. A. 1934. Granny grandiosity. *Southern Medicine and Surgery* 96: 57–59.

Steiner, Roland. 1901. The practice of conjuring in Georgia. *Journal of American Folklore* 14: 173–80.

Stuart, Jesse. 1931. The yarb doctor. *Kentucky Folk-Lore and Poetry Magazine* 6 (1): 4–10.

Sugarman, J., and R. Butters. 1985. Understanding the patient: Medical words the doctor may not know. *North Carolina Medical Journal* 46: 415–17.

Waller, Tom, and Gene Killion. 1972. Georgia folk medicine. *Southern Folklore Quarterly* 36: 71–92.

Webb, J. Y. 1971. Louisiana voodoo and superstitions related to health. *HSMHA Health Reports* 86 (4): 291–301.

Wilson, Gordon. 1966. Talismans and magic in folk remedies in the Mammoth Cave region. *Southern Folklore Quarterly* 30: 192–201.

———. 1967. Swallow it or rub it on: More Mammoth Cave remedies. *Southern Folklore Quarterly* 31: 296–303.

———. 1968a. Local plants in folk remedies in the Mammoth Cave region. *Southern Folklore Quarterly* 32: 320–27.

———. 1968b. "Store-bought" remedies in the Mammoth Cave region. *North Carolina Folklore* 16: 58–62.

Yates, Irene. 1946. Conjures and cures in the novels of Julia Peterkin. *Southern Folklore Quarterly* 10: 137–49.

II.D.   *Midwestern*

Black, Pauline Monette. 1935. *Nebraska folk cures*. Lincoln, Nebraska: University of Nebraska Studies in Language, Literature, and Criticism, no. 15.

Brewster, Paul G. 1939. Folk cures and preventives from southern Indiana. *Southern Folklore Quarterly* 3: 33–43.

———. 1943. Folk beliefs and practices from southern Indiana. *Hoosier Folklore Bulletin* 2: 23–38.

Davenport, Gertrude C. 1898. Folk-cures from Kansas. *Journal of American Folklore* 11: 129–32.

Fox, Ben. 1948. Folk medicine in southern Illinois. *Illinois Folklore* 2: 3–7.

Halpert, Violetta. 1949. Indiana wart cures. *Hoosier Folklore* 8: 37–43.

———. 1950. Folk cures from Indiana. *Hoosier Folklore* 9: 1–12.

Hurty, J. N. 1922. An old Indiana book on medicine. *Journal of the Indiana State Medical Association* 14 (4): 122–24.

Hyatt, Harry Middleton. 1965. *Folklore from Adams County Illinois*. 2nd revised ed. N.p.: Memoirs of the Alma Egan Hyatt Foundation.

Kevin, Mary E. 1947. Indian herbalism and colonial medicine. *Trained Nurse and Hospital Review* 119: 347.

Lathrop, Amy. 1961. Pioneer remedies from western Kansas. *Western Folklore* 20: 1–22.

McAtee, W. L. 1955. Home medication in Grant County, Indiana, in the nineties. *Midwest Folklore* 5: 213–16.

———. 1958. Medical lore in Grant County, Indiana, in the nineties. *Midwest Folklore* 8: 151–53.

O'Dell, Ruth. 1950. Mid-western saliva lore. *Southern Folklore Quarterly* 14: 220–23.

Pickard, Madge E., and R. Carlyle Buley. 1945. *The midwest pioneer, his ills, cures, and doctors*. Crawfordsville, Indiana: R.E. Banta.

Puckett, Newbell Niles. 1981. *Popular beliefs and superstitions: A compendium of American folklore from the Ohio collection of Newbell Niles Puckett*, ed. Wayland D. Hand, Anna Casetta, and Sondra B. Thiederman. 3 vols. Boston: N.p.

Smith, Walter R. 1929. Animals and plants in Oklahoma folk cures. In *Folk-say: A regional miscellany*, ed. Benjamin A. Botkin, 69–78. Norman: University of Oklahoma Press.

Stekert, Ellen J. 1970. Focus for conflict: Southern mountain medical beliefs in Detroit. *Journal of American Folklore* 83: 115–47.

II.E.   *Western*

Anderson, John Q. 1968. Magical transference of disease in Texas folk medicine. *Western Folklore* 27: 191–99.

Appelt, Glenn D. 1985. Pharmacological aspects of selected herbs employed in Hispanic folk medicine in the San Luis Valley of Colorado, U.S.A.: I. *Ligusticum porteri* (osha) and *Matricaria chamomilla* (manzanilla). *Journal of Ethnopharmacology* 13 (1): 51–55.

Baker, Pearl, and Ruth Wilcox. 1948. Folk remedies in early Green River. *Utah Humanities Review* 2: 191–92.

Bushnell, John H. 1947. Medical folklore from California. *Western Folklore* 6: 273–75.

Campa, Arthur L. 1950. Some herbs and plants of early California. *Western Folklore* 9: 338–47.

Cannon, Anthon S. 1984. In *Popular beliefs and superstitions from Utah*, ed. Wayland D. Hand and Jeannine E. Talley. Salt Lake City: University of Utah Press.

Clar, Mimi. 1959. Childhood beliefs from Stockton, California. *Western Folklore* 18: 41–42.

Firestone, Melvin M. 1962. Sephardic folk-curing in Seattle. *Journal of American Folklore* 75: 301–10.

Hatfield, Sadie. 1943. Folklore of Texas plants. *Publications of the Texas Folklore Society* 18: 157–62.

Jordan, Philip D. 1944. Botanic medicine in the western country. *Western Folklore* 40: 143–46.

Kell, Katherine T. 1965. Tobacco in folk cures in Western society. *Journal of American Folklore* 78: 99–114.

Kelley, B. D., Glenn D. Appelt, and J. M. Appelt. 1988. Pharmacological aspects of selected herbs employed in Hispanic folk medicine in the San Luis Valley of Colorado, U.S.A.: II. *Aclepias asperula* (inmortal) and *Achillea lanulosa* (plumajillo). *Journal of Ethnopharmacology* 22 (1): 1–9.

King, Virgil A. 1951. Sandhill remedies and cures. *Western Folklore* 10: 172–73.

Madsen, William. 1955. Hot and cold in the universe of San Francisco Tecospa, Valley of Mexico. *Journal of American Folklore* 68: 123–39.

Marquez, Mary N., and Consuelo Pacheco. 1964. Midwifery lore in New Mexico. *American Journal of Nursing* 64 (9): 81–84.

Newman, Lucille F. 1969. Folklore of pregnancy: Wives' tales in Contra Costa County, California. *Western Folklore* 28: 112–35.

Noall, Claire. 1944. Superstitions, customs, and prescriptions of Mormon midwives. *California Folklore Quarterly* 3: 102–14.

Schedler, Paul W. 1971. Folk medicine in Denton County today: Or, can dermatology displace dishrags? *Publications of the Texas Folklore Society* 35: 11–17.

Smith, Walter R. 1929. Animals and plants in Oklahoma folk cures. In *Folk-say: A regional miscellany*, ed. B. A. Botkin, 69–78. Norman: University of Oklahoma Press.

Wilson, Julius I., M.D. 1967. Pikes Peak or bust: An historical note on the search for health in the Rockies. *Rocky Mountain Medical Journal* 64 (9): 58–62.

II.F.   *Urban*

Becerra, R. M., and A. P. Iglehart. 1995. Folk medicine use: Diverse populations in a metropolitan area. *Social Work in Health Care* 21 (4): 37–58.

Carlisle, D. M., B. D. Leake, R. H. Brook, and M. F. Shapiro. 1996. The effect of race and ethnicity on the use of selected health care procedures: A comparison of south central

Los Angeles and the remainder of Los Angeles County. *Journal of Health Care for the Poor and Underserved* 7 (4): 308–22.

Edgerton, Robert B., Marvin Karno, and Irma Fernandez. 1970. Curanderismo in the metropolis: The diminished role of folk psychiatry among Los Angeles Mexican-Americans. *American Journal of Psychotherapy* 24 (1): 124–34.

Ell, K., L. J. Haywood, M. de Guzman, E. Sobel, S. Norris, D. Blumfield, J. P. Ning, and E. Butts. 1995. Differential perceptions, behaviors, and motivations among African Americans, Latinos, and whites suspected of heart attacks in two hospital populations. *Journal of the Association for Academic Minority Physicians* 6 (2): 60–69.

Fishman, B. M., L. Bobo, K. Kosub, and R. J. Womeodu. 1993. Cultural issues in serving minority populations: Emphasis on Mexican Americans and African Americans. *American Journal of the Medical Sciences* 306 (3): 160–66.

Flaskerud, J. H., and A. M. Nyamathi. 1990. Effects of an AIDS education program on the knowledge, attitudes and practices of low-income black and Latina women. *Journal of Community Health* 15 (6): 343–55.

———. 1996. Home medication injection among Latina women in Los Angeles: Implications for health education and prevention. *AIDS Care* 8 (1): 95–102.

Frankel, Barbara. 1977. *Childbirth in the Ghetto: Folk beliefs of Negro women in a north Philadelphia hospital ward.* San Francisco: R and E Research.

Frerichs, R. R., C. S. Aneshensel, and V. A. Clark. 1981. Prevalence of depression in Los Angeles County. *American Journal of Epidemiology* 113 (6): 691–99.

George, Victoria. 1980. Santería cult and its healers: Beliefs and traditions preserved in Los Angeles. Master's thesis, University of California, Los Angeles.

Gray, S., S. Lawrence, A. Arregui, N. Phillips, R. Bell, T. Richards, T. Fukushima, and H. W. Taeusch. 1995. Attitudes and behaviors of African-American and Mexican-American women delivering newborns in inner-city Los Angeles. *Journal of the National Medical Association* 87 (5): 353–58.

Greenfield, S. M. 1987. The return of Dr. Fritz: Spiritist healing and patronage networks in urban, industrial Brazil. *Social Science and Medicine* 24 (12): 1095–1108.

Gregory, Steven. 1986. *Santería in New York: A study in cultural resistance.* Ph.D. diss., New School for Social Research, New York.

Hayes-Bautista, D. E., L. Baezconde-Garbanati, and M. Hayes-Bautista. 1994. Latino health in Los Angeles: Family medicine in a changing minority context. *Family Practice* 11 (3): 318–24.

Karno, M., R. L. Hough, M. A. Burnam, J. I. Escobar, D. M. Timbers, F. Santana, and J. H. Boyd. 1987. Lifetime prevalence of specific psychiatric disorders among Mexican Americans and non-Hispanic whites in Los Angeles. *Archives of General Psychiatry* 44 (8): 695–701.

Karno, M., J. M. Golding, M. A. Burnam, R. L. Hough, J. I. Escobar, K. M. Wells, and R. Boyer. 1989. Anxiety disorders among Mexican Americans and non-Hispanic whites in Los Angeles. *Journal of Nervous and Mental Disease* 177 (4): 202–9.

Keefe, S. 1979. Folk medicine among urban Mexican Americans: Cultural persistence, change, and displacement. *Hispanic Journal of Behavioral Sciences* 1: 93–115.

Leon, J. J., F. Parra, T. Cheng, and R. E. Flores. 1995. Love-styles among Latino community college students in Los Angeles. *Psychological Reports* 77 (2): 527–30.

Lewin-Epstein, N. 1991. Determinants of regular source of health care in black, Mexican, Puerto Rican, and non-Hispanic white populations. *Medical Care* 29: 543–57.

Mack, T. M., J. Berkel, L. Bernstein, and W. Mack. 1985. Religion and cancer in Los Angeles County. *National Cancer Institute Monographs* 69: 235–45.

Malgady, R. G., and L. H. Rogler. 1993. Mental health status among Puerto Ricans, Mexican Americans, and non-Hispanic whites: The case of the misbegotten hypothesis. *American Journal of Community Psychology* 21 (3): 383–88.

Martinez, Cervando, and Harry W. Martin. 1966. Folk diseases among urban Mexican-Americans. *Journal of the American Medical Association* 196: 161–64.

Press, I. 1977. The urban curandero. In *Culture, disease and healing*, ed. D. Landy. New York: Macmillan.

Rodin, M. B. 1981. Alcoholism as a folk disease: The paradox of beliefs and choice of therapy in an urban American community. *Journal of Studies on Alcohol* 42 (9): 822–35.

Ruiz, Pedro. 1972. Santeros, botánicas and mental health: An urban view. *Transcultural Psychiatric Research Review Journal* 9: 176–77.

Sanders-Phillips, K. 1994. Correlates of healthy eating habits in low-income black women and Latinas. *Preventive Medicine* 23 (6): 781–87.

———. 1996. Correlates of health promotion behaviors in low-income black women and Latinas. *American Journal of Preventive Medicine* 12 (6): 450–58.

Scott, C. S. 1975. Competing health care systems in an inner city area. *Human Organization* 34: 108–10.

Snow, L. F. 1978. Sorcerers, saints and charlatans: Black folk healers in urban America. *Culture, Medicine and Psychiatry* 2 (1): 69–106.

Stekert, Ellen J. 1970. Focus for conflict: Southern mountain medical beliefs in Detroit. *Journal of American Folklore* 83: 115–56.

Takeuchi, D. T., S. Sue, and M. Yeh. Return rates and outcomes from ethnicity-specific mental health programs in Los Angeles. *American Journal of Public Health* 85 (5): 638–43.

Tripp-Reimer, T. 1983. Retention of a folk-healing practice (matiasma) among four generations of urban Greek immigrants. *Nursing Research* 32 (2): 97–101.

Whittemore, A. S., L. N. Kolonel, A. H. Wu, E. M. John, R. P. Gallagher, G. R. Howe, J. D. Burch, J. Hankin, D. M. Dreon, D. W. West, et al. 1995. Prostate cancer in relation to diet, physical activity, and body size in blacks, whites, and Asians in the United States and Canada. *Journal of the National Cancer Institute* 87 (9): 652–61.

Yancey, A. K., and L. Walden. 1994. Stimulating cancer screening among Latinas and African-American women: A community case study. *Journal of Cancer Education* 9 (1): 46–52.

Zambrana, R. E., and S. C. Scrimshaw. 1997. Maternal psychosocial factors associated with substance use in Mexican-origin and African American low-income pregnant women. *Pediatric Nursing* 23 (3): 253–59.

Zambrana, R. E., C. Dunkel-Schetter, and S. Scrimshaw. 1991. Factors which influence use of prenatal care in low-income racial-ethnic women in Los Angeles County. *Journal of Community Health* 16 (5): 283–95.

III.   *Ethnomedical Traditions in North America*

III.A.   *American Indian*

Adams, William R. 1951. Aboriginal American medicine and surgery. *Proceedings of the Indiana Academy of Science* 61: 49–53.

Bean, Lowell John. 1976. California Indian shamanism and folk curing. In *American folk medicine: A symposium*, ed. Wayland D. Hand, 109–23. Berkeley and Los Angeles: University of California Press.

Bourke, John G. 1892. Medicine men of the Apache. In *Ninth annual report of the Bureau of Ethnology, 1887–1888*, 443–603. Washington, D.C.: Governmental Printing Office.

Bracho, F. 1995. Plants, food and civilization: The lessons of indigenous Americans. *Journal of Alternative and Complementary Medicine* 1 (2): 125–30.

Bradley, Will T. 1936. Medical practices of the New England aborigines. *Journal of the American Pharmaceutical Association* 25 (2): 138–46.

Carr, Lloyd G., and Carlos Westez. 1945. Surviving folktales and herbal lore among the Shinnecock Indians of Long Island. *Journal of American Folklore* 58: 113–23.

Cobb, Carolus M. 1917. Some medical practices among the New England Indians and early settlers. *Boston Medical and Surgical Journal* 177 (4): 97–105.

Croom, Edward M., Jr. 1992. Herbal medicine among the Lumbee Indians. In *Herbal and magical medicine: Traditional healing today*, ed. James Kirkland, Holly F. Mathews, C. W. Sullivan III, and Karen Baldwin, 137–69. Durham, North Carolina: Duke University Press.

Darby, George E. 1933. Indian medicine in British Columbia. *Canadian Medical Association Journal* 28: 433–38.

Fenton, William N. 1942. Contacts between Iroquois herbalism and colonial medicine. *Annual Report of the Smithsonian Institution, 1941*, 503–27. Washington, D.C.: Governmental Printing Office.

Garro, L. C. 1988. Resort to folk healers in a Manitoba Ojibwa community. *Arctic Medical Research* 47 (suppl. 1): 317–20.

———. 1990. Continuity and change: The interpretation of illness in an Anishinaabe (Ojibway) community. *Culture, Medicine and Psychiatry* 14 (4): 417–54.

Grinnell, George Bird. 1905. Some Cheyenne plant medicines. *American Anthropologist* 7: 37–43.

———. 1919. A buffalo sweatlodge. *American Anthropologist* 21 (4): 361–75.

Hagey, R. 1984. The phenomenon, the explanations and the responses: Metaphors surrounding diabetes in urban Canadian Indians. *Social Science and Medicine* 18 (3): 265–72.

Herbert, Lester G. 1926. What did the Indians know about medicines and healing treatments? *Medical Journal and Record* 123: 22–24, 117–19.

Johnson, Leslie M. 1997. Health, wholeness, and the land: Gitskan traditional plant use and healing. Ph.D. diss., University of Alberta, Canada.

Kilpatrick, Jack Frederick. 1964. Folk formulas of the Oklahoma Cherokees. *Journal of the Folklore Institute* 1: 214–19.

Kurath, Gertrude P. 1954. The Tutelo fourth night spirit release singing. *Midwest Folklore* 4: 87–103.

La Barre, Weston. 1947. Kiowa folk sciences. *Journal of American Folklore* 60: 105–14.

———. 1951. Aymara biologicals and other medicines. *Journal of American Folklore* 64: 171–78.

Landes, Ruth. 1963. Potawatomi medicine. *Transactions, Kansas Academy of Science* 66: 553–99.

Larson, John A., M.D. 1953. Medicine among the Indians. *Quarterly Bulletin of Northwestern University Medical School* 27: 246–49.

Lee, Joseph G., M.D. 1960. Papago Indian medicine. *Arizona Medicine* 17 (2): 87–89.

MacDermot, J. H., M.D. 1949. Food and medicinal plants used by the Indians of British Columbia. *Canadian Medical Association Journal* 61 (2): 177–83.

MacDonald, Elizabeth. 1959. Indian medicine in New Brunswick. *Canadian Medical Association Journal* 80 (3): 220–24.

Maclean, John. 1961. Blackfoot medical priesthood. *Alberta Historical Review* 9 (2): 1–7.

MacLeish, Kenneth. 1943. Notes on folk medicine in the Hopi village of Moenkopi. *Journal of American Folklore* 56: 62–68.

Mahr, August C. 1951. Materia medica and therapy among the North American Forest Indians. *Ohio State Archaeological and Historical Quarterly* 60: 331–54.

Maxwell, Hu. 1918. Indian medicines: Numerous popular remedies obtained from forest trees. *Scientific American* 86 (suppl. 2224): 100–103.

McAllister, J. Gilbert. 1965. The four quartz rocks medicine bundle of the Kiowa-Apache. *Ethnology* 4: 210–24.

McClintock, Walter. 1909. Materia medica of the Blackfeet. *Zeitschrift für Ethnologie* 11: 273–76.

McElvaine, M. D., E. M. Harder, L. Johnson, R. D. Baer, and R. D. Satzger. 1990. Lead poisoning from the use of Indian folk medicines. Letter. *Journal of the American Medical Association* 264 (17): 2212–23.

Mellinger, Marie B. 1967. Medicine of the Cherokees. *Foxfire* 1 (3): 65–72.

Moerman, Daniel E. 1991a. The medicinal flora of native North America: An analysis. *Journal of Ethnopharmacology* 31: 1–42.

———. 1991b. Poisoned apples and honeysuckles: The medicinal plants of Native America. In *The anthropology of medicine: From culture to method*, ed. Lola Romanucci-Ross, Daniel E. Moerman, and Laurence R. Tancredi, 147–57. New York: Bergin and Garvey.

———. 1998. *Native American ethnobotany*. Portland, Oregon: Timber Press.

Parker, Arthur C. 1909. Secret medicine societies of the Seneca. *American Anthropologist* 2 (2): 161–85.

Rousseau, Jacques. 1947. Ethnobotanique Abénakise. *Les Archives de Folklore* 2: 145–82.

Russell, Frank. 1898. An Apache medicine dance. *American Anthropologist* 11 (12): 367–72.

Speck, Frank G. 1944. Catawba herbals and curative practices. *Journal of American Folklore* 57: 37–50.

Stone, Eric. 1934. Medicine among the Iroquois. *Annals of Medical History* 6 (6): 529–39.

Van Wart, Arthur F. 1948. The Indians of the Maritime Provinces, their diseases and native cures. *Canadian Medical Association Journal* 59 (6): 573–77.

Wallace, Anthony F. C. 1967. Dreams and the wishes of the soul: A type of psychoanalytic theory among the seventeenth century Iroquois. In *Magic, witchcraft, and curing*, ed. John Middleton, 171–91. Austin: University of Texas Press.

Wallis, Wilson D. 1922. Medicines used by the Micmac Indians. *American Anthropologist* 24: 24–30.

Welch, Charles E., Jr. 1964. Some drugs of the North American Indian—Then and now. *Keystone Folklore Quarterly* 9: 83–99.

Wilson, Eddie W. 1951. American Indian concept of saliva. *Midwest Folklore* 1: 229–32.

III.B.   *African, African American, Afro-Caribbean*

Bailey, James A. 1991. *The Yoruba of southwestern Nigeria and Santería in the southeastern United States*. New Bern, North Carolina: Godolphin House.

Bascom, William. 1969. *Sixteen cowries: Yoruba divination from Africa to the New World*. Bloomington: Indiana University Press.

Brandon, George. 1993. *The dead sell memories: Santería from Africa to the New World.* Bloomington: Indiana University Press.

Brown, David H. 1989. Garden in the machine: Afro-Cuban sacred art and performance in New York City. Ph.D. diss., Yale University, New Haven, Connecticut.

———. 1993. Thrones of the orichas: Afro-Cuban altars in New Jersey, New York, and Havana. *African Arts* 26 (4): 44–59, 85.

Canizares, Raul. 1993. *Walking with the night: The Afro-Cuban world of Santería.* Rochester, Vermont: Destiny Books.

Etkin, N. L. 1981. A Hausa herbal pharmacopoeia: Biomedical evaluation of commonly used plant medicines. *Journal of Ethnopharmacology* 4: 75–98.

Evans, David K., Don Stephen Rice, and Joanne Kline Partin. 1968. Parallels in West African, West Indian, and North Carolina folklore. *North Carolina Folklore* 17: 77–84.

Golden, K. M. 1977. Voodoo in Africa and the United States. *American Journal of Psychiatry* 134 (12): 1425–27.

Gonzalez-Wippler, Migene. 1973. *Santería: African magic in Latin America.* New York: Julian Press.

Hielscher, S., and J. Sommerfeld. 1985. Concepts of illness and the utilization of health-care services in a rural Malian village. *Social Science and Medicine* 21 (4): 469–81.

Makanjuola, R. O. 1987. "Ode Ori": A culture-bound disorder with prominent somatic features in Yoruba Nigerian patients. *Acta Psychiatrica Scandinavica* 75 (3): 231–36.

Nunez, Luis Manuel. 1992. *Santería: A practical guide to Afro-Caribbean religion.* Dallas, Texas: Spring Publications.

Oyejide, C. O., and G. A. Aderinokun. 1991. Teething myths in Nigerian rural Yoruba communities. *African Dental Journal* 5: 31–34.

Reynolds, J., and L. Swartz. 1993. Professional constructions of a "lay" illness: "Nerves" in a rural "coloured" community in South Africa. *Social Science and Medicine* 36 (5): 657–63.

Sandoval, Mercedes Cros. 1975. *La religion afrocubana.* Madrid: Coleccion Libre Plaza Mayor.

Sharp, P. T. 1982. Ghosts, witches, sickness and death: The traditional interpretation of injury and disease in a rural area of Papua New Guinea. *Papua New Guinea Medical Journal* 25 (2): 108–15.

Sofowora, A. 1996. Research on medicinal plants and traditional medicine in Africa. *Journal of Alternative and Complementary Medicine* 2 (3): 365–72.

III.C. *Hispanic or Latino*

Acosta, F. X., L. H. Nguyen, and J. Yamamoto. 1994. Using the brief symptom inventory to profile monolingual Spanish-speaking psychiatric outpatients. *Journal of Clinical Psychology* 50 (5): 723–26.

Adolph, C., D. E. Ramos, K. L. Linton, and D. A. Grimes. 1995. Pregnancy among Hispanic teenagers: Is good parental communication a deterrent? *Contraception* 51 (5): 303–6.

Ailinger, R. L. 1988. Folk beliefs about high blood pressure in Hispanic immigrants. *Western Journal of Nursing Research* 10 (5): 629–36.

Ailinger, R. L., and M. E. Causey. 1995. Health concept of older Hispanic immigrants. *Western Journal of Nursing Research* 17 (6): 605–13.

Alegria, D., E. Guerra, C. Martinez, Jr., G. Meyer. 1977. El hospital invisible: A study of curanderismo. *Archives of General Psychiatry* 34: 1354–57.

Appelt, Glenn D. 1985. Pharmacological aspects of selected herbs employed in Hispanic folk medicine in the San Luis Valley of Colorado, U.S.A.: I. *Lingusticum porteri* (osha) and *Matricaria chamomilla* (manzanilla). *Journal of Ethnopharmacology* 13: 51–55.

Applewhite, S. L. 1995. Curanderismo: Demystifying the health beliefs and practices of elderly Mexican Americans. *Health and Social Work* 20 (4): 247–53.

Baca, Josephine Elizabeth. 1969. Some health beliefs of the Spanish speaking. *American Journal of Nursing* 69: 2172–76.

Baer, R. D., and D. Penzell. 1993. Research report: Susto and pesticide poisoning among Florida farmworkers. *Culture, Medicine and Psychiatry* 17 (3): 321–27.

Bailey, James A. 1996. Santería and Palo Mayombe: The presence of Afro-Cuban artifacts at Wrightsville Beach. *North Carolina Folklore Journal* 43: 128–41.

Barnett, E. A. 1989. Notes on nervios: A disorder of menopause. *Journal of Transcultural Nursing* 10 (2–3): 159–69.

Berkanovic, E., and C. Telesky. 1985. Mexican-American, black-American, and white-American differences in reporting illnesses, disability and physician visits for illnesses. *Social Science and Medicine* 20 (6): 567–77.

Bhatt, B. D., M. J. Zuckerman, J. A. Foland, L. G. Guerra, and S. M. Polly. 1988. Rattlesnake meat ingestion—A common Hispanic folk remedy . Letter. *Western Journal of Medicine* 149 (5): 605.

Bird, Hector R., and Ian Canino. 1981. The sociopsychiatry of espiritismo: Findings of a study in psychiatric populations of Puerto Rican and other Hispanic children. *Journal of the American Academy of Child Psychiatry* 20: 725–40.

Borrello, Mary Ann, and Elizabeth Mathias. 1977. Botanicas: Puerto Rican folk pharmacies. *Natural History* 86 (7): 64–72, 116–17.

Brooks, T. R. 1992. Pitfalls in communication with Hispanic and African-American patients: Do translators help or harm? *Journal of the National Medical Association* 84: 941–47.

Canino, G. 1982. The Hispanic woman: Sociocultural influences on diagnosis and treatment. In *Mental health and Hispanic Americans*, ed. R. M. Becerra, M. Karno, and J. I. Escobar. New York: Grune and Stratton.

Carrasco, S. 1974. Curanderismo in south Texas. *School Health Review* 5 (5): 7.

Castro, F. G., P. Furth, and H. Karlow. 1984. The health beliefs of Mexican, Mexican American and Anglo American women. *Hispanic Journal of Behavioral Sciences* 6: 365–83.

Chavez, L. R. 1984. Doctors, curanderos, and brujas: Healthcare delivery and Mexican immigrants in San Diego. *Medical Anthropology Quarterly* 15: 31–37.

Chesney, A. P., B. L. Thompson, A. Guevara, A. Vela, and M. F. Schottstaedt. 1980. Mexican-American folk medicine: Implications for the family physician. *Journal of Family Practice* 11 (4): 567–74.

Clark, Margaret. 1959. *Health in the Mexican American culture: A community study.* Berkeley: University of California Press.

Cohen, Lucy M. 1979. *Culture, disease and stress among Latino immigrants.* Washington, D.C.: Smithsonian Institution, Research Institute on Immigration and Ethnic Studies.

Currier, Richard L. 1966. The hot-cold syndrome and symbolic balance in Mexican and Spanish-American folk medicine. *Ethnology* 5: 251–63.

Delgado, Melvin. 1978. Folk medicine in the Puerto Rican culture. *International Social Work* 21: 45–54.

————. 1979a. Herbal medicine in the Puerto Rican community. *Health and Social Work* 4: 5–40.

————. 1979b. Puerto Rican folk healers in big cities. *Forum on Medicine* 2: 784–93.

Deyo, R. A., A. K. Diehl, H. Hazuda, and M. P. Stern. 1985. A simple language-based acculturation scale for Mexican Americans: Validation and application to health care research. *American Journal of Public Health* 75 (1): 51–55.

Dodson, Ruth. 1932. Folk curing among the Mexicans. *Proceedings of the Texas Folklore Society* 10: 82–98.

————. 1951. Don Pedrito Jaramillo: The curandero of Los Olmos. *Publications of the Texas Folklroe Society* 24: 9–70.

Edgerton, Robert B., Marvin Karno, and Irma Fernandez. 1970. Curanderismo in the metropolis: The diminishing role of folk psychiatry among Los Angeles Mexican Americans. *American Journal of Psychotherapy* 24 (1): 124–34.

Erickson, P. I. 1996. Contraceptive methods: Do Hispanic adolescents and their family planning care providers think about contraceptive methods the same way? *Medical Anthropology* 17 (1): 65–82.

Espín, Olivia. 1988. Spiritual power and the mundane world: Hispanic female healers in urban U.S. communities. *Women's Studies Quarterly* 16 (3–4): 33–47.

————. 1996. *Latina healers.* Encino California: Floricanto Press.

Flaskerud, J. H., and A. M. Nyamathi. 1996. Home medication injection among Latina women in Los Angeles: Implications for health education and prevention. *AIDS Care* 8 (1): 95–102.

Flaskerud, J. H., and E. R. Calvillo. 1991. Beliefs about AIDS, health and illness among low-income Latina women. *Research in Nursing and Health* 14: 431–38.

Flaskerud, J. H., and G. Uman. 1993. Directions for AIDS education for Hispanic women based on analyses of survey findings. *Public Health Reports* 108 (3): 298–304.

Flores, Glenn, and Luis R. Vega. 1998. Barriers to health care access for Latino children: A review. *Family Medicine* 30: 196–205.

Ford, Daren Cowan. 1975. *Las yerbas de la gente: A study of Hispano-American medicinal plants.* Ann Arbor: University of Michigan.

Formenti, S. C., B. E. Meyerowitz, K. Ell, L. Muderspach, S. Groshen, B. Leedham, V. Klement, and P. C. Morrow. 1995. Inadequate adherence to radiotherapy in Latina immigrants with carcinoma of the cervix: Potential impact on disease free survival. *Cancer* 75 (5): 1135–40.

Foster, George M. 1953. Relationships between Spanish and Spanish-American folk medicine. *Journal of American Folklore* 66: 201–17.

Fox, S. A., and R. G. Roetzheim. 1994. Screening mammography and older Hispanic women: Current status and issues. *Cancer* 74 (suppl. 7): 2028–33.

Garrison, Vivian. 1974. Sectarianism and psychological adjustment: A controlled comparison of Puerto Rican Pentecostals and Catholics. In *Religious movements in contemporary America,* ed. I. R. Zaretzky and M. P. Leone. Princeton, New Jersey: Princeton University Press.

————. 1977a. Doctor, espiritista or psychiatrist? Health-seeking behavior in a Puerto Rican neighborhood in New York City. *Medical Anthropology* 1: 65–191.

————. 1977b. The "Puerto Rican syndrome" in psychiatry and espiritismo. In *Case studies in spirit possession,* ed. V. Crapanzano and V. Garrison, 383–449. New York: John Wiley and Sons.

————. 1978. Support systems of schizophrenic and non-schizophrenic Puerto Rican migrant women in New York City. *Schizophrenia Bulletin* 4: 591–96.

Gaviria, M., and R. M. Wintrob. 1976. Supernatural influence in psychopathology: Puerto Rican folk beliefs about mental illness. *Canadian Psychiatric Association Journal* 21 (6): 361–69.

Giachello, A., R. Bell, L. Aday, and R. Anderson. 1983. Uses of the 1980 census for Hispanic health research. *American Journal of Public Health* 73: 266–74.

Gloria, A. M., and J. J. Peregoy. Counseling Latino alcohol and other substance users/abusers: Cultural considerations for counselors. *Journal of Substance Abuse Teatment* 13 (2): 119–26.

Golding, J. M., and M. A Burnam. 1990. Immigration, stress, and depressive symptoms in a Mexican-American community. *Journal of Nervous and Mental Disease* 178 (3): 161–71.

Golding, J. M., M. Karno, and C. M. Rutter. 1990. Symptoms of major depression among Mexican-Americans and non-Hispanic Whites. *American Journal of Psychiatry* 147 (7): 861–66.

Golding, J. M., M. A. Burnam, and K. B. Wells. 1990. Alcohol use and depressive symptoms among Mexican Americans and non-Hispanic whites. *Alcohol and Alcoholism* 25 (4): 421–32.

Gomez, G. E., and E. A. Gomez. 1985. Folk healing among Hispanic Americans. *Public Health Nursing* 2 (4): 245–49.

Gonzalez-Swafford, M. J., and M. G. Gutierrez. 1983. Ethno-medical beliefs and practices of Mexican-Americans. *Nurse Practitioner* 8 (10): 29–30, 32, 34.

Gordon, S. M. 1994. Hispanic cultural health beliefs and folk remedies. *Journal of Holistic Nursing* 12 (3): 307–22.

Graham, Joe S. 1976. The role of the curandero in the Mexican American folk medicine system in west Texas. In *American folk medicine: A symposium*, ed. Wayland D. Hand, 175–89. Berkeley and Los Angeles: University of California Press.

————. 1985. Folk medicine and intracultural diversity among west Texas Mexican Americans. *Western Folklore* 44: 168–93.

Granger, Byrd Howell. 1976. Some aspects of folk medicine among Spanish-speaking people in southern Arizona. In *American folk medicine: A symposium*, ed. Wayland D. Hand, 191–202. Berkeley and Los Angeles: University of California Press.

Gray, S., S. Lawrence, A. Arregui, N. Phillips, R. Bell, T. Richards, T. Fukushima, and H. W. Taeusch. 1995. Attitudes and behaviors of African-American and Mexican-American women delivering newborns in inner-city Los Angeles. *Journal of the National Medical Association* 87 (5): 353–58.

Guarnaccia, Peter J. 1993. Ataques de nervios in Puerto Rico: Culture-bound syndrome or popular illness? *Medical Anthropology* 15 (2): 157–70.

Guarnaccia, Peter J., V. DeLaCancela, and Emilio Carillo. 1989. The multiple meanings of ataques de nervios in the Latino community. *Medical Anthropology* 11: 47–62.

Harwood, Alan. 1971. The hot-cold theory of disease: Implications for treatment of Puerto Rican patients. *Journal of the American Medical Association* 216: 1153–58.

————. 1981. Mainland Puerto Ricans. In *Ethnicity and medical care*, ed. Alan Harwood, 397–481. Cambridge: Harvard University Press.

Hatch, E. Le Roy. 1969. Home remedies Mexican style. *Western Folklore* 28: 163–68.

Hayes-Bautista, D. E., L. Baezconde-Garbanati, and M. Hayes-Bautista. 1994. Latino health in Los Angeles: Family medicine in a changing minority context. *Family Practice* 11 (3): 318–24.

Higginbotham, J. C., F. M. Trevino, and L. A. Ray. 1990. Utilization of curanderos by Mexican Americans: Prevalence and predictors. Findings from HHANES 1982–84. *American Journal of Public Health* 80 (suppl.): 32–35.

Holland, William R. 1963. Mexican-American medical beliefs: Science or magic. *Arizona Medicine* 20 (5): 89–101.

Holloway, G. 1994. Susto and the career path of the victim of an industrial accident: A sociological case study. *Social Science and Medicine* 38 (7): 989–97.

Hovey, J. D., and C. A. King. 1996. Acculturative stress, depression, and suicidal ideation among immigrant and second-generation Latino adolescents. *Journal of the American Academy of Child and Adolescent Psychiatry* 35 (9): 1183–92.

Jenkins, J. H. 1988. Ethnopsychiatric Interpretations of schizophrenic illness: The problem of nervios within Mexican-American families. *Culture, Medicine and Psychiatry* 12 (3): 301–29.

Karno, M., J. M. Golding, M. A. Burnam, R. L. Hough, J. I. Escobar, K. M. Wells, and R. Boyer. 1989. Anxiety disorders among Mexican Americans and non-Hispanic whites in Los Angeles. *Journal of Nervous and Mental Disease* 177 (4): 202–9.

Kay, Margarita Artschwager. 1972. Health and illness in the barrio: Women's point of view. Ph.D. diss., University of Arizona, Tucson.

Keefe, S. E. 1979. Folk medicine among urban Mexican Americans: Cultural persistence, change, and displacement. *Hispanic Journal of Behavioral Sciences* 1: 93–115.

Keefe, S. E., and J. M. Casas. 1980. Mexican Americans and mental health: A selected review and recommendations for mental health service delivery. *American Journal of Community Psychology* 8 (3): 303–26.

Keegan, L. 1996. Use of alternative therapies among Mexican Americans in the Texas Rio Grande Valley. *Journal of Holistic Nursing* 14 (4): 277–94.

Kelley, B. D., G. D. Appelt, and J. M. Appelt. 1988. Pharmacological aspects of selected herbs employed in Hispanic folk medicine in the San Luis Valley of Colorado, USA: II. *Asclepias asperula* (inmortal) and *Achillea lanulosa* (plumajillo). *Journal of Ethnopharmacology* 22: 1–9.

Kiev, Ari. 1962. The psychotherapeutic aspects of primitive medicine. *Human Organization* 21: 25–29.

———. 1968. *Curanderismo: Mexican-American folk psychiatry*. New York: Free Press.

Kosko, D. A., and J. H. Flaskerud. 1987. Mexican American, nurse practitioner, and lay control group beliefs about cause and treatment of chest pain. *Nursing Research* 36 (4): 226–31.

Koss-Chioino, J. D., and J. M. Canive. 1993. The interaction of popular and clinical diagnostic labeling: The case of embrujado. *Medical Anthropology* 15 (2): 171–88.

Krajewski-Jaime, E. R. 1991. Folk-healing among Mexican-American families as a consideration in the delivery of child welfare and child health care services. *Child Welfare* 70 (2): 157–67.

Kriesman, J. J. 1975. The curandero's perspective: A therapeutic integration of folk and medicinal healing. *American Journal of Psychiatry* 132 (1): 81–83.

Leon, C. A. 1975. "El duende" and other incubi: Suggestive interactions between culture, the devil, and the brain. *Archives of General Psychiatry* 32 (2): 155–62.

Leon, J. J., F. Parra, T. Cheng, and R. E. Flores. 1995. Love-styles among Latino community college students in Los Angeles. *Psychological Reports* 77 (2): 527–30.

Lewin-Epstein, N. 1991. Determinants of regular source of health care in black, Mexican, Puerto Rican, and non-Hispanic white populations. *Medical Care* 29: 543–57.

Lewis, M. A., C. E. Lewis, B. Leake, G. Monahan, and G. Rachelefsky. 1996. Organizing the community to target poor Latino children with asthma. *Journal of Asthma* 33 (5): 289–97.

Logan, M. H. 1993. New lines of inquiry on the illness of susto. *Medical Anthropology* 15 (2): 189–200.

Macklin, June. 1974. Belief, ritual, and healing: New England spiritualism and Mexican-American spiritism compared. In *Religious movements in contemporary America*, ed. I. I. Zaretsky and M. P. Leone, 383–417. Princeton, New Jersey: Princeton University Press.

Madsen, William. 1955. Hot and cold in the universe of San Francisco Tecospa, Valley of Mexico. *Journal of American Folklore* 68: 123–39.

———. 1964. *The Mexican-Americans of south Texas*. New York: Holt, Rinehart, and Winston.

Maduro, R. 1983. Curanderismo and Latino views of disease and curing. *Western Journal of Medicine* 139 (6): 868–74.

Malgady, R. G., and L. H. Rogler. 1993. Mental health status among Puerto Ricans, Mexican Americans, and non-Hispanic whites: The case of the misbegotten hypothesis. *American Journal of Community Psychology* 21 (3): 383–88.

Marks, G., J. Solis, J. L. Richardson, L. M. Collins, L. Birba, and J. C. Hisserich. 1987. Health behavior of elderly Hispanic women: Does cultural assimilation make a difference? *American Journal of Public Health* 77 (10): 1315–19.

Marsh, W. W., and M.. Eberle. 1987. Curanderismo associated with fatal outcome in a child with leukemia. *Texas Medicine* 83 (2): 38–40.

Martinez, R., and C. V. Wetli. 1989. Tattoos of the Marielitos. *American Journal of Forensic Medicine and Pathology* 10 (4): 315–25.

Martinez, Cervando, and Harry W. Martin. 1966. Folk diseases among urban Mexican-Americans. *Journal of the American Medical Association* 196: 161–64.

Mason, Michael Atwood. 1993. The blood-that-runs-through-the-veins: The creation of identity and a client's experience of Cuban-American Santería-dilogun divination. *Drama Review* 37: 119–30.

———. 1994. "I bow my head to the ground": The creation of bodily experience in a Cuban American Santería initiation. *Journal of American Folklore* 107: 23–39.

Mayers, Raymond Sanchez. 1989. Use of folk medicine by elderly Mexican-American women. *Journal of Drug Issues* 19: 283–95.

Mickley, J., and K. Soeken. 1993. Religiousness and hope in Hispanic- and Anglo-American women with breast cancer. *Oncology Nursing Forum* 20 (8): 1171–77.

Mikhail, B. I. 1994. Hispanic mothers' beliefs and practices regarding selected children's health problems. *Western Journal of Nursing Research* 16 (6): 623–38.

Monteiro, L. A. 1982. Folk remedies of Rhode Island's Portuguese-American immigrants. *Rhode Island Medical Journal* 65 (8): 324–28.

Mull, J. D. 1983. A visit with a curandero. *Western Journal of Medicine* 139: 730–36.

Munoz, J. A. 1986. Countertransference and its implementation in the treatment of a Hispanic adolescent boy. *Psychiatry* 49 (2): 169–79.

Murphy, R. S. 1990. At last—A view of Hispanic health and nutritional status. *American Journal of Public Health* 80 (12): 1429–30.

Nall, Frank C., II, and Joseph Speilberg. 1967. Social and cultural factors in the responses of Mexican-Americans to medical treatment. *Journal of Health and Social Behavior* 8 (4): 299–308.

Nations, M. 1992. The child's disease (doenca de crianca): Popular paradigm of persistent diarrhea? *Acta Paediatrica Supplement* 381: 55–65.

Newell, G. R., and P. K. Mills. 1986. Low cancer rates in Hispanic women related to social and economic factors. *Women and Health* 11 (3–4): 23–35.

Norris, S. L., M. de Guzman, E. Sobel, S. Brooks, and L. J. Haywood. 1993. Risk factors and mortality among black, Caucasian, and Latina women with acute myocardial infarction. *American Heart Journal* 126 (6): 1312–19.

Novo Pena, Silvia. 1993. Religion. In *The Hispanic-American almanac*, 367–86. Detroit: Gale Research.

Nyamathi, A. M., J. Flaskerud, C. Bennett, B. Leake, and C. Lewis. 1994. Evaluation of two AIDS education programs for impoverished Latina women. *AIDS Education and Prevention* 6 (4): 296–309.

Pachter, L. M. 1993. Introduction: Latino folk illnesses: Methodological considerations. *Medical Anthropology* 15 (2): 103–8.

Pachter, L. M., B. Bernstein, and A. Osorio. 1992. Clinical implications of a folk illness: Empacho in mainland Puerto Ricans. *Medical Anthropology* 13 (4): 285–99.

Pachter, L. M., M. M. Cloutier, and B. A. Bernstein. 1995. Ethnomedical (folk) remedies for childhood asthma in a mainland Puerto Rican community. *Archives of Pediatrics and Adolescent Medicine* 149 (9): 982–88.

Perez y Mena, Andres Isidoro. 1991. *Speaking with the dead: Development of Afro-Latin religion among Puerto Ricans in the United States: A study into the interpenetration of civilizations in the New World.* New York: AMS Press.

Perrone, B., H. Stockel, and V. Krueger. 1989. *Medicine women, curanderas, and women doctors.* Norman: University of Oklahoma Press.

Press, I. 1977. The urban curandero. In *Culture, disease, and healing,* ed. D. Landy. New York: Macmillan.

Quesada, G. M., and P. L. Heller. 1977. Sociocultural barriers to medical care among Mexican Americans in Texas: A summary report of research conducted by the Southwest Medical Sociology Ad Hoc Committee. *Medical Care* 15 (suppl. 5): 93–101.

Richardson, L. 1982. Folk medicine in the Hispanic population. Part 2 of Breakthrough to nursing: Caring through understanding. *Imprint* 29 (2): 21, 72–77.

Ring, J. M., and P. Marquis. 1991. Depression in a Latino immigrant medical population: An exploratory screening and diagnosis. *American Journal of Orthopsychiatry* 61 (2): 298–302.

Ripley, G. D. 1986. Mexican-American folk remedies: Their place in health care. *Texas Medicine* 82 (11): 41–44.

Risser, A. L., and L. J. Mazur. 1995. Use of folk remedies in a Hispanic population. *Archives of Pediatrics and Adolescent Medicine* 149 (9): 978–81.

Roberts, R. E. 1992. Manifestation of depressive symptoms among adolescents: A comparison of Mexican Americans with the majority and other minority populations. *Journal of Nervous and Mental Disease* 180 (10): 627–33.

Rodriguez, Josie. 1983. Mexican American factors influencing health practices. *Journal of School Health* 53: 136–39.

Roeder, Beatrice. 1988. *Chicano folk medicine from Los Angeles*. Berkeley: University of California Press.

Rogler, Lloyd H., and August B. Hollingshead. 1961. The Puerto Rican spiritualist as psychiatrist. *American Journal of Sociology* 67: 17–22.

Rubel, Arthur J. 1960. Concepts of disease in Mexican-American culture. *American Anthropologist* 62: 795–814.

———. 1966. *Across the tracks: Mexican Americans in a Texas city*. Austin: University of Texas Press.

———. 1978. The epidemiology of a folk illness: Susto in Hispanic America. In *Hispanic culture and health care*, ed. R. Martinez. St. Louis, Missouri: C. V. Mosby.

———. 1993. The study of Latino folk illnesses. *Medical Anthropology* 15 (2): 209–13.

Ruiz, Pedro. 1972. Santeros, botánicas and mental health: An urban view. *Transcultural Psychiatric Research Review Journal* 9: 176–77.

Sanchez, Mabel S. 1997. Pathways to health: A naturalistic study of Mexican-American women's lay health behaviors. Ph.D. diss., University of Texas, Austin.

Sandler, A. P., and L. S. Chan. 1978. Mexican-American folk belief in a pediatric emergency room. *Medical Care* 16 (9): 778–84.

Sandoval, Mercedes Cros. 1977. Afrocuban concepts of disease and its treatment in Miami. *Journal of Operational Psychiatry* 8: 52–63.

Schreiber, Janet M., and John P. Homiak. 1981. Mexican Americans. In *Ethnicity and medical care*, ed. Alan Harwood, 264–336. Cambridge: Harvard University Press.

Shapiro, E. R. 1995. Grief in family and cultural context: Learning from Latino families. *Cultural Diversity in Mental Health* 1 (2): 159–76.

Shrout, P. E., G. J. Canino, H. R. Bird, M. Rubio-Stipec, M. Bravo, and M. A. Burnam. 1992. Mental health status among Puerto Ricans, Mexican Americans, and non-Hispanic whites. *American Journal of Community Psychology* 20 (6): 729–52.

Singer, Merrill. 1984. Indigenous treatment for alcoholism: The case of Puerto Rican spiritism. *Medical Anthropology* 8 (4): 246–73.

Smithers, W. D. 1961. Nature's pharmacy and the curanderos. *Sul Ross State College Bulletin* 41 (3).

Stolley, J. M., and H. Koenig. 1997. Religion/spirituality and health among elderly African Americans and Hispanics. *Journal of Psychosocial Nursing and Mental Health Services* 35 (11): 32–38.

Suarez, M., M. Raffaelli, and A. O'Leary. 1996. Use of folk healing practices by HIV-infected Hispanics living in the United States. *AIDS Care* 8 (60): 683–90.

Tamez, E. G. 1978. Curanderismo: Folk Mexican-American health care system. *Journal of Psychiatric Nursing and Mental Health Services* 16 (12): 34–39.

Thiel de Bocanegra, H., F. Gany, and R. Fruchter. 1993. Available epidemiologic data on New York's Latino population: A critical review of the literature. *Ethnicity and Disease* 3 (4): 413–26.

Tigerman, N. S. 1989. Health beliefs, knowledge, and health seeking behaviors of recently immigrated Central American mothers in Los Angeles. Ph.D. diss., University of California, Los Angeles.

Tousignant, M. 1979. Espanto: A dialogue with the Gods. *Culture, Medicine and Psychiatry* 3 (4): 347–61.

Trotter, Robert T., II. 1981. Folk remedies as indicators of common illnesses: Examples from the United States-Mexico border. *Journal of Ethnopharmacology* 4 (2): 207–21.

Trotter, Robert T., II, and Juan Antonio Chavira. 1980. Curanderismo: An emic theoretical perspective of Mexican-American folk medicine. *Medical Anthropology* 4: 423–87.

———. 1981. *Curanderismo: Mexican American folk healing.* Athens: University of Georgia Press.

Van Oss Marin, B., G. Marin, A. Padilla, and C. de la Rocha. 1983. Utilization of traditional and non-traditional sources of health care among Hispanics. *Hispanic Journal of Behavioral Sciences* 5: 65–80.

Vega, W. A. 1980. The Hispanic natural healer—A case study: Implications for prevention. In *Hispanic natural support systems: Mental health promotion perspectives,* ed. R. Valle and W. Vega, 65–74. Sacramento: California Department of Mental Health.

Vega, W. A., B. Kolody, S. Aguilar-Gaxiola, E. Alderete, R. Catalano, and J. Caraveo-Anduaga. 1998. Lifetime prevalence of DSM-III-R psychiatric disorders among urban and rural Mexican Americans in California. *Archives of General Psychiatry* 55 (9): 771–78.

Wakefield, Dan. 1975. *Island in the city: The world of Spanish Harlem.* New York: Corinth Books, 1959. Reprint, New York: Arno Press.

Waterman, S. H., G. Juarez, S. J. Carr, and L. Kilman. 1990. Salmonella Arizona infections in Latinos associated with rattlesnake folk medicine. *American Journal of Public Health* 80 (3): 286–89.

Weclew, R. V. 1975. The nature, prevalence, and level of awareness of "curanderismo" and some of its implications for community mental health. *Community Medical Health Journal* 11 (2): 145–54.

Weller, S. C., L. M. Pachter, R. T. Trotter, II, and R. D. Baer. 1992. Empacho in four Latino groups: A study of intra- and inter-cultural variation in belief. *Medical Anthropology* 15: 109–36.

Wells, K. B., R. L. Hough, J. M. Golding, M. A. Burnam, and M. Karno. 1987. Which Mexican-Americans underutilize health services? *American Journal of Psychiatry* 144 (7): 918–22.

Woodhull, Frost. 1930. Ranch remedies. *Publications of the Texas Folklore Society* 8: 9–73.

Yancey, A. K., and L. Walden. 1994. Stimulating cancer screening among Latinas and African-American women: A community case study. *Journal of Cancer Education* 9 (1): 46–52.

Zaldivar, A., and J. Smolowitz. 1994. Perceptions of the importance placed on religion and folk medicine by non-Mexican-American Hispanic adults with diabetes. *Diabetes Educator* 20 (4): 303–6.

Zambrana, R. E., and S. C. Scrimshaw. 1997. Maternal psychosocial factors associated with substance use in Mexican-origin and African American low-income pregnant women. *Pediatric Nursing* 23 (3): 253–59.

Zayas, L. H., and P. O. Ozuah. 1996. Mercury use in espiritismo: A survey of botanicas. *American Journal of Public Health* 86 (1): 111–12.

Zuckerman, M. J., L. G. Guerra, D. A. Drossman, J. A. Foland, and G. G. Gregory. 1996. Health-care-seeking behaviors related to bowel complaints: Hispanics versus non-Hispanic whites. *Digestive Diseases and Sciences* 41 (1): 77–82.

Zuniga, M. E. 1992. Using metaphors in therapy: Dichos and Latino clients. *Social Work* 37 (1): 55–60.

III.D.   Pennsylvania German

Aurand, A. Monroe, Jr. 1941. *Popular home remedies and superstitions of the Pennsylvania Germans.* Harrisburg, Pennsylvania: n.p.

Brendle, Thomas R., and Claude W. Unger. 1935. *Folk medicine of the Pennsylvania Germans: The Non-Occult cures,* 45. Norristown: Proceedings of the Pennsylvania German Society.

Doering, J. Frederick. 1936. Pennsylvania German folk medicine in Waterloo County, Ontario. *Journal of American Folklore* 49: 194–98.

Gifford, Edward S., Jr. 1960. The evil eye in Pennsylvania medical history. *Keystone Folk Quarterly* 5 (3): 3–8.

Hoffman, W. J., M.D. 1893. Notes on Pennsylvania German folk medicine. *Science* 21: 355.

Jack, Phil R. 1964. Folk medicine from western Pennsylvania. *Pennsylvania Folklife* 14 (1): 35–37.

Lick, David E., and Thomas R. Brendle. 1922. Plant names and plant lore among the Pennsylvania Germans. *Proceedings and Addresses of the Pennsylvania German Society* 33.

Long, Amos, Jr. 1964. Bakeovens in Pennsylvania folk culture. *Pennsylvania Folklife* 14 (2): 16–29.

White, Emma Gertrude. 1897. Folk-medicine among Pennsylvania Germans. *Journal of American Folklore* 10: 78–80.

III.E.   Asian American

Adler, Shelley R. 1995. Refugee stress and folk belief: Hmong sudden deaths. *Social Science and Medicine* 40 (12): 1623–29.

Bartholomew, R. E. 1994. The social psychology of "epidemic" koro. *International Journal of Social Psychiatry* 40 (1): 46–60.

Cheon-Klessig, Y., D. D. Camilleri, B. J. McElmurry, and V. M. Ohlson. 1988. Folk medicine in the health practice of Hmong refugees. *Western Journal of Nursing Research* 10 (5): 647–60.

Chowdhury, A. N. 1996. The definition and classification of koro. *Culture, Medicine and Psychiatry* 20 (1): 41–65.

Clarvit, S. R., F. R. Schneier, and M. R. Liebowitz. 1996. The offensive subtype of Taijin-kyofu-sho in New York City: The phenomenology and treatment of a social anxiety disorder. *Journal of Clinical Psychiatry* 57 (11): 523–27.

Coin rubbing and related folk medicine. Letter. 1981. *Journal of the American Medical Association* 245 (18): 1819.

Dwyer, Philip. 1987. Herbalism and ritual: Folk medical practices among Asian immigrants in Southern California. Ph.D. diss., University of California, Los Angeles.

Etsuko, M. 1991. The interpretations of fox possession: Illness as metaphor. *Culture, Medicine and Psychiatry* 15 (4): 453–77.

Fishman, C., R. Evans, and E. Jenks. 1988. Warm bodies, cool milk: Conflicts in post partum food choice for Indochinese women in California. *Social Science and Medicine* 26 (11): 1125–32.

Kendall, L. 1987. Cold wombs in balmy Honolulu: Ethnogynecology among Korean immigrants. *Social Science and Medicine* 25 (4): 367–76.

Lin, K. M., K. J. Lau, J. Yamamoto, Y. P. Zheng, H. S. Kim, K. H. Cho, and G. Nakasaki. 1992. Hwa-byung: A community study of Korean Americans. *Journal of Nervous and Mental Disease* 180 (6): 386–91.

Oberg, C. N., and A. Deinard. 1984. Marasmus in a seventeen-month-old Laotian: Impact of folk beliefs on health. *Pediatrics* 73 (2): 254–57.

Oubre, A. 1995. Traditional Chinese medicine and HIV illness. Part 2 of Social context of complementary medicine in Western society. *Journal of Alternative and Complementary Medicine* 1 (2): 161–85.

Pang, K. Y. 1989. The practice of traditional Korean medicine in Washington, D.C. *Social Science and Medicine* 28 (8): 875–84.

———. 1990. Hwabyung: The construction of a Korean popular illness among Korean elderly immigrant women in the United States. *Culture, Medicine and Psychiatry* 14 (4): 495–512.

Reinhart, M. A., and H. Ruhs. 1985. Moxibustion: Another traumatic folk remedy. *Clinical Pediatrics* 24 (1): 58–59.

Rubio, E. L., B. R. Ekins, P. D. Singh, and J. Dowis. 1987. Hmong opiate folk remedy toxicity in three infants. *Veterinary and Human Toxicology* 29 (4): 323–25.

Snyder, P. 1981. Ethnicity and folk healing in Honolulu, Hawaii. *Social Science and Medicine.* 15B (2): 125–32.

———. 1984. Health service implications of folk healing among older Asian Americans and Hawaiians in Honolulu. *Gerontologist* 24 (5): 471–76.

III.F. *Canadian*

Brandon, Elizabeth. 1955. La médicine populaire dans la paroisse de Vermillion en Louisiane. Ph.D. diss., Universite Laval, Quebec.

Cantero, Antonio, M.D. 1929. Occult healing practices in French Canada. *Canadian Medical Association Journal* (Canadian Medical Association), n.s., 20: 303–6.

Crellin, John K. 1994. *Home medicine: The Newfoundland experience.* Montreal and Kingston: McGill-Queen's University Press.

Davis, D.L. 1988. Folk images of health and menstrual patterns among Newfoundland outport women. *Health Care for Women International* 9 (3): 211–23.

———. 1989. The variable character of nerves in a Newfoundland fishing village. *Medical Anthropology* 11 (1): 63–78.

Doering, John Frederick, and Eileen Elita Doering. 1938. Some western Ontario folk beliefs and practices. *Journal of American Folklore* 51: 60–68.

———. 1941. Some western Ontario folk beliefs and practices. *Journal of American Folklore* 54: 197.

Riddell, William Rensick. 1934. Some old Canadian folk medicine. *Canada Lancet and Practitioner* 83: 41–44.

Rosenbaum, J. N. 1991. The health meanings and practices of older Greek-Canadian widows. *Journal of Advanced Nursing* 16 (11): 1320–27.

Street, Anne C. 1959. Medicine populaire des Iles Saint-Pierre et Miquelon. *Arts et Traditions Populaires* 7: 75–85.

IV. *World ethnomedical traditions*

IV.A. *Latin American*

Baer, R. D., and A. Ackerman. 1988. Toxic Mexican folk remedies for the treatment of empacho: The case of Azarcon, Greta, and Albayalde. *Journal of Ethnopharmacology* 24 (1): 31–39.

Barrett, B. 1995. Herbal knowledge on Nicaragua's Atlantic Coast: Consensus within diversity. *Journal of Community Health* 20 (5): 403–21.

Bascom, William. 1950. The focus of Cuban Santería. *Southwestern Journal of Anthropology* 6: 64–68.

Benedetti, M. D. 1989. *Earth and spirit: Healing lore and more from Puerto Rico.* New Jersey: Waterfront Press.

Cabrera, Lydia. 1975. *El monte: Notas sobre las religiones, la magia, las supersticiones, y el folklore de Pueblo de Cuba.* 1940. Reprint, Miami: Ediciones Universal.

———. 1994–1995. Religious syncretism in Cuba. *Journal of Caribbean Studies* 10 (1–2): 84–94.

Canizares, Raul. 1993. *Walking with the night: The Afro-Cuban world of Santería.* Rochester, Vermont: Destiny Books.

Carbajal, D., A. Casaco, L. Arruzazabala, R. Gonzalez, and V. Fuentes. 1991. Pharmacological screening of plant decoctions commonly used in Cuban folk medicine. *Journal of Ethnopharmacology* 33 (1–2): 21–24.

Colson, A. B., and C. de Armellada. 1983. An Amerindian derivation for Latin American Creole illnesses and their treatment. *Social Science and Medicine* 17 (17): 1229–48.

Cortes-Gallo, G., M. A. Hernandez-Gonzalez, M. A. Ayala-Garcia, A. Rocha-Moreles, F. Aguinaga-Jasso, J. J. Morales-Aguirre, and J. A. Bribiesca-Lopez. 1993. The indigestion cure: A common and dangerous practice (trans. from Spanish). *Boletin Medico del Hospital Infantil de Mexico* 50 (1): 44–47.

Curtis, James R. 1982. Santería: Persistence and change in an Afrocuban cult religion. In *Objects of special devotion: Fetishism in popular culture,* 336–51. Bowling Green, Ohio: Bowling Green Popular Press.

Dal , R. A. 1996. New developments in Cuban holistic medicine: A personal view. *Journal of Alternative and Complementary Medicine* 2 (2): 299–305.

Dobkin, Maralene. 1968. Folk curing with a psychedelic cactus in the north coast of Peru. *International Journal of Social Psychiatry* 15 (1): 23–32.

———. 1969. Fortune's malice: Divination, psychotherapy, and folk medicine in Peru. *Journal of American Folklore* 82: 132–41.

———. 1981. Saladerra—A culture-bound misfortune syndrome in the Peruvian Amazon. *Culture, Medicine and Psychiatry* 5 (2): 193–213.

———. 1989. A modern-day shamanistic healer in the Peruvian Amazon: Pharmacopoeia and trance. *Journal of Psychoactive Drugs* 21 (1): 91–99.

Fabrega, H., and H. Nutini. 1993. Witchcraft-explained childhood tragedies in Tlaxcala, and their medical sequelae. *Social Science and Medicine* 36 (6): 793–805.

Finkler, Kaja. 1985. *Spiritualist healers in Mexico: Successes and failures of alternative therapeutics.* New York: Praeger.

Frei, Barbara. 1997. Medical ethnobotany of the Isthmus-Sierra Zapotecs (Oaxaca, Mexico) and biological-phytochemical investigation of selected plants. Ph.D. diss., Eidgenoessische Technische Hochschule, Zurich, Switzerland.

Gonzales-Wippler, Migene. 1973. *Santería: African magic in Latin America.* Garden City, New York: Doubleday and Anchor.

Greenfield, S. M. 1987. The return of Dr. Fritz: Spiritist healing and patronage networks in urban, industrial Brazil. *Social Science and Medicine* 24 (12): 1095–1108.

———. 1992. Spirits and spiritist therapy in southern Brazil: A case study of an innovative, syncretic healing group. *Culture, Medicine and Psychiatry* 16 (1): 23–51.

Heinrich, Michael. 1994. Herbal and symbolic medicines of the Lowland Mixe (Oaxaca, Mexico): Disease concepts, healer's roles, and plant use. *Anthropos* 89: 73–83.

Hess, David J. 1994. *Samba in the night: Spiritism in Brazil.* New York: Columbia University Press.

Kelly, Isabel. 1965. Folk practices in north Mexico: Birth customs, folk medicine, and spiritualism in the Laguna Zone. In *Institute of Latin American Studies.* Austin: University of Texas Press.

Low, S. M. 1981. The meaning of nervios: A sociocultural analysis of symptom presentation in San Jose, Costa Rica. *Culture, Medicine and Psychiatry* 5 (1): 25–47.

Macklin, June. 1980. "All the good and bad in this world": Women, traditional medicine, and Mexican culture. In *Twice a minority: Mexican American women,* ed. M. B. Melville, 127–54. St. Louis, Missouri: C. V. Mosby.

Madsen, William. 1955. Hot and cold in the universe of San Francisco Tecospa, Valley of Mexico. *Journal of American Folklore* 68: 123–39.

Mandel-Campbell, Andrea. 1996. Cuba's visa seekers try an animist faith. *Christian Science Monitor,* 15 February, 6.

Marsh, W. W., and K. Hentges. 1988. Mexican folk remedies and conventional medical care. *American Family Physician* 37 (3): 257–62.

Mena, Aipy. 1998. Cuban Santería, Haitian vodun, Puerto Rican spiritualism: A multiculturalist inquiry into syncretism. *Journal for the Scientific Study of Religion* 37: 15–27.

Morton, Julia F. 1981. *Atlas of medicinal plants of Middle America: Bahamas to Yucatan.* Springfield, Illinois: Charles C. Thomas.

Nations, M. K., and L. A. Rebhun. 1988. Angels with wet wings won't fly: Maternal sentiment in Brazil and the image of neglect. *Culture, Medicine and Psychiatry* 12 (2): 141–200.

Ngokwey, N. 1995. Naming and grouping illnesses in Feira (Brazil). *Culture, Medicine and Psychiatry* 19 (3): 385–408.

Nunez, Luis Manuel. 1992. *Santería: A practical guide to Afro-Caribbean religion.* Dallas, Texas: Spring Publications.

Ortiz de Montellano, B. R., and C. H. Browner. 1985. Chemical bases for medicinal plant use in Oaxaca, Mexico. *Journal of Ethnopharmacology* 13: 57–88.

Pedersen, D., and V. Baruffati. 1985. Health and traditional medicine cultures in Latin America and the Caribbean. *Social Science and Medicine* 21 (1): 5–12.

Sharon, Douglas C. 1974. The symbol system of a north Peruvian shaman. Ph.D. diss., University of California, Los Angeles.

Simmons, Ozzie G. 1955. Popular and modern medicine in mestizo Communities of coastal Peru and Chile. *Journal of American Folklore* 68: 57–71.

Simpson, S. H. 1988. Some preliminary considerations on the sobada: A traditional treatment for gastrointestinal illness in Costa Rica. *Social Science and Medicine* 27 (1): 69–73.

Smith, Lovisa V. 1951. Folk remedies in Andes. *New York Folklore Quarterly* 7: 295–98.

Tousignant, M. 1984. Pena in the Ecuadorian Sierra: A psychoanthropological analysis of sadness. *Culture, Medicine and Psychiatry* 8 (4): 381–98.

Van Oss Marin, B., G. Marin, A. Padilla, and C. de la Rocha. 1983. Utilization of traditional and non-traditional sources of health care among Hispanics. *Hispanic Journal of Behavioral Sciences* 5: 65–80.

Vega, W. 1980. The Hispanic natural healer—A case study: Implications for prevention. In *Hispanic natural support systems: Mental health promotion perspectives*, ed. R. Valle and W. Vega, 65–74. Sacramento: California Department of Mental Health.

Weller, S. C., T. K. Ruebush III, and R. E. Klein. 1991. An epidemiological description of a folk illness: A study of empacho in Guatemala. *Medical Anthropology* 13 (1–2): 19–31.

IV.B.   *Caribbean*

Beckwith, Martha W. 1927. *Notes on Jamaican ethnobotany*. Poughkeepsie, New York: Vassar College.

Benedek, C., and L. Rivier. 1989. Evidence for presence of tetrodotoxin in a powder used in Haiti for zombification. *Toxicon* 27 (4): 473–80.

Benedetti, M. D. 1989. *Earth and spirit: Healing lore and more from Puerto Rico*. New Jersey: Waterfront Press.

Borrello, Mary Ann, and Elizabeth Mathias. 1977. Botanicas: Puerto Rican folk pharmacies. *Natural History* 86 (7): 64–72, 116–17.

Bourguignon, Erika. 1959. The persistence of folk belief: Some notes on cannibalism and zombis in Haiti. *Journal of American Folklore* 72: 36–45

Bram, Joseph. 1958. Spirits, mediums and believers in contemporary Puerto Rico. *Transactions of the New York Academy of Sciences* 20: 340–47.

Brandon, George. 1989–1990. African religious influences in Cuba, Puerto Rico, and Hispaniola. *Journal of Caribbean Studies* 7 (2–3): 201–31.

Brodwin, Paul. 1996. *Medicine and morality in Haiti: The contest for healing power*. New York: Cambridge University Press.

Cabrera, Lydia. 1975. *El monte: Notas sobre las religiones, la magia, las supersticiones, y el folklore de Pueblo de Cuba*. 1940. Reprint, Miami: Ediciones Universal.

———. 1994–1995. Religious syncretism in Cuba. *Journal of Caribbean Studies* 10 (1–2): 84–94.

Camas-Diaz, L. 1981. Puerto Rican espiritismo and psychotherapy. *American Journal of Orthopsychiatry* 138 (11): 1477–81.

Carbajal, D., A. Casaco, L. Arruzazabala, R. Gonzalez, and V. Fuentes. 1991. Pharmacological screening of plant decoctions commonly used in Cuban folk medicine. *Journal of Ethnopharmacology* 33 (1–2): 21–24.

Coreil, J. 1983. Parallel structures in professional and folk health care: A model applied to rural Haiti. *Culture, Medicine and Psychiatry* 7 (2): 131–51.

Costantino, G., R. G. Malgady, and L. H. Rogler. 1988. Folk hero modeling therapy for Puerto Rican adolescents. *Journal of Adolescence* 11 (2): 155–65.

Craan, A. G. 1988. Toxicological aspects of voodoo in Haiti. *Biomedical and Environmental Sciences* 1 (4): 372–81.

Dale , R. A. 1996. New developments in Cuban holistic medicine: A personal view. *Journal of Alternative and Complementary Medicine* 2 (2): 299–305.

Davis, E. W. 1983. The ethnobiology of the Haitian zombi. *Journal of Ethnopharmacology* 9 (1): 85–104.

Delgado, Melvin. 1978. Folk medicine in the Puerto Rican culture. *International Social Work* 21: 45–54.

DeSantis, Lydia, and Janice T. Thomas. 1990. The immigrant Haitian mother: Transcultural nursing perspective on preventive health care for children. *Journal of Transcultural Nursing* 2 (1): 2–15.

Dorta-Morales, José 1976. *Puerto Rican espiritismo: Religion and psychotherapy*. New York: Vantage Press.

Fredrich, B. E. Research note: A prospective St. Lucian folk medicine survey. *Social Science and Medicine*. Part D. *Medical Geography* 15 (4): 435–37.

Galli, N. 1975. The influence of cultural heritage on the health status of Puerto Ricans. *Journal of School Health* 45 (1): 10–15.

Gaviria, M., and R. M. Wintrob. 1976. Supernatural influence in psychopathology: Puerto Rican folk beliefs about mental illness. *Canadian Psychiatric Association Journal* 21 (6): 361–69.

Guarnaccia, P. J. 1993. Ataques de nervios in Puerto Rico: Culture-bound syndrome or popular illness? *Medical Anthropology* 15 (2): 157–70.

Halberstein, R. A. 1997. Traditional botanical remedies on a small Caribbean island: Middle (Grand) Caicos, West Indies. *Journal of Alternative and Complementary Medicine* 3 (3): 227–39.

Halberstein, R. A., and A. B. Saunders. 1978. Traditional medical practices and medicinal plant usage on a Bahamian island. *Culture, Medicine and Psychiatry* 2 (2): 177–203.

Harwood, Alan. 1977a. *Rx: Spiritist as needed: A study of Puerto Rican community mental health resource*. New York: Wiley.

———. 1977b. Description and analysis of an alternative psychotherapeutic approach. Part 1 of Puerto Rican spiritism. *Culture, Medicine and Psychiatry* 1: 69–95.

———. 1977c. An institution with preventive and therapeutic functions in community psychiatry. Part 2 of Puerto Rican spiritism. *Culture, Medicine and Psychiatry* 1: 135–53.

———. 1981. Mainland Puerto Ricans. In *Ethnicity and medical care*, ed. Alan Harwood, 397–481. Cambridge: Harvard University Press.

Hohmann, A. A., M. Richeport, B. M. Marriott, G. J. Canino, M. Rubio-Stipec, and H. Bird. 1990. Spiritism in Puerto Rico: Results of an island-wide community study. *British Journal of Psychiatry* 156: 328–35.

Koss, Joan D. 1970. Therapy of a system of a sect in Puerto Rico. *Revista de Ciencias Sociales* 14: 259–75.

———. 1975. Therapeutic aspects of Puerto Rican cult practices. *Psychiatry* 38: 160–71.

———. 1977a. Religion and science divinely related: A case history of spiritism in Puerto Rico. *Caribbean Studies* 16: 22–43.

———. 1977b. Social process, healing and self-defeat among Puerto Rican spiritualists. *American Ethnologist* 4: 453–69.

———. 1980. The therapist spiritist training project in Puerto Rico: An experiment to relate the traditional healing system to the public health system. *Social Science and Medicine* 14B: 255–66.

———. 1987. Expectations and outcomes for patients given mental health care or spiritist healing in Puerto Rico. *American Journal of Psychiatry* 144: 56–61.

Koss-Chioino, Joan. 1992. *Women as healers, women as patients: Mental health care and traditional healing in Puerto Rico*. Boulder, Colorado: Westview Press.

Laguerre, M. S. 1987. *Afro-Caribbean folk medicine*. South Hadley, Massachusetts: Bergin and Garvey Publishers.

Lefever, Harry G. 1996. When the saints go riding in: Santería in Cuba and the United States. *Journal for the Scientific Study of Religion* 35: 318–30.

Lubchansky, Isaac, Gladys Egri, and Janet Stokes. 1970. Puerto Rican spiritualists view mental illness: The faith healer as paraprofessional. *American Journal of Psychiatry* 127: 312–21.

Mills, J., K. O. Pascoe, J. Chambers, and G. N. Melville. 1986. Preliminary investigations of the wound-healing properties of a Jamaican folk medicinal plant (Justicia pectoralis). *West Indian Medical Journal* 35 (3): 190–93.

Newell, William Wells. 1888. Voodoo worship and child sacrifice in Hayti. *Journal of American Folklore* 1: 16–30.

———. 1889. Reports of voodoo worship in Hayti and Louisiana. *Journal of American Folklore* 2: 41–47.

Oakes, A. J., and M. P. Morris. 1958. The West Indian weedwoman of the United States Virgin Islands. *Bulletin of the History of Medicine* 32: 164–69.

Ortiz, Fernando. 1906. *Hampa Afro-Cubana: Los negros brujos.* Madrid: Editorial America.

Pachter, L. M., B. Bernstein, and A. Osorio. 1992. Clinical implications of a folk illness: Empacho in mainland Puerto Ricans. *Medical Anthropology* 13 (4): 285–99.

Pachter, L. M., M. M. Cloutier, and B. A. Bernstein. 1995. Ethnomedical (folk) remedies for childhood asthma in a mainland Puerto Rican community. *Archives of Pediatrics and Adolescent Medicine* 149 (9): 982–88.

Rousseau, Jacques. 1946. Notes sur l'ethnobotanique d'Anticosti. *Les Archives de Folklore* 1: 60–69.

———. 1948. Ethnobotanique et ethnozoologie Gaspésiennes. *Les Archives de Folklore* 3: 51–63.

Sandoval, Mercedes Cros. 1975. *La religion afrocubana.* Madrid: Coleccion Libre Plaza Mayor.

Schwartz, Dorothy. 1985. Caribbean folk beliefs and Western psychiatry. *Journal of Psychosocial Nursing and Mental Health Services* 23: 26–30.

Simpson, George E. 1954. Magical practices in northern Haiti. *Journal of American Folklore* 67: 395–403.

Singer, Merrill. 1984. Indigenous treatment for alcoholism: The case of Puerto Rican spiritism. *Medical Anthropology* 8 (4): 246–73.

Vilayleck, E. 1996. The Bles, a Caribbean Creole disease (trans. from French). *Bulletin de la Societe de Pathologie Exotique* 89 (1): 57–67.

Weniger, B., M. Haag-Berrurier, and R. Anton. 1982. Plants of Haiti used as infertility agents. *Journal of Ethnopharmacology* 6 (1): 67–84.

Wong, W. 1976. Some folk medicinal plants from Trinidad. *Economic Botany* 30: 103–42.

IV.C. *African*

Bailey, James A. 1991. *The Yoruba of southwestern Nigeria and Santería in the southeastern United States.* New Bern, North Carolina: Godolphin House.

Bascom, William. 1969. *Sixteen cowries: Yoruba divination from Africa to the New World.* Bloomington: Indiana University Press.

Brandon, George. 1993. *The dead sell memories: Santería from Africa to the New World.* Bloomington: Indiana University Press.

Brown, David H. 1989. Garden in the machine: Afro-Cuban sacred art and performance in New York City. Ph.D. diss., Yale University, New Haven, Connecticut.

———. 1993. Thrones of the orichas: Afro-Cuban altars in New Jersey, New York, and Havana. *African Arts* 26 (4): 44–59, 85.

Canizares, Raul. 1993. *Walking with the night: The Afro-Cuban world of Santería.* Rochester, Vermont: Destiny Books.

Etkin, N. L. 1981. A Hausa herbal pharmacopoeia: Biomedical evaluation of commonly used plant medicines. *Journal of Ethnopharmacology* 4: 75–98.

Evans, David K., Don Stephen Rice, and Joanne Kline Partin. 1968. Parallels in West African, West Indian, and North Carolina Folklore. *North Carolina Folklore* 17: 77–84.

Golden, K. M. 1977. Voodoo in Africa and the United States. *American Journal of Psychiatry* 134 (12): 1425–27.

Gonzalez-Wippler, Migene. 1973. *Santería: African magic in Latin America.* New York: Julian Press.

Hielscher, S., and J. Sommerfeld. 1985. Concepts of illness and the utilization of health-care services in a rural Malian village. *Social Science and Medicine* 21 (4): 469–81.

Macklin, June. 1974. Belief, ritual and healing: New England spiritualism and Mexican-American spiritism compared. In *Religious movements in contemporary America*, ed. I. I. Zaretsky and M. P. Leone, 383–417. Princeton, New Jersey: Princeton University Press.

Makanjuola, R.O. 1987. "Ode Ori": A culture-bound disorder with prominent somatic features in Yoruba Nigerian patients. *Acta Psychiatrica Scandinavica* 75 (3): 231–36.

Nunez, Luis Manuel. 1992. *Santería: A practical guide to Afro-Caribbean religion.* Dallas, Texas: Spring Publications.

Oyejide, C. O., and G. A. Aderinokun. 1991. Teething myths in Nigerian rural Yoruba communities. *African Dental Journal* 5: 31–34.

Reynolds, J., and L. Swartz. 1993. Professional constructions of a "lay" illness: "Nerves" in a rural "coloured" community in South Africa. *Social Science and Medicine* 36 (5): 657–63.

Sandoval, Mercedes Cros. 1975. *La religion afrocubana.* Madrid, Spain: Coleccion Libre Plaza Mayor.

Sharp, P. T. 1982. Ghosts, witches, sickness and death: The traditional interpretation of injury and disease in a rural area of Papua New Guinea. *Papua New Guinea Medical Journal* 25 (2): 108–15.

Sofowora, A. 1996. Research on medicinal plants and traditional medicine in Africa. *Journal of Alternative and Complementary Medicine* 2 (3): 365–72.

IV.D. *Asian*

Ashikaga, Ensho. 1954. Votive pictures: A Japanese superstition. *Western Folklore* 13: 29–33.

Bhopalm, R. S. 1986. The inter-relationship of folk, traditional and Western medicine within an Asian community in Britain. *Social Science and Medicine* 22 (1): 99–105.

Castillo, R. J. 1994. Theoretical background. Part 1 of Spirit possession in south Asia, dissociation or hysteria? *Culture, Medicine and Psychiatry* 18 (1): 1–21.

Cheng, S. T. 1996. A critical review of Chinese koro. *Culture, Medicine and Psychiatry* 20 (1): 67–82.

Cheung, F. M. 1989. The indigenization of neurasthenia in Hong Kong. *Culture, Medicine and Psychiatry* 13 (2): 227–41.

Eguchi, S. 1991. Between folk concepts of illness and psychiatric diagnosis: Kitsune-tsuki (fox possession) in a mountain village of western Japan. *Culture, Medicine and Psychiatry* 15 (4): 421–51.

Fukunishi, I., T. Nakagawa, H. Nakamura, M. Kikuchi, and M. Takubo. 1997. Is alexithymia a culture-bound construct? Validity and reliability of the Japanese versions of the twenty-item Toronto alexithymia scale and modified Beth Israel Hospital psychosomatic questionnaire. *Psychological Reports* 80 (3): 787–99.

Good, B. J. 1977. The heart of what's the matter: The semantics of illness in Iran. *Culture, Medicine and Psychiatry* 1 (1): 25–58.

Hiruta, G. 1984. A study of Goyodomecho (an official record) of Mutsu-Moriyama-domain (Japan, the Edo Period) from a psychiatric viewpoint; with special regard to folk concepts of mental illness. *Seishin Shinkeigaku Zasshi* 86 (9): 699–735.

Kang, J. T., C. F. Chen, and P. Chou. 1996. Factors related to the choice between traditional Chinese medicine and modern Western medicine among patients with two-method treatment. *Chung Hua I Hsueh Tsa Chih (Taipei)* 57 (6): 405–12.

Kim, Y. K., D. Sich, T. K. Park, and D. H. Kang. 1980. Naeng: A Korean folk illness, its ethnography and its epidemiology. *Yonsei Medical Journal* 21 (2): 147–55.

Kleinman, A. M. 1975. The symbolic context of Chinese medicine: A comparative approach to the study of traditional medical and psychiatric forms of care in Chinese culture. *American Journal of Chinese Medicine* 3 (2): 103–24.

Kleinman, A., and J. L. Gale. 1982. Patients treated by physicians and folk healers: A comparative outcome study in Taiwan. *Culture, Medicine and Psychiatry* 6 (4): 405–23.

Kohda, H., K. Kozai, N. Nagasaka, Y. Miyake, H. Suginaka, K. Hidaka, and K. Yamasaki. 1986. Prevention of dental caries by Oriental folk medicines—Active principles of zizyphi fructus for inhibition of insoluble glucan formation by cariogenic bacterium streptococcus mutans. *Planta Medica* April (2): 119–20.

Koo, L. C. 1987. Concepts of disease causation, treatment and prevention among Hong Kong Chinese: Diversity and eclecticism. *Social Science and Medicine* 25 (4): 405–17.

Kua, E. H., L. P. Sim, and K. T. Chee. 1986. A cross-cultural study of the possession-trance in Singapore. *Australian and New Zealand Journal of Psychiatry* 20 (3): 361–64.

Lambert, H. 1992. The cultural logic of Indian medicine: Prognosis and etiology in Rajasthani popular therapeutics. *Social Science and Medicine* 34 (10): 1069–76.

Lee, S. 1997. How lay is lay? Chinese students' perceptions of anorexia nervosa in Hong Kong. *Social Science and Medicine* 44 (4): 491–502.

Li, S. X., and M. R. Phillips. 1990. Witch doctors and mental illness in mainland China: A preliminary study. *American Journal of Psychiatry* 147 (2): 221–24.

Lieban, R. W. 1983. Gender aspects of illness and practitioner use among Filipinos. *Social Science and Medicine* 17 (13): 853–59.

Lin, K. M. 1983. Hwa-byung: A Korean culture-bound syndrome? *American Journal of Psychiatry* 140 (1): 105–107.

Lock, M. M. 1978. Scars of experience: The art of moxibustion in Japanese medicine and society. *Culture, Medicine and Psychiatry* 2 (2): 151–75.

Malhotra, H. K., and N. N. Wig. 1975. Dhat syndrome: A culture-bound sex neurosis of the orient. *Archives of Sexual Behavior* 4 (5): 519–28.

McNee, A., N. Khan, S. Dawson, J. Gunsalam, V. L. Tallo, L. Manderson, and I. Riley. 1995. Responding to cough: Boholano illness classification and resort to care in response to childhood ARI. *Social Science and Medicine* 40 (9): 1279–89.

Morinis, A. 1985. Sanctified madness: The God-intoxicated saints of Bengal. *Social Science and Medicine* 21 (2): 211–20.

Mushtaque, A., R. Chowdhury, and Z. N. Kabir. 1991. Folk terminology for diarrhea in rural Bangladesh. *Reviews of Infectious Diseases* 13 (suppl. 14): S252–54.

Palgi, P. 1979. Persistent traditional Yemenite ways of dealing with stress in Israel. *Mental Health and Society* 5 (3–4): 113–40.

Pang, K. Y., and M. H. Lee. 1994. Prevalence of depression and somatic symptoms among Korean elderly immigrants. *Yonsei Medical Journal* 35 (2): 155–61.

Rauyajin, O., B. Kamthornwachara, and P. Yablo. 1995. Socio-cultural and behavioural aspects of mosquito-borne lymphatic filariasis in Thailand: A qualitative analysis. *Social Science and Medicine* 41 (12): 1705–13.

Rosca-Rebaudengo, P., R. Durst, and S. Minuchin-Itzigsohn. 1996. Transculturation, psychosis and koro symptoms. *Israel Journal of Psychiatry and Related Sciences* 33 (1): 54–62.

Russell, J. G. 1989. Anxiety disorders in Japan: A review of the Japanese literature on shinkeishitsu and taijinkyofusho. *Culture, Medicine and Psychiatry* 13 (4): 391–403.

Shawyer, R. J., A. S. bin Gani, A. N. Punufimana, and N. K. Seuseu. 1996. The role of clinical vignettes in rapid ethnographic research: A folk taxonomy of diarrhoea in Thailand. *Social Science and Medicine* 42 (1): 111–23.

Shields, N. K. 1987. Healing spirits of South Kanara. *Culture, Medicine and Psychiatry* 11 (4): 417–35.

Shimoji, A. 1991. Interface between shamanism and psychiatry in Miyako Islands, Okinawa, Japan: A viewpoint from medical and psychiatric anthropology. *Japanese Journal of Psychiatry and Neurology* 45 (4): 767–74.

Simon, Gwladys Hughes. 1952. Some Japanese beliefs and home remedies. *Journal of American Folklore* 65: 281–94.

Smith, R. M., and L. A. Nelsen. 1991. Hmong folk remedies: Limited acetylation of opium by aspirin and acetaminophen. *Journal of Forensic Sciences* 36 (1): 280–87.

Sugaya, E., A. Sugaya, K. Kajiwara, N. Yuyama, T. Tsuda, M. Motoki, K. Shimizu-Nishikawa, and M. Kimura. 1997. Nervous diseases and kampo (Japanese herbal) medicine: A new paradigm of therapy against intractable nervous diseases. *Brain and Development* 19 (2): 93–103.

Swagman, C. F. 1989. Fijac: Fright and illness in highland Yemen. *Social Science and Medicine* 28 (4): 381–88.

Tonai, S., M. Maezawa, M. Kamei, T. Satoh, and T. Fukui. 1989. Illness behavior of housewives in a rural area in Japan: A health diary study. *Culture, Medicine and Psychiatry* 13 (4): 405–17.

Tseng, W. S., K. M. Mo, J. Hsu, L. S. Li, L. W. Ou, G. Q. Chen, and D. W. Jiang. 1988. A sociocultural study of koro epidemics in Guangdong, China. *American Journal of Psychiatry* 145 (12): 1538–43.

Uba, L. 1992. Cultural barriers to health care for southeast Asian refugees. *Public Health Reports* 107 (5): 544–58.

Weiner, M. A. 1986. Stomach cancer in Japan: Relationship to a common folk remedy? *Medical Hypotheses* 20 (4): 357–58.

Weiss, M. G., S. D. Sharma, R. K. Gaur, J. S. Sharma, A. Desai, and D. R. Doongaji. 1986. Traditional concepts of mental disorder among Indian psychiatric patients: Preliminary report of work in progress. *Social Science and Medicine* 23 (4): 379–86.

Westermeyer, J., and R. Wintrob. 1979. "Folk" criteria for the diagnosis of mental illness in rural Laos: On being insane in sane places. *American Journal of Psychiatry* 136 (6): 755–61.

Wikan, U. 1989. Illness from fright or soul loss: A north Balinese culture-bound syndrome? *Culture, Medicine and Psychiatry* 13 (1): 25–50.

IV.E.   *British*

Bhopalm, R. S. 1986. The inter-relationship of folk, traditional and western medicine within an Asian community in Britain. *Social Science and Medicine* 22 (1): 99–105.

Davidson, T. D. 1960. A survey of some British veterinary folklore. *Bulletin of the History of Medicine* 34: 199–232.

Helman, Cecil G. 1978. "Feed a cold, starve a fever"—Folk models of infection in an English suburban community, and their relationship to medical treatment. *Culture, Medicine and Psychiatry* 2: 107–37.

Logan, Patrick. 1972. *Making the cure: A look at Irish folk medicine.* Dublin: Talbot Press.

IV.F.   *European*

Angermeyer, M. C., and H. Matschinger. 1994. Lay beliefs about schizophrenic disorder: The results of a population survey in Germany. *Acta Psychiatrica Scandinavica,* suppl. 382: 39–45.

Blum, Richard H. and Eva. 1965. *Health and healing in rural Greece.* Stanford, California: Stanford University Press.

Bonser, W. 1956. Medical folklore of Venice and Rome. *Folklore* 67: 1–15.

Cattermole-Tally, Frances M. 1978. From the mystery of conception to the miracle of birth: An historical survey of beliefs and rituals surrounding the pregnant woman in Germanic folk tradition, including modern American folklore. Ph.D. diss., University of California, Los Angeles.

Clark, M. H. 1989. Nevra in a Greek village: Idiom, metaphor, symptom, or disorder? *Health Care for Women International* 10 (2–3): 195–218.

Dunk, P. 1989. Greek women and broken nerves in Montreal. *Medical Anthropology* 11 (1): 29–45.

Foster, George M. 1953. Relationships between Spanish and Spanish-American folk medicine. *Journal of American Folklore* 66: 201–17.

Gunda, Bela. 1949. Wandering healers, medicine hawkers in Slovakia and Transylvania. *Southwestern Journal of Anthropology* 5: 147–50.

———. 1962. Gypsy medical folklore in Hungary. *Journal of American Folklore* 75: 131–46.

Jones, Louis C. 1951. The evil eye among European-Americans. *Western Folklore* 10: 11–25.

Kay, M. 1987. Lay theory of healing in northwestern New Spain. *Social Science and Medicine* 24 (12): 1051–60.

Kemp, Phyllis. 1935. *Healing ritual in the technique and tradition of the southern Slavs.* London: Faber and Faber.

Kerewsky-Halpern, B. 1985. Trust, talk and touch in Balkan folk healing. *Social Science and Medicine* 21 (3): 319–25.

Mathiessen, C. C. 1962–1963. Learned and popular tradition in Nordic veterinary folk-medicine. *Arv* 18–19: 312–24.

Moss, Leonard W., and Stephen C. Cappannari. 1960. Folklore and medicine in an Italian village. *Journal of American Folklore* 73: 95–102.

Ozturk, O. M. 1965. Folk interpretation of illness in Turkey and its psychological significance. *Turkish Journal of Pediatrics* 7 (4): 165–79.

Pedrabissi, L., J. P. Rolland, and M. Santinello. 1993. Stress and burnout among teachers in Italy and France. *Journal of Psychology* 127 (5): 529–35.

Petulengro, Gipsy. 1935. *Romany remedies and recipes.* London, n.p.

Pitré, Giuseppe. 1971. *Sicilian folk medicine.* Trans. Phyllis H. Williams. Lawrence, Kansas: Coronado Press.

Romanucci-Ross, L. 1986. Creativity in illness: Methodological linkages to the logic and language of science in folk pursuit of health in central Italy. *Social Science and Medicine* 23 (1): 1–7.

Scheiber, Alexander. 1954. The catechism song in Hungary. *Western Folklore* 13: 27–28.

Simpson, George E. 1962. Folk medicine in Trinidad. *Journal of American Folklore* 75: 326–40.

Tavenner, Eugene. The amulet in Roman curative medicine. Washington University Studies, *Humanistic Series* 9 (2): 185–209.

Williams, Phyllis H. 1938. *South Italian folkways in Europe and America—A handbook for social workers, visiting nurses, school teachers, and physicians.* New Haven, Connecticut: Yale University Press.

IV.G. *Judaic and biblical*

Bilu, Y. 1988. Rabbi Yaacov Wazana: A Jewish healer in the Atlas Mountains. *Culture, Medicine and Psychiatry* 12 (1): 113–35.

Callcott, Maria. 1842. *A scripture herbal.* London: n.p.

Davis, C. Truman, M.D. 1966. Medicine and the Bible. *Arizona Medicine* 23: 173–79.

Hess, Joseph, M.D. 1963. Treatment of mental ailments among the Jews in Yemen. *Hebrew Medical Journal* 2: 224–28.

Jakobovits, Immanuel. 1957. Irrational medical beliefs in Jewish law. Superstitious, occult and scatological cures. *Hebrew Medical Journal* 31 (2): 187–201.

Kamsler, Harold M. 1938. Hebrew menstrual taboos. *Journal of American Folklore* 51: 76–82.

Krause, Louis A. M. 1959. Medicine and the Bible. *West Virginia Medical Journal* 55.

Shepherd, P. M. 1955. The Bible as a source book for physicians. *Glasgow Medical Journal* 36: 348–75

V. *History of medicine*

Ackernecht, Erwin H. 1942. Problems of primitive medicine. *Bulletin of the History of Medicine* 11: 503–21.

Aikman, Lonnelle. 1977. Nature's healing arts: From folk medicine to modern drugs. Washington, D.C.: National Geographic Society.

Alvarez, Walter C., M.D. 1937. The emergence of modern medicine from ancient folkways. *Annual Report of the Smithsonian Institution,* 409–30. Washington, D.C.: Governmental Printing Office.

———. 1943. The impact of the introduction of iron on medical and religious thought. In *Essays in biology in honor of Herbert M. Evans,* 27–32. Berkeley: University of California Press.

Anderson, Urban. 1937. A comparative study of some of the older beliefs and usages of east Tennessee. *Tennessee Folklore Society Bulletin* 3: 1–7.

Babcock, J. W., M.D. 1895. Communicated insanity and Negro witchcraft. *American Journal of Insanity* 51: 518–23.

Bergen, Fanny D. 1890. Some saliva charms. *Journal of American Folklore* 3: 51–59.

———. 1892. Some bits of plant lore. *Journal of American Folklore* 5: 19–22.

———. 1899. Animal and plant lore collected from the oral tradition of English speaking folk. *Memoirs of the American Folk-Lore Society*. Vol. 7. Boston and New York: n.p.

Bergen, Fanny D., W. M. Beauchamp, and W. W. Newell. 1889. Current superstitions. *Journal of American Folklore* 2: 12–22, 105–12, 203–8.

Berman, Alex. 1956. A striving for scientific respectability: Some American botanics and the nineteenth century plant materia medica. *Bulletin of the History of Medicine* 30 (1): 7–31.

Black, William George. 1883. Folk-medicine: A chapter in the history of culture. *Publications of the Folk-Lore Society*, 12.

Bourke, John G. 1892.The medicine-men of the Apache. In *Ninth Annual Report of the Bureau of Ethnology, 1887–1888*, 443–603. Washington D.C.: Governmental Printing Office.

———. 1894. Popular medicine, customs, and superstitions of the Rio Grande. *Journal of American Folklore* 7: 119–46.

Brown, T. H. 1988. The African connection: Cotton Mather and the Boston Smallpox Epidemic of 1721–1722. *Journal of the American Medical Association* 260 (15): 2247–49.

Bryan, Leon S. 1964. Blood-letting in American medicine, 1830–1892. *Bulletin of the History of Medicine* 38(6)516–29.

Cadwallader, D. E., and F. J. Wilson. 1965. Folklore medicine among Georgia's Piedmont Negroes after the Civil War. *Collections of the Georgia Historical Society* 49: 217–27.

Cartwright, Samuel A. 1854a. Some further remarks on the sugar-house cure for bronchial, dyseptic, and consumptive complaints. *Boston Medical and Surgical Journal* 51 (8): 149–56.

———. 1854b. The sugar-house cure for bronchial, dyseptic and consumptive complaints. *Boston Medical and Surgical Journal* 51 (10): 195–202.

———. 1854c. The case of the strong-minded woman from Boston in a sugar house with bronchitis and illustrating the therapeutic power of the vapor of boiling cane juice. *Boston Medical and Surgical Journal* 51 (12): 229–36.

———. 1854d. The case of a lady in a sugar house with aphonic, haemorrhagic, tubercular phthisis in the softening stage. *Boston Medical and Surgical Journal* 51 (14): 269–77.

Cayleff, S. E. 1988. "Prisoners of their own feebleness": Women, nerves and Western medicine—An historical overview. *Social Science and Medicine* 26 (12): 1199–1208.

Clements, Forrest E. 1932. Primitive concepts of disease. *University of California Publications in American Archaeology and Ethnology*. Vol. 32, 185–252. Berkeley: University of California.

Cobb, Carolus M. 1917. Some medical practices among the New England Indians and early settlers. *Boston Medical and Surgical Journal* 177 (4): 97–105.

Craddock, S. 1995. Sewers and scapegoats: Spatial metaphors of smallpox in nineteenth century San Francisco. *Social Science and Medicine* 41 (7): 957–68.

Culin, Stewart. 1890. Concerning Negro sorcery in the United States. *Journal of American Folklore* 3: 281–87.

Curtin, L. S. M. 1930. Pioneer medicine in New Mexico. *Folk-Say* 186–96.

Davenport, Gertrude C. 1898. Folk-cures from Kansas. *Journal of American Folklore* 11: 129–32.

Davis, D. L. 1989. George Beard and Lydia Pinkham: Gender, class, and nerves in late nineteenth century America. *Health Care for Women International* 10(2–3): 93–114.

de Laszlo, Henry, and Paul S. Henshaw. 1954. Plant materials used by primitive peoples to affect fertility. *Science* 119: 626–30.

Denninger, Henry Stearns. 1940. A history of substances known as aphrodisiacs. *Annals of Medical History* 2: 383–93.

DeVoto, Bernard. 1955. Frontier family medicine. *What's New* 192: 3–5, 41–42.

Dougherty, Thomas M. 1956. Epilepsy: The history of folklore in its treatment. *Journal of the Kansas Medical Society* 57 (4): 304–17.

Edgar, Irving I. 1960. Origins of the healing art. *Journal of the Michigan State Medical Society* 59 (7): 1035–39.

Eggleston, Edward. 1899. Some curious colonial remedies. *American Historical Review* 5: 199–206.

Engelhardt, H. Tristram, Jr. 1974. The disease of masturbation: Values and the concept of disease. *Bulletin of the History of Medicine* 48: 234–48.

Fenton, William N. 1942. Contacts between Iroquois herbalism and colonial medicine. *Annual Report of the Smithsonian Institution*, 1941, 503–27. Washington, D.C.: Governmental Printing Office.

Fife, Austin E. 1957. Pioneer Mormon remedies. *Western Folklore* 16: 153–62.

Fletcher, Robert, M.D. 1896. The witches' pharmacopoeia. *Bulletin, John Hopkins Hospital* 7 (65): 147–56.

Forbes, Thomas R. 1946. The origin of "freemartin." *Bulletin of the History of Medicine* 20: 461–66.

———. 1953. The social history of the caul. *Yale Journal of Biology and Medicine* 25: 495–508.

———. 1954. The origin of the term "ridgeling." *Yale Journal of Biology and Medicine* 27: 20–25.

———. 1962. Perette the midwife: A fifteenth century witchcraft case. *Bulletin of the History of Medicine* 36: 124–29.

———. 1964. The regulation of English midwives in the sixteenth and seventeenth centuries. *Medical History* 8: 235–44.

Gifford, Edward S., Jr., M.D. 1957. The evil eye in medical history. *American Journal of Ophthalmology* 44 (2): 237–43.

———. 1960. The evil eye in Pennsylvania medical history. *Keystone Folk Quarterly* 5 (3): 3–8.

Gordon, Benjamin Lee. 1957. The roots of Russian medicine. *Journal of the Medical Society of New Jersey (Orange)* 54: 79–84.

———. 1958a. Lay medicine during the early Middle Ages. *Journal of the Michigan State Medical Society* 57 (7): 1001–1007.

———. 1958b. Medieval medicine in England. *Journal of the Medical Society of New Jersey (Orange)* 55: 444–53.

Gordon, R. 1995. The healing event in Graeco-Roman folk-medicine. *Clio Medica* 28: 363–76.

Guerra, Francisco. 1961. Medical almanacs of the American colonial period. *Journal of the History of Medicine* 16: 234–55.

Harding, T. Swann, M.D. 1934. Curious remedies—Old and new. *American Journal of Pharmacy* 106: 211–26.

Harris, David. 1939. Medicine in colonial America. *California and Western Medicine* 51: 35–38.

Hetrick, George. 1957. Practice of medicine in Berks from time of early settlers to 1824. *Medical Record (Berks County, Pennsylvania, Medical Society)* 48 (8): 247–50.

Hispanius, Petrus. 1585. *The treasury of health, containing many profitable medicines, gathered out of Hippocrates, Galen, and Avicen, by one Petrus Hispanius and translated into English by Humfrie Lloyd.* London: n.p.

Hoffman, W. J., M.D. 1893. Notes on Pennsylvania German folk medicine. *Science* 21: 355.

Hurty, J. N. 1922. An old Indiana book on medicine. *Journal of the Indiana State Medical Association* 14 (4): 122–24.

Idler, E. L. 1989. Moral medicine: Symbolic content in nineteenth century Shaker therapeutics. *Culture, Medicine and Psychiatry* 13 (1): 1–24.

Jankovic, S. M., D. V. Sokic, Z. M. Levic, V. Susic, N. Stojsavljevic, and J. Drulovic. 1996. Epilepsy, eponyms and patron saints (history of Western civilization). *Rpski Arhiv Za Celokokupino Lekarstvo* 124 (5–6): 162–65.

Jones, Ida B. 1937. Popular medical knowledge in fourteenth century English literature. *Bulletin of the Institute of the History of Medicine* 5: 405–51, 538–88.

Kanner, Leo. 1930. The folklore and cultural history of epilepsy. *Medical Life* 37: 167–214.

———. 1931. The teeth of gods, saints, and kings: Mythologic and historical contributions to dental folklore. *Medical Life* 38: 506–18.

Lathrop, Amy. 1961. Pioneer remedies from western Kansas. *Western Folklore* 20: 1–22.

Lee, Charles O. 1960. The Shakers as pioneers in the American herb and drug industry. *American Journal of Pharmacy* 132 (5): 178–93.

Lipton, May. 1969. The history and superstitions of birth defects. *Journal of School Health* 39: 579–82.

Lorenz, Anthony J. 1957. Scurvy in the Gold Rush. *Journal of the History of Medicine* 12: 473–510.

Lucas, E. H. 1959. The role of folklore in discovery and rediscovery of plant drugs. *Centennial Review of Arts and Science* 3: 173–88.

Maddox, John Lee. 1930. Spirit theory in early medicine. *American Anthropologist* 32: 503–21.

McAtee, W. L. 1955. Home medication in Grant County, Indiana, in the nineties. *Midwest Folklore* 5: 213–16.

———. 1958. Medical lore in Grant County, Indiana, in the nineties. *Midwest Folklore* 8: 151–53.

McCullen, J. T. 1962. The tobacco controversy, 1571–1961. *North Carolina Folklore* 10 (1): 30–35.

McDaniel, Walton Brooks. 1948. The medical and magical significance in ancient medicine of things connected with reproduction and its organs. *Journal of the History of Medicine* 3: 525–46.

Moncrief, John. 1716. *The poor man's physician or the receipts of the famous John Moncrief of Tippermalloch being a choice collection of simple and easy remedies for most distempers. Very useful for all persons, especially those of a poorer condition.* 2nd ed., enlarged and corrected. Edinburgh: n.p.

Newell, William W. 1888. Voodoo worship and child sacrifice in Hayti. *Journal of American Folklore* 1: 16–30.

———. 1889. Reports of voodoo worship in Hayti and Louisiana. *Journal of American Folklore* 2: 41–47.

Oritz, Fernando. 1906. *Hampa Afro-Cuban: Los negros brujos.* Madrid, Spain: Editorial America.

Pendleton, Louis. 1890. Notes on Negro folk-lore and witchcraft in the South. *Journal of American Folklore* 3: 201–7.

Pettigrew, Thomas Joseph. 1844. *On superstitions connected with the history and practice of medicine and surgery.* London: n.p.

Pichot, P. 1994. Neurasthenia, yesterday and today (trans. from French). *Encephale* 20 (3): 545–49.

Pizer, Irwin H. 1965. Medical aspects of the westward migrations, 1830–1860. *Bulletin of the Medical Library Association* 53: 1–14.

Pockrein, G. A. 1981. Humoralism and social development in colonial America. *Journal of the American Medical Association* 245 (17): 1755–57.

Potts, Albert M. 1960. The mind's eye: Some concepts of vision in the ancient and primitive world. *Bulletin of the Cleveland Medical Library* 7 (1): 5–14.

Riddell, William Renwick. 1931. Historical medicine (some early Spanish American remedies: A soldier's letter to Monardes). *Medical Journal and Record* 83: 401–3.

———. 1934. Some old Canadian folk medicine. *Canada Lancet and Practitioner* 83: 41–44.

Rogers, E. G. 1941. *Early folk medical practices in Tennessee.* Murfreesboro, Tennessee: n.p.

Rogers, Spencer L. 1942. Primitive theories of disease. *Ciba Symposia* 4 (1): 1190–1200.

Shier, M. 1916. The woundsuckers of the seventeenth and eighteenth centuries. *Medical Pickwick* 2: 125–26.

Sledzik, P. S., and N. Bellantoni. 1994. Brief communication: Bioarcheological and biocultural evidence for the New England vampire folk belief. *American Journal of Physical Anthropology* 94 (2): 269–74.

Snively, W. D., Jr. 1962. Down strange byways of our medical past. *Journal of the Indiana State Medical Association* 55 (12): 1814–23.

Stromberg, W. H. 1989. Helmholtz and Zoellner: Nineteenth-century empiricism, spiritism, and the theory of space perception. *Journal of the History of the Behavioral Sciences* 25 (4): 371–83.

Talbot, C. H. 1965. Some notes on Anglo-Saxon medicine. *Medical History* 9: 156–69.

Temkin, Owsei. 1945. *The falling sickness. A history of epilepsy from the Greeks to the beginnings of modern neurology.* Baltimore: n.p.

Thiederman, Sondra B. 1984. The use of opium by women in nineteenth-century Britain. Ph.D. diss., University of California, Los Angeles.

Thomas, S. J. 1982. Nostrum advertising and the image of women as invalid in late Victorian America. *Journal of American Culture* 5: 104–12.

Thorington, J. Monroe. 1944. The ibex and chamois in ancient medicine. *Bulletin of the History of Medicine* 15 (1): 65–78.

Vance, Lee J. 1891. Evolution of patent medicine. *Popular Science Monthly* 39: 76–83.

Van Wart, Arthur F. 1948. The Indians of the maritime provinces: Their diseases and native cures. *Canadian Medical Association Journal* 59 (6): 573–77.

Welch, Charles E., Jr. 1964. Some drugs of the North American Indian—Then and now. *Keystone Folklore Quarterly* 9: 83–99.

White, Emma Gertrude. 1897. Folk-medicine among Pennsylvania Germans. *Journal of American Folklore* 10: 78–80.

Willis, Thomas. 1684. *Dr. Willis's practice of physick, being the works of that renowned and famous physician.* London: n.p.

Wilson, Julius I., M.D. 1967. Pikes Peak or bust: An historical note on the search for health in the Rockies. *Rocky Mountain Medical Journal* 64 (9): 58–62.

Wright, Jonathan. 1927. The medicine of primitive man. *Medical Life* 34: 363–408.

Young, James Harvey. 1967. *The medical messiahs: A social history of health quackery in twentieth-Century America.* Princeton, New Jersey: Princeton University Press.

VI.   *General studies*

Autotte, P. A. 1995. Folk medicine. Editorial. *Archives of Pediatrics and Adolescent Medicine* 149 (9): 949–50.

Bagley, S. P., R. Angel, P. Dilworth-Anderson, W. Liu, and S. Schinke. 1995. Adaptive health behaviors among ethnic minorities. *Health Psychology* 14 (7): 632–40.

Becerra, R. M., and A. P. Iglehart. 1995. Folk medicine use: Diverse populations in a metropolitan area. *Social Work in Health Care* 21 (4): 37–58.

Begbie, G. H. 1985. Health messages through folk media: A critical review. *Nursing Journal of India* 76 (11): 287–95.

Blumhagen, D. 1980. Hyper-tension: A folk illness with a medical name. *Culture, Medicine and Psychiatry* 4: 197–217.

Bodner, A., and M. Leininger. 1992. Transcultural nursing care values, beliefs, and practices of American (USA) Gypsies. *Journal of Transcultural Nursing* 4 (1): 17–28.

Bolton, J. 1995. Medical practice and anthropological bias. *Social Science and Medicine* 40 (12): 1655–61.

Bond, J. 1974. Health care problems for minorities. 1974. *Medical Arts and Sciences* 28 (3): 23–28.

Breslin, E. T. 1996. Metaphorical communication as aesthetic method for nursing practice. *Issues in Mental Health Nursing* 17 (6): 507–16.

Briggs, Charles. 1986. *Learning how to ask: A sociolinguistic appraisal of the role of the interview in social science research.* Cambridge: Cambridge University Press.

Brorsson, A., M. Troein, E. Lindbladh, S. Selander, M. Widlund, and L. Rastam. 1995. My family dies from heart attacks: How hypercholesterolaemic men refer to their family history. *Family Practice* 12 (4): 433–37.

Browner, C. H., B. R. Ortiz de Montellano, and A. J. Rubel. 1988. A methodology for cross-cultural ethnomedical research. *Current Anthropology* 29: 681–702.

Bushy, A. 1992. Cultural considerations for primary health care: Where do self-care and folk medicine fit? *Holistic Nursing Practice* 6 (3): 10–18.

Carlisle, D. M., B. D. Leake, and M. F. Shapiro. 1995. Racial and ethnic differences in the use of invasive cardiac procedures among cardiac patients in Los Angeles County, 1986 through 1988. *American Journal of Public Health* 85: 352–56.

———. 1997. Racial and ethnic disparities in the use of cardiovascular procedures: Associations with type of health insurance. *American Journal of Public Health* 87: 263–67.

Cassell, Eric J. 1976. *The healer's art; A new approach to the doctor-patient relationship.* New York: Lippincott.

Cassidy, Claire M. 1995. Social science theory and methods in the study of alternative and complementary medicine. *Journal of Alternative and Complementary Medicine* 1: 19–40.

Cattermole-Tally, Frances M. 1979–82. Interrelationship of folk medicine, magical healing, religious healing and holistic medicine: Verbal charms and visualization (in Spanish). *Cuadernos* 9: 293–303.

Chrisman, N. J. 1977. The health seeking process: An approach to the natural history of illness. *Culture, Medicine and Psychiatry* 1 (4): 351–77.

Cockerham, W. C., M. C. Creditor, U. K. Creditor, and P. B. Imrey. 1980. Minor ailments and illness behavior among physicians. *Medical Care* 18 (2): 164–73.

Dacher, E. S. 1995. A systems theory approach to an expanded medical model: A challenge for biomedicine. *Journal of Alternative and Complementary Medicine* 1 (2): 187–96.

Dean, Kathryn. 1981. Self-care responses to illnesses: A selected review. *Social Science and Medicine* 15A: 673–87.

———. 1986. Lay care in illness. *Social Science and Medicine* 22 (2): 275–84

Dines, A. 1994. A review of lay health beliefs research: Insights for nursing practice in health promotion. *Journal of Clinical Nursing* 3 (6): 329–38.

Dodier, N. 1985. Social uses of illness at the workplace: Sick leave and moral evaluation. *Social Science and Medicine* 20 (2): 123–28.

Eisenberg, L. 1977. Disease and illness. Distinctions between professional and popular ideas of sickness. *Culture, Medicine and Psychiatry* 1 (1): 9–23.

Engebretson, J. 1994. Folk healing and biomedicine: Culture clash or complementary approach? *Journal of Holistic Nursing* 12 (3): 240–50.

Etkin, Nina L. 1993. Anthropological methods in ethnopharmacology. *Journal of Ethnopharmacology* 38: 93–104.

Fabrega, H. Jr. 1977. Group differences in the structure of illness. *Culture, Medicine and Psychiatry* 1 (4): 379–94.

Fife, B. L. 1994. The conceptualization of meaning in illness. *Social Science and Medicine* 38 (2): 309–16.

———. 1995. The measurement of meaning in illness. *Social Science and Medicine* 40 (8): 1021–28.

Finkler, Kaja. 1986. The social consequence of wellness: A view of healing outcomes from micro and macro perspectives. *International Journal of Health Services* 16: 627–42.

Flack, J. M., H. Amaro, W. Jenkins, S. Kunitz, J. Levy, M. Mixon, and E. Yu. 1995. Epidemiology of minority health. *Health Psychology* 14 (7): 592–600.

Foster, George M., and Barbara G. Anderson. 1978. *Medical anthropology*. New York: Wiley.

Freer, C. B. 1980. Self-care: A health diary study. *Medical Care* 18 (8): 853–61.

Furnham, A. 1994. Explaining health and illness: Lay perceptions on current and future health, the causes of illness, and the nature of recovery. *Social Science and Medicine* 39 (5): 715–25.

Furnham, A., C. Vincent, and R. Wood. 1995. The health beliefs and behaviors of three groups of complementary medicine and a general practice group of patients. *Journal of Alternative and Complementary Medicine* 1: 347–59.

Gannik, D., and M. Jespersen. 1984. Lay concepts and strategies for handling symptoms of disease: A sample of adult men and women experiencing back pain symptoms. *Scandinavian Journal of Primary Health Care* 2 (2): 67–76.

Gerhardt, U. 1989. Ideas about illness: An intellectual and political history of medical sociology. New York: New York University Press.

Gevitz, Norman, ed. 1988. *Other healers: Unorthodox medicine in America*. Baltimore: Johns Hopkins University Press.

Gums, J. G., and D. S. Carson. 1987. Influence of folk medicine on the family practitioner. *Southern Medical Journal* 80 (2): 209–12.

Hand, Wayland D., ed. 1961, 1964. *The Frank C. Brown collection of North Carolina folklore*. Vols. 6 and 7. Durham, North Carolina: Duke University Press.

———, ed. 1976. *Folk medicine: A symposium*. Berkeley and Los Angeles: University of California Press.

Harwood, Alan, ed. 1981. *Ethnicity and medical care*. Cambridge: Harvard University Press.

Hentges, K. 1987. Folk medicine: Economics, biology, and culture. Letter. *Texas Medicine* 83 (4): 9.

Heurtin-Roberts, S. 1993. "High-pertension": The uses of a chronic folk illness for personal adaptation. *Social Science of Medicine* 37: 285–94.

Heurtin-Roberts, S., and E. Reisin. 1992. The relation of culturally influenced lay models of hypertension to compliance with treatment. *American Journal of Hypertension* 5: 787–92.

Honko, Lauri. 1962–63. On the effectivity of folk-medicine. *Arv* 18–19: 290–300.

Hopper, S. V. 1993. The influence of ethnicity on the health of older women. *Clinics in Geriatric Medicine* 9 (1): 231–59.

Hufford, David J. 1983. Folk healers. In *Handbook of American folklore*, ed. Richard M. Dorson, 306–13. Bloomington: Indiana University Press.

———. 1992. Folk medicine in contemporary America. In *Herbal and magical medicine: Traditional healing today*, ed. James Kirkland, Holly F. Mathews, C. W. Sullivan III, and Karen Baldwin, 14–32. Durham, North Carolina: Duke University Press.

———. 1994. Folklore and medicine. In *Putting folklore to use*, ed. Michael Owen Jones, 117–35. Lexington: University Press of Kentucky.

Hughes, Charles C. 1968. Ethnomedicine. *International Encyclopaedia of the Social Sciences* 10: 87–93. New York: Free Press and MacMillan.

Johnson, K. W., N. B. Anderson, E. Bastida, B. J. Kramer, D. Williams, and M. Wong. 1995. Macrosocial and environmental influences on minority health. *Health Psychology* 14 (7): 601–12.

Johnson, A. E., and G. V. Baboila. 1996. Integrating culture and healing: Meeting the health care needs of a multicultural community. *Minnesota Medicine* 79 (5): 41–45.

Jones, Michael Owen. 1967. Climate and disease: The traveler describes America. *Bulletin of the History of Medicine* 41: 254–66.

Kelner, M., and B. Wellman. 1997. Who seeks alternative health care?: A profile of the users of five modes of treatment. *Journal of Alternative and Complementary Medicine* 3: 127–40.

Kleinman, A., L. Eisenberg, and B. Good. 1978. Culture, illness, and care: Clinical lessons from anthropological and cross-cultural research. *Annals of Internal Medicine* 88: 251–58.

Kleinman, Arthur, and Lilias H. Sung. 1979. Why do indigenous practitioners successfully heal? *Social Science and Medicine* 13B: 7–26.

Kleinman, Arthur. 1980. *Patients and healers in the context of culture*. Berkeley: University of California Press.

Krippner, S. 1995. A cross-cultural comparison of four healing models. *Alternative Therapies in Health and Medicine*. Health and Social Work 1 (1): 21–29.

Lau, B. W. 1988. An appraisal of lay and medical concepts of illness. *Journal of the Royal Society of Health* 108 (5): 185–87.

Levine, R. E., and A. C. Gaw. 1995. Culture-bound syndromes. *Psychiatric Clinics of North America* 18 (3): 523–36.

Lupton, D. 1992. Discourse analysis: A new methodology for understanding the ideologies of health and illness. *Australian Journal of Public Health* 16 (2): 145–50.

Maida, C. A. 1985. Social support and learning in preventive health care. *Social Science and Medicine* 21 (3): 335–39.

Mechanic, D. 1992. Health and illness behavior and patient-practitioner relationships. *Social Science and Medicine* 34 (12): 1345–50.

Meininger, J. C. 1986. Sex differences in factors associated with use of medical care and alternative illness behaviors. *Social Science and Medicine* 22 (3): 289–92.

Micozzi, M. S. 1983. Anthropological study of health beliefs, behaviors, and outcomes: Traditional folk medicine and ethnopharmacology. *Human Organization* 42 (4): 351–53.

Millstein, S. G., and C. E. Irwin Jr. 1987. Concepts of health and illness: Different constructs or variations on a theme? *Health Psychology* 6 (6): 515–24.

Money, J. 1989. Paleodigms and paleodigmatics: A new theoretical construct applicable to Munchausen's Syndrome by Proxy, child-abuse dwarfism, paraphilias, anorexia nervosa, and other syndromes. *American Journal of Psychotherapy* 43 (1): 15–24.

Morgan, S. 1996. Gods, daemons, and banshees on the journey to the magic scroll: The use of myth as a framework for reflective practice in nurse education. *Nurse Education Today* 16 (2): 144–48.

Morris, B. 1984. The pragmatics of folk classification. *Journal of Ethnobiology* 4: 45–60.

Myers, H. F., M. Kagawa-Singer, S. K. Kumanyika, B. W. Lex, and K. S. Markides. 1995. Behavioral risk factors related to chronic diseases in ethnic minorities. *Health Psychology* 14 (7): 613–21.

Nations, M. K., L. A. Camino, and F. B. Walker. 1985. "Hidden" popular illnesses in primary care: Residents' recognition and clinical implications. *Culture, Medicine and Psychiatry* 9: 223–40.

———. 1988. "Nerves": Folk idiom for anxiety and depression? *Social Science and Medicine* 26 (12): 1245–59.

Ness, R. C. 1978. The Old Hag phenomenon as sleep paralysis: A biocultural interpretation. *Culture, Medicine and Psychiatry* 2 (1): 15–39.

———. and R. M. Wintrob. 1981. Folk healing: A description and synthesis. *American Journal of Psychiatry* 138 (11): 1477–81.

Newman, Leslie F. 1948. Some notes on the pharmacology and therapeutic value of folk-medicine. 2 parts. *Folk-Lore* 59: 118–35, 145–56.

O'Connor, Bonnie B. 1995. *Healing traditions: Alternative medicine and the healing professions*. Philadelphia: University of Pennsylvania Press.

O'Reilly, Kevin R. 1985. Applied anthropology and public health. In *Training manual in medical anthropology*, ed. Carole E. Hill, 8–20. Washington, D.C.: American Anthropological Association.

Pachter, L. M. 1994. Culture and clinical care: Folk illness beliefs and behaviors and their implications for health care delivery. *Journal of the American Medical Association* 271: 690–94.

Pedersen, P. B., R. T. Carter, and J. G. Ponterotto. 1996. The cultural context of psychology: Questions for accurate research and appropriate practice. *Cultural Diversity and Mental Health* 2: 205–16.

Richardson, J. L., B. Langholz, L. Bernstein, C. Burciaga, K. Danley, and R. K. Ross. 1992. Stage and delay in breast cancer diagnosis by race, socioeconomic status, age, and year. *British Journal of Cancer* 65: 922–26.

Rubel, Arthur J. 1988. Lessons for biomedicine from folk medicine. In *Rituales y fiestas de las Americas. 45th Congreso Internacional de Americanistas*, 342–47. Bogota: Ediciones Uniandes.

Santino, Jack. 1985. On the nature of healing as a folk event. *Western Folklore* 44: 153–67.

Scott, C. J. 1997. Enhancing patient outcomes through an understanding of intercultural medicine: Guidelines for the practitioner. *Maryland Medical Journal* 46 (4): 175–80.

Scott, C. S. 1974. Health and healing practices among five ethnic groups in Miami, Florida. *Public Health Reports* 89: 524–53.

Sensky, T. 1996. Eliciting lay beliefs across cultures: Principles and methodology. *British Journal of Cancer*, suppl. 29: S63–65.

Todd, Harry F., Jr., and M. Margaret Clark. 1985. Medical anthropology and the challenge of medical education. In *Training manual in medical anthropology*, ed. Carole E. Hill, 40–57. Washington, D.C.: American Anthropological Association.

Winkelman, Michael J. 1990. Shamans and other "magico-religious" healers: A cross-cultural study of their origins, nature, and social transformations. *Ethos* 18: 305–52.

Yoder, Don. 1972. Folk medicine. In *Folklore and folklife: An introduction*, ed. Richard M. Dorson, 191–215. Chicago: University of Chicago Press.

VII.   *"Quackery"*

Fishbein, Morris. 1930. *Shattering health superstitions*. New York: n.p.

———. 1938. Modern medical charlatans. Parts 1 and 2. *Hygeia* 16: 21–24.

King, R. F. H. 1890. *Quakery: American, Anglo-American, and quackery in all its various forms as it appears in the medical and dental profession at the present time*. London: n.p.

Knight, Robert P. 1939. Why people go to cultists. *Journal of the Kansas Medical Society* 40 (7): 285–89.

Quen, Jacques M. 1963. Elisha Perkins: Physician, nostrum-vendor, or charlatan? *Bulletin of the History of Medicine* 37 (2): 159–66.

Trimmer, Eric J. 1965. Medical folklore and quackery. *Folklore* 76: 161–75.

Walker, Jack D. 1956. The goat gland surgeon: The story of the late John R. Brinkley. *Journal of the Kansas Medical Society* 57 (12): 749–55.

Walsh, James J. 1924. The cures that have failed. *Illinois Medical Journal* 45: 392–401.

Young, James Harvey. 1965. Device quackery in America. *Bulletin of the History of Medicine* 34: 154–62.

———. 1967. *The medical messiahs: A social history of health quackery in twentieth-century America*. Princeton, New Jersey: Princeton University Press.

VIII.   *Specific Pathologies*

Baer, R. D., and D. Penzell. 1993. Research report: Susto and pesticide poisoning among Florida farmworkers. *Culture, Medicine and Psychiatry* 17 (3): 321–27.

Bartholomew, R. E. 1994. The social psychology of "epidemic" Koro. *International Journal of Social Psychiatry* 40 (1): 46–60.

Burstein, Sona Rosa. 1949. Aspects of the psychopathology of old age. *British Medical Society Bulletin* 6(1–2): 63–72.

Cheng, S. T. 1996. A critical review of Chinese Koro. *Culture, Medicine and Psychiatry* 20 (1): 67–82.

Chowdhury, A. N. 1996. The definition and classification of Koro. *Culture, Medicine and Psychiatry* 20 (1): 41–65.

Courville, Cyril B., M.D. 1951. Epilepsy in mythology, legend, and folktale. *Bulletin of the Los Angeles Neurological Society* 16 (2): 213–24.

Cramp, Arthur J. 1935. Some diabetes "cures" and "treatments." *Hygeia* 13: 916–20.

Davis, D. L., and S. M. Low. 1989. *Gender, health, and illness: The case of nerves*. New York: Hemisphere.

Dickie, W. R., and N. C. Hughes. 1961. Caustic pastes: Their survival as quack cancer remedies. *British Journal of Plastic Surgery* 14 (2): 97–109.

Doering, J. Frederick. 1944. Folk remedies for diverse allergies. *Journal of American Folklore* 57: 140–41.

Elvin-Lewis, M. 1982. The therapeutic potential of plants used in dental folk medicine. *Odonto-Stomatologie Tropicale* 5 (3): 107–17.

Fukunishi, I., T. Nakagawa, H. Nakamura, M. Kikuchi, and M. Takubo. 1997. Is alexithymia a culture-bound construct? Validity and reliability of the Japanese versions of the twenty-item Toronto alexithymia scale and modified Beth Israel Hospital psychosomatic questionnaire. *Psychological Reports* 80 (3): 787–99.

Garland, L. H. 1958. The pursuit of the unorthodox: Some observations on certain forms of cancer therapy. *Journal of the Michigan State Medical Society* 57: 525–31.

Granger, Byrd Howell. 1961. Of the teeth. *Journal of American Folklore* 74: 47–56.

Kanner, Leo. 1942. Contemporary folk-treatment of sternutation. *Bulletin of the History of Medicine* 11: 273–90.

Kraus, A., G. Guerra-Bautista, and D. Alarcon-Segovia. 1991. Salmonella Arizona arthritis and septicemia associated with rattlesnake ingestion by patients with connective tissue diseases: A dangerous complication of folk medicine. *Journal of Rheumatology* 18 (9): 1328–31.

Lin, K. M. 1983. Hwa-Byung: A Korean culture-bound syndrome? *American Journal of Psychiatry* 140 (1): 105–7.

Long, Eleanor. 1973. Aphrodisiacs, charms, and philtres. *Western Folklore* 32: 153–63.

Loomis, C. Grant. 1949. Indications of miners' medicine. *Western Folklore* 8: 117–22.

Mack, T. M., J. Berkel, L. Bernstein, and W. Mack. 1985. Religion and cancer in Los Angeles County. *National Cancer Institute Monographs* 69: 235–45.

Makarius, Laura. 1968. The blacksmith's taboos from the man of iron to the man of blood. *Diogenes* 62: 25–48.

Malhotra, H. K., and N. N. Wig. 1975. Dhat syndrome: A culture-bound sex neurosis of the orient. *Archives of Sexual Behavior* 4 (5): 519–28.

McGowan, Virginia. 1996. Evaluating and planning cancer screening programs. *Practicing Anthropology* 18 (fall): 12–15.

Morgan, Edward A. 1934. Some traditional beliefs encountered in the practice of pediatrics. *Canadian Medical Association Journal* 31: 666–69.

Morgan, Edwin Lee. 1912. Snakestones and madstones in the treatment of lyssa and other poisons. *Medical Era* 21: 92–100.

Pandey, R., M. K. Mandal, G. J. Taylor, and J. D. Parker. 1996. Cross-cultural alexithymia: Development and validation of a Hindi translation of the twenty-item Toronto alexithymia scale. *Journal of Clinical Psychology* 52 (2): 173–76.

Poma, P. A. 1984. A dangerous folk therapy. *Journal of the National Medical Association* 76 (4): 387–89.

Raaf, John E. 1932. Hernia healers. *Annals of Medical History*, n.s., 4: 377–89.

Radbill, Samuel X. 1943. Whooping cough in fact and fancy. *Bulletin of the History of Medicine* 13: 33–54.

Ritenbaugh, C. 1982. Obesity as a culture-bound syndrome. *Culture, Medicine and Psychiatry* 6 (4): 347–64.

Rochford, E. B., Jr. 1983. Stutterers' practices: Folk remedies and therapeutic intervention. *Journal of Communication Disorders* 16 (5): 373–84.

Rolleston, J. D., M.D. 1941. The folk-lore of pulmonary tuberculosis. *Tubercle* 22: 55–65.

———. 1942a. The folk-lore of venereal disease. *British Journal of Venereal Diseases* 18 (1–2): 1–13.

———. 1942b. Otology and folk-lore. *Journal of Laryngology and Otology* 57: 311–18.

———. 1942c. Laryngology and folk-lore. *Journal of Laryngology and Otology* 57: 527–32.

———. 1942d. Ophthalmic folk-lore. *British Journal of Ophthalmology* 26: 481–502.

———. 1942e. Folklore of acute exanthemata. *Proceedings of the Royal Society of Medicine* 35: 535–38.

———. 1943. Rhinology and folk-lore. *Journal of Laryncology and Otology* 58: 272–79.

———. 1944. Respiratory folk-lore. *Tubercle* 25: 7–12.

———. 1945. Cardiac folklore. *Proceedings of the Royal Society of Medicine* 39: 119–22.

Schroeder, Theodore. 1930. Witchcraft and the erotic life. *Journal of Nervous and Mental Disease* 72: 640–51.

Sigerist, Henry E. 1943. Impotence as a result of witchcraft. In *Essays in biology in honor of Herbert M. Evans*, 541–46. Berkeley: n.p.

Swetnam, George. 1965. Sex—The missing fascicle. *Keystone Folklore Quarterly* 10: 155–71.

Tanner, Jeri. 1968. The teeth in folklore. *Western Folklore* 27: 97–105.

Townsend, B. R. 1944. The story of the tooth-worm. *Bulletin of the History of Medicine* 15 (1): 37–58.

Tseng, W. S., K. M. Mo, J. Hsu, L. S. Li, L. W. Ou, G. Q. Chen, and D. W. Jiang. 1988. A Sociocultural study of koro epidemics in Guangdong, China. *American Journal of Psychiatry* 145 (12): 1538–43.

Walsh, H. P., and J. C. Dorgan. 1988. Etiology of Freiberg's disease: Trauma. *Journal of Foot Surgery* 27 (3): 243–44.

Ware, N. C., and A. Kleinman. 1992. Culture and somatic experience: The social course of illness in neurasthenia and chronic fatigue syndrome. *Psychosomatic Medicine* 54 (5): 546–60.

Waterman, S. H., G. Juarez, S. J. Carr, and L. Kilman. 1990. Salmonella Arizona infections in Latinos associated with rattlesnake folk medicine. *American Journal of Public Health* 80 (3): 286–89.

Williams, G. H. 1986. Lay beliefs about the causes of rheumatoid arthritis: Their implications for rehabilitation. *International Rehabilitation Medicine* 8 (2): 65–68.

Wilson, Gordon W., and L. Y. Lancaster. 1968. Folklore in certain professions: The biologist and folklore. *Tennessee Folklore Society Bulletin* 34: 10–17.

Winslow, David J. 1968. Occupational superstitions of Negro prostitutes in an upstate New York city. *New York Folklore Quarterly* 24: 294–301.

Wittwer, B. 1978. Self-treatment among employees of the Swiss railroad and postal systems (trans. from German). *Sozial- und Praventivmedizin* 23 (4): 267–68.

Ziment, I. 1991. History of the treatment of chronic bronchitis. *Respiration* 58 (suppl. 1): 37–42.

Contributors

SHELLEY R. ADLER, PH.D., is assistant professor in the Department of Anthropology, History, and Social Medicine at the University of California, San Francisco. She conducts research and teaches graduate and medical students in the areas of complementary and alternative medicine, ethnomedicine, women's health (primarily with regard to breast cancer and menopause), patient-physician communication, cultural issues in U.S. health care, and qualitative research methodology. Dr. Adler's current projects include directing a National Institutes of Health–funded study of alternative and biomedical treatment decision-making in women with breast cancer, designing a mixed-method approach to clinical trials of alternative treatments, and developing alternative medicine and culture educational components for medical school curricula.

RICHARD BLAUSTEIN, PH.D., is professor of sociology and anthropology and adjunct professor of family medicine at East Tennessee State University. Blaustein and his colleague Anthony P. Cavender have been researching traditional healers and medical belief systems of Southern Appalachia since the mid-1970s. Blaustein first met Knoxville folk healer Tim Waggoner when the two were employed as performers and interpreters at the Stokeley Folklife Festival at the 1982 Knoxville World's Fair.

ERIKA BRADY, PH.D., holds degrees in folklore from Harvard, UCLA, and Indiana University. She is currently associate professor and director of folk studies and anthropology at Western Kentucky University. A former chaplain associate at Southeast Hospital in Cape Girardeau, Missouri, she is an adjunct associate professor in the Department of Family Practice and Community Medicine at University of South Alabama and is affiliated with the South Central Kentucky Area Health Education Center. She presents monthly faculty conferences on medicine, region, and culture as a faculty member of the University of Louisville Family Medicine Residency located at T. J. Samson Hospital in Glasgow, Kentucky, as well as conducting the residency's Balint program. Her book *A Spiral Way: How the Phonograph Changed Ethnography* appeared in 1999 (University Press of Mississippi).

ANTHONY CAVENDER, PH.D., is a medical anthropologist and associate professor of anthropology at East Tennessee State University. His primary area of research interest is ethnomedicine, traditional medical practitioners, and health care policy. He has conducted research on these and other topics in Southern Appalachia, Zimbabwe, and Ecuador.

WILLIAM M. CLEMENTS, PH.D., teaches folklore, anthropology, and literature at Arkansas State University. His research interests include American religious folklife—on which he has published articles in *Journal of American Folklore, Western Folklore, Indiana Folklore, International Folklore Review,* and other periodicals—and American Indian oral literature, treated in his book *Native American Verbal Art: Texts and Contexts* (University of Arizona Press, 1996) as well as in several periodical articles.

ROBERTA J. EVANCHUK, PH.D., is administrative assistant and graduate advisor to the UCLA Folklore and Mythology Program and Archives. Her dissertation, "When the Curtain Goes Up, the Gods Come Down: Aspects of Performance in Public Ceremonies of Orisha Worship" (UCLA, 1996), examines the aesthetic, symbolic, and performative aspects of Lucumí religious behavior. Several of her more than thirty papers and articles focus on cultural and aesthetic aspects of orisha worship. She is co-author with Ysamur Flores-Peña of *Santería Garments and Altars: Speaking Without a Voice* (University Press of Mississippi, 1994).

YSAMUR FLORES-PEÑA, PH.D., is a research associate with the UCLA Folklore and Mythology Program and Archives. His dissertation, "'The Tongue Is the Whip of the Body': Identity and Appropriation through Narrative in Lucumí Religious Culture" (UCLA, 1998) focuses on the use of *pataki*, or sacred stories, in Lucumí. He has authored nearly a dozen papers on issues of syncretism, identity, and meaning in Afro-Caribbean religions. Publications include "'Fit For a Queen': Analysis of a Consecration Outfit in the Cult of Yemaya," *Folklore Forum* (1990) and, co-authored with Roberta J. Evanchuk, *Santería Garments and Altars: Speaking Without a Voice* (University Press of Mississippi, 1994). He has worked for U.S.

departments on health and aging and served as consultant on several health-related projects.

DIANE GOLDSTEIN, PH.D., is associate professor of folklore at Memorial University of Newfoundland and is cross-appointed to Memorial University's faculty of medicine. She is the editor of one of the earliest interdisciplinary anthologies on AIDS, *Talking AIDS: Interdisciplinary Perspectives on Acquired Immune Deficiency Syndrome* (Memorial University of Newfoundland, 1991) and is co-editor of *Reckless Vectors: AIDS and the Infecting "Other" in Law, Ethics, Policy and Narrative* (University of Pennsylvania Press, 2001). She has been extensively involved in AIDS priority-setting and policy-making initiatives over the last ten years, including an appointment from 1994–1997 to the Canadian National Planning Forum for HIV/AIDS operated by the AIDS Secretariat. Her ongoing interests include stigmatized illnesses; AIDS and HIV; health beliefs and cultural issues in health care; risk perception and management; public health law; rumor and epidemic control; and health narratives.

BONNIE GLASS-COFFIN received her Ph.D. in anthropology from UCLA in 1992. She has conducted extensive fieldwork with female shamans (called *curanderas*) and has studied the transformation of healing practices in Northern Peru over the last five hundred years. Her recently published book, *The Gift of Life: Female Spirituality and Healing in Northern Peru* (University of New Mexico, 1998) describes the results of this research. In addition to her book, she has published in scholarly journals such as *Ethnohistory* and the *Journal of Ritual Studies*. Her opinion piece "Anthropology, Shamanism, and the 'New Age.'" appeared in *The Chronicle of Higher Education* in 1994. Currently, she is associate professor of anthropology and anthropology program director at Utah State University, where she has been employed since 1993.

DAVID J. HUFFORD, PH.D., is professor of medical humanities, director of The Doctors Kienle Center for Humanistic Medicine, and academic director of the Medical Ethnography Collection at Penn State College of Medicine, the Milton S. Hershey Medical Center, Hershey, Pennsylvania, with joint appointments in behavioral science and family and community medicine. At the College of Medicine he has taught on alternative and folk medicine, spirituality and health, and human diversity since 1974. At the University of Pennsylvania he is also adjunct professor of religious studies and a member of the principal faculty in the Bioethics Master's Degree Program and the

Folklore and Folklife Program, teaching courses on belief systems, folk medicine, and human diversity and health care. He has published extensively in both medical and ethnographic literature and is a founding member of the editorial boards of *Alternative Therapies in Health and Medicine* (1995) and *Alternative Health Practitioner* (1999).

MICHAEL OWEN JONES is professor of folklore, history, and world arts and cultures at UCLA where he has taught folklore courses since 1968. Among his publications are *Why Faith Healing?* (Canadian Centre for Folk Culture Studies, 1972), *People Studying People: The Human Element in Fieldwork* (co-authored, University of California Press, 1980), *Exploring Folk Art: Twenty Years of Thought on Craft, Work, and Aesthetics* (1987; rpt., Utah State University Press, 1993), *Inside Organizations* (co-edited, Sage Publications, 1988), *Craftsman of the Cumberlands* (University Press of Kentucky, 1989), *Folkloristics: An Introduction* (co-authored, Indiana University Press, 1995), and *Studying Organizational Symbolism* (Sage Publications, 1996). He has also served as principal investigator of a five-year project funded by the National Library of Medicine to digitize holdings in the UCLA Archive of American Folk Medicine.

FRANCES M. MALPEZZI, PH.D., professor of English at Arkansas State University, has published essays on sixteenth- and seventeenth-century devotional literature as well as on numerous women writers. She co-edited *John Donne's Religious Imagination: Essays in Honor of John T. Shawcross* (UCA Press, 1995) and with William M. Clements is co-author of *Italian American Folklore* (August House, 1992).

BONNIE O'CONNOR, PH.D., is a folklorist and medical educator specializing in cultural and cross-cultural issues in health care; health belief systems, including what is now called complementary/alternative medicine; patients' experiences and viewpoints on health, illness, and care; and the aspects of patient-physician communication and relationship-building in which these matters are involved. She was a postdoctoral fellow in medical humanities at the Medical College of Pennsylvania (now MCP-Hahnemann School of Medicine), subsequently becoming a member of the school's faculty for eight years. She has recently joined the faculty of the Division of Pediatric Ambulatory Medicine at Rhode Island Hospital/Brown University School of Medicine where she is an associate professor and education coordinator for faculty development in pediatrics. Her book, *Healing Traditions: Alternative Medicine and the Health Professions*, was released in 1995 by the University of

Pennsylvania Press, and she has published on the subjects of both complementary medicine and cultural issues in health care in medical and health professions journals and reference works.

PATRICK A. POLK is the archivist for the UCLA Folklore and Mythology Program and Archives and a Ph.D. candidate in the program completing his dissertation on Haitian Vodou. Several of his papers and publications concern Haitian Vodou religious beliefs, practices, and art. He has authored African Religion and Christianity in Grenada," *Caribbean Quarterly* (1993); Sacred Banners and the Divine Cavalry Charge," *The Sacred Arts of Vodou*, ed. Donald J. Cosentino (University Press of Mississippi, 1995), and *Haitian Vodou Flags* (University Press of Mississippi, 1997). He has also served as research consultant for the book *Alternative Medicine, A Definitive Guide* and has mounted museum exhibits on various arts in Southern California, including *Botánica*: Art and Spirit in Los Angeles" (1998).

JACKIE SLUDER has a master's degree in sociology and currently serves as a case manager with the Tennessee Department of Children's Services. She is currently involved in research in Southern Appalachia on folk medical beliefs and practices related to women's health. Jackie Sluder was born and raised in Johnson County, Tennessee. Under the supervision of Richard Blaustein and Anthony Cavender, she wrote a master's thesis in sociology based on extensive taped interviews recorded in Tillman Waggoner's home in the Third Creek section of Knoxville.

BARRE TOELKEN, PH.D., is professor of English and history at Utah Sate University, where he is director of both the Graduate Program in American Studies and the interdisciplinary Folklore Program. His professional focus has been primarily on vernacular expression (especially in occupational and ethnic folklore) and on intercultural studies. He has served as editor of the *Journal of American Folklore*, was founding editor of *Northwest Folklore*, and has been an associate editor for other professional journals. He held a six-year congressional appointment to the Board of Trustees of the American Folklife Center in the Library of Congress. He is past president of the American Folklore Society, the Oregon Folklore Society, and the Utah Folklore Society. He is former chair of the Folk Arts Panel for the National Endowment for the Arts, and for twenty years was director of the Folklore and Ethnic Studies Program at the University of Oregon. His publications include *The Dynamics of Folklore* (1979; revised and expanded edition, Utah State University Press, 1996), *The Ballad and the Scholars* (with D. K. Wilgus,

UCLA, 1986), *Ghosts and the Japanese: Cultural Experience in Japanese Death Legends* (with Michiko Iwasaka, Utah State University, 1994), *Morning Dew and Roses: Nuance, Metaphor and Meaning in Folksongs* (University of Illinois Press, 1995), and a number of scholarly and popular essays on folklore, balladry, world view, medieval literature, intercultural perspective, and Native American traditions.

TILLMAN WAGGONER was born and raised in the Third Creek section of Knoxville,where he and his family still live today. A self-taught herbalist and collector of local folk traditions, Tillman Waggoner compiled and published *The Poor Man's Medicine Bag* in 1983, based upon cures and remedies collected from his own family members and neighbors. In 1982, he appeared at the Stokelely Folk Festival, and in 1986 he represented Tennessee at the 1986 Smithsonian Festival of American Folklife.

Index

A

acupuncture, 6, 8, 95, 123
addiction. *See* drug use
advertising. *See* folk medicine: in media
African traditions, 3, 43, 45, 53–54, 56, 131–38
African-American traditions, 21, 23–24, 39–43, 55, 71–72
Afro-Cuban traditions. *See* Santería, El Palo Mayombe
AIDS, 42, 129–40, 155
alcoholism. *See* drug use
American Medical Association, 5
anthropology. *See* ethnography
Asian traditions, 19, 23, 30, 58, 71, 148, 153–54. *See also* Buddhism
authority, methods of obtaining, 7–8, 16, 26–27, 55, 59, 149, 165, 173

B

balance. *See* harmony and balance
biomedicine. *See* conventional medicine
Black Elk, Wallace, 145, 148, 155, 157–58
blood stopping, 26, 96, 107
botánicas, 39–40, 43–60, 70, 73–75, 78–79. *See also* herbal remedies
Bräuche. See Pennsylvania-German traditions
Brazil, 43
Buddhism, 47, 54, 154

C

calling. *See* authority, methods of obtaining
cancer, 58, 65, 97–98, 104–5, 116–22, 125–26, 155, 173

Caribbean traditions, 19, 40, 43, 45, 47–48, 54. *See also botánicas; diloggun*
Catholicism. *See* religious-medical traditions
charms, 15, 21, 23, 66, 169, 174, 191. *See also* rituals
chiropractic care, 8, 30–31
coining. *See* physical therapies
communication. *See* folk medicine: transmission of
complementary and alternative medicine (CAM), 14, 69, 74–75, 115–26. *See also* folk medicine
Compton, California, 40
Conjure. *See* Hoodoo
consciousness, states of, 10, 27, 57, 144, 193, 205
conventional medicine
    described, 4, 6, 9, 56–57, 139
    history of, 4–6, 13–14, 91, 94, 117–18, 152–54, 173. *See also* folk medicine
credentials. *See* authority, methods of obtaining
Cuba, 40, 43, 47, 52–53
Culpeper, Nicholas, 10
cupping. *See* physical therapies
Curanderismo, 21, 39, 42–44, 55, 57, 74, 77, 184–85, 187
curses, 20, 22–25, 51–56, 58, 64, 183–89, 192–94. *See also* skinwalkers

D

dead, communication with the, 27, 53–54, 59, 185. *See also* El Palo Mayombe

diagnosis. *See* etiology
diloggun, 48–50, 68
Dominican Republic, 47
drug use, 93–94, 129, 143–44, 185, 193,
    195

E

education. *See* folk medicine: economic
    factors in using
El Monte, California, 40, 78
El Palo Mayombe, 43–44, 53–54, 56, 61
El Salvador, 40, 48–50, 72
empacho. See folk illnesses: *empacho*
Espiritismo, 43–44, 54–55, 57, 59, 77
ethnography, 3–4, 7–9, 42, 58, 116, 131–39,
    183–86, 190–93, 198–99
etiology, 20–25, 42, 52, 54–58, 64–66, 70, 74,
    194
evil eye. *See* curses

F

fate. *See* religious-medical traditions
Fife Conference, vii–viii
first aid, 26, 95–96, 99, 109–10
Flexner, Abraham, 5, 7, 11–12
folk illnesses, 24–25
    empacho, 55, 58
    susto, 20, 25, 55, 58–60, 66–67
    traveling diseases, 22–23, 51, 64, 69,
        184
folk medicine
    defined, 6, 10, 13–23, 28, 32, 75, 115–17, 154
    economic factors in using, 6–7, 40–42,
        66, 71, 73–74, 78, 115, 118, 194
    in media, 8, 10–11, 31, 78, 90, 92, 152, 156,
        163
    relationship with conventional
        medicine, 4, 6, 21–22, 32, 40, 55,
        57, 63–65, 70–74, 96, 115–25,
        203–4
    transmission of, 10, 14–16, 56, 74, 88–89,
        95, 145, 204
foodways, 7, 15, 19, 22, 26, 29, 58, 64. *See
    also* Waggoner, Tillman

G

Guatemala, 40

H

Haiti, 20, 43, 47, 51, 129
Hand, Wayland, 3, 9
hantavirus, 206
harmony and balance, 18–25, 29–31, 52,
    57–58, 68, 98, 153, 157, 167–69, 175, 201–2,
    205–7
Heckewelder, John, 147
herbal remedies, 28–29, 58, 60–70, 75,
    94–110, 151, 154, 173–74, 199
heroic medicine. *See* conventional medi-
    cine: history of
Hildegard of Bingen, 153, 163–78
Hispanic traditions, 15, 19–20, 29, 39–44,
    46–47, 54–55, 57, 71–74, 78
history. *See* conventional medicine:
    history of
Hoodoo, 21, 55–56
hospitals. *See* conventional medicine
hot and cold. *See* foodways; harmony and
    balance; herbal remedies
humors. *See* harmony and balance
Huntington Park, California, 40

I

illness, meaning of. *See* etiology; folk illnesses

J

Jaramillo, Don Pedrito, 55
Jung, Carl G., 176

K

Kardec, Allan. *See* Rivail, Hippolyte

L

Lakota traditions, 143–46, 150. *See also*
    sweat lodges
Latino traditions. *See* Hispanic traditions
Los Angeles, California, 39–44, 47, 54,
    59–60, 72
Lucumí. *See* Santería

M

magic. *See* curses; supernatural
magical contagion. *See* folk illnesses: trav-
    eling diseases
mandalas. *See* supernatural

mash. *See* physical therapies

massage. *See* physical therapies

media. *See* folk medicine: in media

Mexican traditions. *See* Hispanic traditions

Miami, Florida, 47, 61

moxibustion, 29

music, 7, 56, 74, 163–64, 167, 174–76, 202

N

Native American traditions. *See* Lakota traditions; Navajo traditions; sweat lodges

Nature. *See* harmony and balance; Hildegard of Bingen; Waggoner, Tillman

Navajo traditions, 197–208. *See also* harmony and balance; skinwalkers

new age medicine. *See* sweat lodges

New York City, New York, 47

Nicaragua, 40

nonconventional medicine. *See* folk medicine

numbers, significance of, 68, 70

O

omieros. See herbal remedies

oncology, 3, 121–22

orichas. See Santería

P

paleros. See El Palo Mayombe

Pennsylvania-German traditions, 15, 21, 23

physical therapies, 23, 28–30, 69

preventative medicine, 57, 91–92. *See also* Waggoner, Tillman

Puerto Rico, 40, 43, 47, 61, 77–78

R

Red Road group, 143–45, 149–50

reincarnation, 54, 164

relaxation techniques, 6, 30, 62

religious-medical traditions, 3, 5, 15, 22, 24, 28, 42–45, 51–55, 57–59, 70, 90–93, 99–102, 104–108, 155, 165, 168–71, 189. *See also specific religions*

rituals, 28, 45–48, 53–54, 56–57, 64, 185–87, 201–3. *See also* charms; *diloggun*; sweat lodges

Rivail, Hippolyte, 43, 54

rootwork. *See* Hoodoo

S

sacramental objects. *See* charms; rituals

Santería, 52–53, 57, 59–70, 74

scarification. *See* African traditions

seances. *See* dead, communication with the; supernatural

shamanism, 21, 27, 152, 184, 187, 189, 191, 200

skinwalkers, 200–203, 205

sociology. *See* ethnography

sorcery. *See* curses

Spiritism. *See* Espiritismo

Stephens, G. Gayle, 7, 11–12

supernatural, 20–23, 28, 30, 47, 54, 58–59, 97, 99, 169, 176, 186–88, 190–92. *See also* curses

surgery, decision to have, 5, 61, 72, 93, 123

susto. See folk illnesses: *susto*

sweat lodges, 29, 143–51, 153–59

T

thrush, 26–27, 97

trauma. *See* folk illnesses: *susto*

V

Vodou, 43

W

Waggoner, Tillman, 88–111

witchcraft. *See* curses

Y

yin and yang. *See* harmony and balance